T0206216

Register Now for Online Access to Your Book!

SPRINGER PUBLISHING
CONNECT™

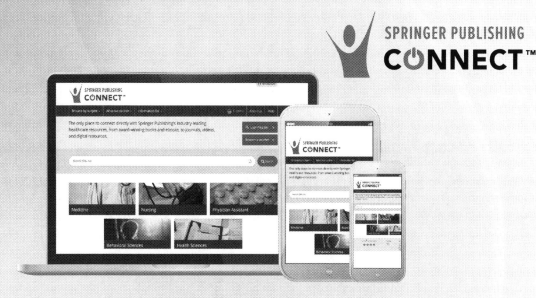

Your print purchase of *Advanced Practice Nursing Roles, Sixth Edition,* **includes online access to the contents of your book**—increasing accessibility, portability, and searchability!

Access today at:
http://connect.springerpub.com/content/book/978-0-8261-6153-6
or scan the QR code at the right with your smartphone. Log in or register, then click "Redeem a voucher" and use the code below.

B401UP4C

Scan here for quick access.

Having trouble redeeming a voucher code?
Go to https://connect.springerpub.com/redeeming-voucher-code

If you are experiencing problems accessing the digital component of this product, please contact our customer service department at cs@springerpub.com

The online access with your print purchase is available at the publisher's discretion and may be removed at any time without notice.

Publisher's Note: New and used products purchased from third-party sellers are not guaranteed for quality, authenticity, or access to any included digital components.

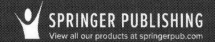
SPRINGER PUBLISHING
View all our products at springerpub.com

Advanced Practice Nursing Roles

Kathryn A. Blair, PhD, FNP-BC, FAANP, is professor and family nurse practitioner (FNP) coordinator at the University of Colorado–Colorado Springs, practices as an FNP at the William Storms Allergy and Asthma Clinic (also in Colorado Springs), and is subinvestigator at the Storms Clinical Research Institute. Dr. Blair has published in peer-reviewed journals and as a book and chapter author. Additionally, she serves on multiple editorial boards, including *American Journal of Nurse Practitioners, Journal for Nurse Practitioners, Journal of the American Academy of Nurse Practitioners*, and *McMaster Online Rating of Evidence*. Dr. Blair has presented nationally and internationally (Australia, Canada, England, Ireland, and Russia) and has participated in many professional development workshops and seminars, both in the United States and abroad. She has served as an expert witness for the state of Colorado and as a consultant for several universities, including Western Governors' University, the University of Missouri (DNP program development), and as external examiner for the University of Botswana FNP program. She is a fellow of the American Academy of Nurse Practitioners and is an active member of numerous professional organizations, including the National Organization of Nurse Practitioner Faculties, the American Association of Nurse Practitioners, and Sigma Theta Tau International.

Advanced Practice Nursing Roles

Core Concepts for Professional Development

Sixth Edition

Kathryn A. Blair, PhD, FNP-BC, FAANP
Editor

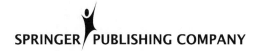

SPRINGER PUBLISHING COMPANY

Springer Publishing Company, LLC
11 West 42nd Street
New York, NY 10036
www.springerpub.com

Acquisitions Editor: Margaret Zuccarini
Production Manager: Kris Parrish
Compositor: Newgen Digital Works Pvt Ltd

ISBN: 978-0-8261-6152-9
ebook ISBN: 978-0-8261-6153-6
Instructor's Manual: 978-0-8261-6155-0
Instructor's PowerPoints: 978-0-8261-6154-3

Instructor's Materials: Qualified instructors may request supplements by emailing textbook@springerpub.com.

Printed by BnT

The author and the publisher of this Work have made every effort to use sources believed to be reliable to provide information that is accurate and compatible with the standards generally accepted at the time of publication. The author and publisher shall not be liable for any special, consequential, or exemplary damages resulting, in whole or in part, from the readers' use of, or reliance on, the information contained in this book. The publisher has no responsibility for the persistence or accuracy of URLs for external or third-party Internet websites referred to in this publication and does not guarantee that any content on such websites is, or will remain, accurate or appropriate.

Library of Congress Cataloging-in-Publication Data
Data Names: Blair, Kathryn A., editor.
Title: Advanced practice nursing roles : core concepts for professional
    development / Kathryn A. Blair, editor.
Other titles: Advanced practice nursing (Mirr Jansen)
Description: Sixth edition. | New York, NY : Springer Publishing Company,
    LLC, [2019] | Includes bibliographical references and index.
Identifiers: LCCN 2018038646| ISBN 9780826161529 (pbk.) | ISBN 9780826161550
    (instructor's manual) | ISBN 9780826161536 (ebook) | ISBN 9780826161543
    (instructor's manual PowerPoints)
Subjects: | MESH: Advanced Practice Nursing | Nurse's Role
Classification: LCC RT82.8 | NLM WY 128 | DDC 610.7306/92—dc23
LC record available at https://lccn.loc.gov/2018038646

Contact us to receive discount rates on bulk purchases.
We can also customize our books to meet your needs.
For more information please contact: sales@springerpub.com

Publisher's Note: New and used products purchased from third-party sellers are not guaranteed for quality, authenticity, or access to any included digital components.

Printed in the United States of America.

CONTENTS

II: Implementation of the APRN Role

III: Transitions to the Advanced Practice Role

CONTRIBUTORS

Kathryn A. Blair, PhD, FNP-BC, FAANP, Professor, FNP Option Coordinator, University of Colorado-Colorado Springs, Colorado Springs, Colorado

Vicki J. Brownrigg, PhD, FNP, Retired Associate Professor, Clinical Track, University of Colorado–Colorado Springs (Retired), Rio Grande Hospital System, Del Norte Colorado, Creede, Colorado

Patricia A. Ducklow, MSN, ACNS-BC, Acute Care Clinical Nurse Specialist, University Colorado Health Memorial Hospital, Colorado Springs, Colorado

Evelyn G. Duffy, DNP, AGPCNP-BC, FAANP, Associate Professor, Associate Director of the University Center on Aging and Health, Case Western Reserve University, Frances Payne Bolton School of Nursing, Cleveland, Ohio

Andra Fjone, DrPH, MN, RN, Clinical Associate Professor, University of Minnesota, Minneapolis, Minnesota

Cheri Friedrich, DNP, RN, CNP, Clinical Associate Professor, Coordinator of DNP Pediatric Specialties, University of Minnesota, Minneapolis, Minnesota

Deborah J. Kenny, PhD, RN, FAAN, Associate Professor, Helen and Arthur E. Johnson College of Nursing and Health Sciences, University of Colorado– Colorado Springs, Colorado Springs, Colorado

Patricia Biller Krauskopf, PhD, FNP-BC, FAANP, Professor and Helen Zebarth Chair in Nursing, Eleanor Wade Custer School of Nursing, Shenandoah University, Winchester, Virginia

Ruth Ludwick, PhD, RN-BC, APRN-CNS, FAAN,   Professor Emerita, Kent State University, College of Nursing, Kent, Ohio

Rebecca M. Patton, DNP, RN, CNOR, FAAN,   Lucy Jo Atkinson Scholar in Perioperative Nursing, Case Western Reserve University Frances Payne Bolton School of Nursing; Past President, American Nurses Association, Cleveland, Ohio

Maria N. Ruud, DNP, APRN, WHNP-C,   Clinical Assistant Professor, University of Minnesota School of Nursing, Minneapolis, Minnesota

Melissa A. Saftner, PhD, CNM, FACNM,   Clinical Associate Professor, University of Minnesota School of Nursing, Minneapolis, Minnesota

Lorna L. Schumann, PhD, FNP-C, ACNP-BC, ENP-C, ACNS-BC, FAAN, FAANP,   Vice Chair, American Academy of Nurse Practitioners, Certification Board, Austin, Texas

Carole G. Traylor, DNP, APRN, CPNP,   Assistant Professor, NP Practicum Coordinator, Helen and Arthur E. Johnson College of Nursing and Health Sciences, University of Colorado–Colorado Springs, Colorado Springs, Colorado

Kathy J. Wheeler, PhD, RN, APRN, NP-C, FNAP, FAANP,   Assistant Professor, Interim Coordinator Primary Care NP Track, University of Kentucky College of Nursing, Lexington, Kentucky

Patricia A. White, PhD, ANP-BC, FAANP,   Associate Professor, DNP Program, Graduate School of Nursing, University of Massachusetts Medical School, Worcester, Massachusetts

Margarete L. Zalon, PhD, RN, ACNS-BC, FAAN,   Professor, Department of Nursing; Director, Online MS in Health Informatics Program, University of Scranton, Scranton, Pennsylvania

Jana G. Zwilling, MS, APRN, FNP-C,   Clinical Instructor, Director FNP Program, University of North Dakota, College of Nursing and Professional Disciplines, Grand Forks, North Dakota

PREFACE

The sixth edition of *Advanced Practice Nursing Roles: Core Concepts for Professional Development* carries on the tradition of the previous five editions: updating current trends in practice; reviewing the origins, standards, and competencies of the advanced practice registered nurses (APRNs) in the United States; discussing APRN roles within a nursing context; identifying organizational roles for APRNs; and examining ethics in guiding APRN clinical decision making. This edition examines and addresses all four APRN roles. As with similar texts, this edition offers a synopsis of translating research into practice with emphasis on implementing evidence-based practice and how to stay up-to-date with current research. Useful tools in advanced clinical decision making, practice issues (regulation, certification prescriptive authority, credentialing, and liability), and the exploration of employment opportunities and strategies are reviewed. Content assisting the novice APRN in developing entrepreneur models of care and in transitioning from a professional nursing role to an advanced practice role is included. As advanced practice nursing continues to evolve and expand, new material addressing the upcoming challenges for APRNs has been incorporated into this edition.

For decades the mantra in healthcare has been the need for collaborative interprofessional teams (IPTs). Chapter 5 explores the role of the APRN in the team's formation and leadership. This chapter discusses the composition of IPTs that will include a variety of healthcare providers, but in some cases, community leaders, chief executive officers (CEOs), technology experts, and others as well. The author challenges APRNs to assume more prominent leadership roles in healthcare delivery systems.

With the movement toward expanding the APRN role in collaborative IPTs, new skills and understanding of leadership competencies are needed. These concepts are explored in Chapter 7. This revised chapter emphasizes the importance of leadership competencies necessary for the delivery of quality care, evidence-based practice, and patient safety. Different leadership development models and curricula related to leadership in master's and doctor of nursing practice (DNP) programs are considered.

Health issues have become global, as evidenced by recent infectious disease outbreaks and by the prominence of organizations such as the World Health Organization, Doctors Without Borders, Sigma Theta Tau International Nursing Society, and International Council of Nursing.

The demand for APRNs is extending beyond the borders of the United States. Chapter 6 describes the multifaceted roles of APRNs internationally. As the advanced practice role emerges and evolves internationally, new opportunities for APRNs have surfaced. Roles such as (a) developing programs of study for U.S. students, (b) instituting cross-cultural exchange programs, (c) providing direct patient care in the form of mission trips, (d) assisting in the design and evaluation of educational programs for the advanced nursing practice role in developing countries, (e) identifying research partnerships and conducting research, and (f) influencing policies that improve health are presented.

The Patient Protection and Affordable Care Act (ACA) has placed APRNs on the front lines of healthcare reform; however, it was not the panacea to fix the healthcare system. Although this legislation has resulted in an increased demand for APRNs to meet the healthcare needs of those previously uninsured or underinsured, the necessary infrastructure to implement the ACA is lacking. The Institute of Medicine (IOM) reports have argued that the time is right for all nurses to function to their full capacity and that the barriers to advanced practice nursing need to be removed. Chapter 9 argues that this is the "golden age" for APRNs, despite all the changes in healthcare and APRNs being continually identified as "midlevel providers." This chapter reviews the critical events that have sculpted the APRN policy role in influencing and creating legislation and discusses how to become an engaged citizen in directing change.

Chapter 14 has been revised and expanded and discusses health information technology (HIT) competencies for nurses and APRNs, as well as common information management resources that APRNs are using or likely to encounter in the near future. The chapter explores "meaningful use" as described in HIT for economic and clinical health legislation and includes a discussion of select HIT controversies and failures.

All APRNs are scholars. APRNs should therefore be actively engaged in the scholarship of practice. Chapter 15 explores the multiple modalities that are incorporated into the scholarship of practice, such as sharing tricks of the trade, completing quality improvement projects, collaborating with nursing researchers, and being an active member in professional organizations. The chapter highlights the tools to disseminate knowledge, which is critical for the scholarship of practice.

In this edition, Chapters 16 and 17 from the previous edition have been merged to provide strategies for the emerging APRN to find a place in the healthcare system, whether as an employee or entrepreneur. Practical approaches to designing a practice or becoming part of an existing practice are included.

Woven throughout the text is the evolution of nursing education for APRNs in the context of the DNP. The future of APRN education will be the

DNP as the norm rather than as the exception. The DNP-educated APRN will be able to bring to the table a broader knowledge base of population-based healthcare, organizational systems, leadership skills, utilization of best practices or evidence-based practice, and meaningful use of electronic information systems.

With the goal to enhance student engagement, the sixth edition includes resources for instructors, including an instructor's manual and PowerPoint slides. **Qualified instructors may obtain access to ancillary materials by emailing textbook@springerpub.com.**

As with previous editions, this text equips the APRN student for success in the multidimensional advanced practice role.

Kathryn A. Blair, PhD, FNP-BC, FAANP

FOUNDATIONS OF ADVANCED NURSING PRACTICE

Melissa A. Saftner and Maria N. Ruud

OVERVIEW OF ADVANCED PRACTICE REGISTERED NURSING

Advanced practice registered nurses (APRNs) are at the forefront of the rapidly changing healthcare system, filling myriad roles in organizations where they provide cost-effective, high-quality care. APRNs are found in virtually every area of the American healthcare system: clinics, hospitals, community health, government, administration, policy-making boards, and private practice. In addition, APRNs have expanded practice into international and transglobal arenas. They serve the most economically disadvantaged as well as the elite. APRNs are deans, educators, consultants, researchers, policy experts, and, of course, outstanding clinicians.

Advanced practice registered nursing is an exciting career choice with many opportunities and challenges. The challenges are often related to the rapidly changing healthcare environment that is contingent on funding decisions made at the state and federal levels of governmental funding. Prospective payment systems, health inequities, required outcome measures, and spiraling costs are daily APRN practice realities. Technology improves diagnostic and treatment results; genetic research is unraveling complex pathophysiology and immunotherapy; and sophisticated "big data" electronic infrastructures change the way information is gathered, stored, analyzed, and shared. Innovative care models are common and include telehealth programs, integrated or complementary modalities, and retail clinics. These and other trends result in a rapidly changing healthcare system, ready for the influence and influx of APRNs.

Graduate education prepares APRNs to be key players in these complex systems. Midrange nursing theories provide strong conceptual foundations for APRN practice and nurse scholars. Nursing research uncovers scientific evidence for best practice, and research utilization skills enable APRNs to bring fresh ideas and proven interventions to healthcare consumers.

Complex policies and laws require that APRNs routinely navigate insurance reimbursement, management, and health policy regulations. Although APRNs were traditionally educated to provide advanced nursing care in specific clinics or hospital units, they now often work across system boundaries as they follow their patients through transitions of care. For example, APRNs care for patients in outpatient clinics, admit them to the hospital, assist in coordinating discharge plans, and collaborate with long-term care organizations, perhaps working with public health agencies to return their patients to their home communities. These new cross-system care models result in regulatory complexity for APRNs. They must be able to legally provide care across systems. Working across state lines results in even more complexity due to each state's laws and regulations. In addition, each healthcare organization can interpret state and federal laws and regulations in its own professional staff policies. Organizations can be more restrictive than laws, but they cannot be less restrictive. For example, state law may not require a signed collaboration agreement between a physician and APRN, but the healthcare system may mandate such an agreement. Given considerable variations among practice environments, APRNs must be experts and proactive in the business and regulatory policies and processes. Staying current is best accomplished by participation in role-specific APRN professional organizations.

ADVANCED PRACTICE REGISTERED NURSING: THEN AND NOW

Advanced specialization of nurses beyond their formal entry-level education has a long and proud history of innovative risk-takers and key events. To capture that history and unify the advanced nursing specialists, the term "advanced practice registered nurse" (APRN) became the common umbrella term used to designate four specialty roles of nurses with formal postbaccalaureate preparation: certified nurse-midwives (CNMs), certified registered nurse anesthetists (CRNAs), nurse practitioners (NPs), and clinical nurse specialists (CNSs).

Nurse anesthetists and nurse-midwives organized nearly a century ago and were the first APRNs to develop national standards for educational programs, professional organizations, and certification. NPs and CNSs standardized their preparation, certification, and licensing incrementally in recent decades. Various scholars and professional organizations have documented the unique history of each APRN role.

A number of factors led nursing leaders to delineate these four APRN roles. A critical factor was obtaining legal status to be directly reimbursed for their nursing services, a gradual process first achieved by nurse-midwives more than 35 years ago and subsequently expanded through federal and state legislation for the other three roles. Reimbursement laws and regulations require that nursing be able to specify the qualifications of these reimbursable APRNs, which contributed to increased standardization of titling, education, and national certification.

Public protection was another factor that led to the delineation of the APRN roles. State boards of nursing are mandated by state legislatures to safeguard the public from unsafe practice, and over time, all states have implemented laws and regulations to ensure that nurses in the four roles have specific expertise and skills. Some states have accomplished this through a second-level licensure process. In other states, APRNs are regulated through title protection and scope of practice laws. In 2008, APRNs reached an agreement defining a desired national model of regulation for the United States. This agreement, the Consensus Model for APRN Regulation: Licensure, Accreditation, Certification, and Education, is known as the LACE model (APRN Consensus Workgroup & APRN Joint Dialogue Group, 2008). The National Council of State Boards of Nursing (NCSBN) created a map in 2011 to track the implementation of the consensus model by the United States. A numerical point system to rate implementation of the LACE model was created by NCSBN with 28 points indicating full consensus adaptation by a state and 0 points indicating no adaptation (NCSBN, 2017b). By 2017, 15 states had fully implemented the LACE model and received a score of 28, 10 states and the District of Columbia enacted 75% to 96% (21–27 points) of the LACE model, 17 states scored 14–20 points, and 8 states received fewer than 14 points (NCSBN, 2017b). The changes in state laws required complex legislative initiatives led by APRNs (Kopanos, 2014). Most other states' APRN groups are working toward amending state nurse practice laws by adopting the LACE model of regulation.

A final factor influencing APRN standardization has been the adoption of national APRN curricular guidelines and program standards. These standards were developed by many specialty organizations and brought through negotiations to consensus by nursing organizations such as the American Association of Colleges of Nursing (AACN), the American Nurses Association (ANA), and the National Organization of Nurse Practitioner Faculties (NONPF). APRN educational standards have been endorsed by numerous nursing specialty organizations in the past decade and are used for national program accreditation.

Nursing's Scope and Standards of Practice (ANA, 2015b) defines APRNs as having advanced specialized clinical knowledge and skills through master's or doctoral education that prepares them for specialization, expansion, and advancement of practice. "Specialization" is concentrating or limiting one's focus to part of the whole field of nursing. "Expansion" refers to the acquisition of new practice knowledge and skills, including knowledge and skills legitimizing role autonomy within areas of practice that overlap traditional boundaries of medical practice. "Advancement" involves both specialization and expansion and is characterized by the integration of theoretical, research-based, and practical knowledge that occurs as part of graduate education in nursing. This APRN definition, which is regulated by state and federal laws, does not include nurses with advanced preparation for administration, informatics, education, public health, or research; those roles are considered "advanced nursing practice" and are not regulated, a fine but important legal distinction.

APRNs are educated within master's or doctoral nursing programs. Although CNSs have always required master's nursing degrees, in the past nurse-midwives, nurse anesthetists, and NPs were not all prepared in graduate nursing programs. Now, however, NPs must receive their education in graduate master's or clinical doctoral programs in nursing. CRNAs are prepared in master's or doctoral graduate programs. Although the majority of CNMs are prepared in graduate nursing programs, some nurse-midwifery programs are located in health-related professional schools.

Because of their unique historical underpinnings, members of each APRN category have strong allegiance to their titles and their professional organizations. At times, this allegiance has been a barrier to the development of consistent language regarding APRN roles because each group has developed its own education, history, and titles. However, significant progress continues to be made in identifying commonalities and working together in coalitions to improve regulations and policies restricting APRN practice.

Research-based practice (sometimes called "evidence-based" practice) is a key characteristic of APRN practice. Clinical doctoral nursing programs emphasize and expand the utilization of evidence-based practice, especially in terms of preparing APRNs to be organizational change agents. Graduates of clinical doctoral programs complete quality improvement projects to hone their skills at implementing research-based practice into all levels of the healthcare system.

Through a consensus-building process, the AACN formulated curricular elements for graduate APRN education (AACN, 2011), specifying the content of the graduate core curriculum and the advanced practice nursing core curriculum in master's programs (Exhibit 1.1). Practice doctoral nursing programs are based on the *Essentials of Doctoral Nursing Education for Advanced Practice Nurses* (AACN, 2006; Exhibit 1.2). The role-specific professional nursing organizations have further delineated specialized core competencies; documents are readily available on their websites and are frequently updated.

The core clinical content requires advanced health and physical assessment, advanced physiology and pathology, and advanced pharmacology (often referred to as "the three Ps"). These courses must be taught across the life span, with additional specific content required for students in each specialty area. For example, nurse-midwifery students need additional content on assessment of pregnant women and newborn infants, nurse anesthetist students require extensive content on anesthetic agents, and psychiatric/mental health students need additional content on antipsychotic medications.

There are also professional ethics standards for APRNs. In addition to issues related to confidentiality and relationships, APRNs must provide support to patients and their families in making ethical decisions related to treatment options (ANA, 2015a). Although ethical issues appear to be more prominent in tertiary care settings, issues such as abuse and neglect are

Exhibit 1.1 ESSENTIAL ELEMENTS OF MASTER'S CURRICULUM FOR ADVANCED PRACTICE NURSING

I.   Background for Practice From Sciences and Humanities

II. Organizational and Systems Leadership

III. Quality Improvement and Safety

IV. Translating and Integrating Scholarship Into Practice

V.   Informatics and Healthcare Technologies

VI. Health Policy and Advocacy

VII. Interprofessional Collaboration for Improving Patient and Population Health Outcomes

VIII. Clinical Prevention and Population Health for Improving Health

IX. Master's-Level Nursing Practice

Source: American Association of Colleges of Nursing. (2011). *The essentials of master's education for advanced practice nursing.* Washington, DC: Author.

Exhibit 1.2 ESSENTIALS OF DOCTORAL EDUCATION AND COMPETENCIES FOR ADVANCED NURSING PRACTICE

I.   Scientific Underpinnings for Practice

II. Organizational and Systems Leadership for Quality Improvement and Systems Thinking

III. Clinical Scholarship and Analytical Methods for Evidence-Based Practice

IV. Information Systems/Technology and Patient Care Technology for the Improvement and Transformation of Healthcare

V.   Healthcare Policy for Advocacy in Healthcare

VI. Interprofessional Collaboration for Improving Patient and Population Health Outcomes

VII. Clinical Prevention and Population Health for Improving the Nation's Health

VIII. Advanced Practice Nursing

Source: American Association of Colleges of Nursing. (2006). *The essentials of doctoral education for advanced nursing practice.* Washington, DC: Author. Retrieved from http://www.aacnnursing.org/Portals/42/Publications/DNPEssentials.pdf

present in all settings. APRNs are frequently called on to work with professional colleagues, patients, and their families to resolve ethical dilemmas.

All APRNs collaborate with other healthcare professionals to promote patient-centered care. Collaboration is a standard of APRN care and is also referenced in state and federal laws. Interprofessional and interdisciplinary teams require APRNs to clearly identify their unique contributions to patient outcomes. APRNs also collaborate with patients and their families in planning care and making decisions about the most acceptable treatments.

Recent scholarship emphasizes the benefits of APRN care including cost-effective, safe outcomes with positive patient satisfaction (Newhouse et al., 2011; Rantz, Birtley, Flesner, Crecelius, & Murray, 2017; Woo, Lee, & Tam, 2017), especially essential in an era of rapidly changing insurance and health system reform. In fact, the literature supports the use of APRNs in all aspects of healthcare delivery including anesthesia administrations, primary care, elder care, maternity and newborn care, and acute care (Edkins, Cairns, & Hultman, 2014; Newhouse et al., 2011; Rantz et al., 2017; Woo et al., 2017).

APRNs and Doctoral Education

The previous description of content in APRN educational and professional standards demonstrates the complexity and depth of APRN preparation and practice. Some nurse leaders question whether APRNs can be fully prepared for their scope of practice in 2-year master's programs. This has prompted discussion of the feasibility of doctoral preparation being required for APRN practice (Edwardson, 2004).

Doctoral APRN education existed in nursing doctorate (ND) programs as early as the mid-1980s at Rush University, Case Western Reserve University, and the University of Colorado, all of which awarded ND degrees to students completing NP programs. These NP programs have now discontinued the ND degrees; they have been replaced by doctorate of nursing practice (DNP) degrees. The DNP is a new degree first advocated by the AACN and the NONPF. In October 2004, the nation's nursing deans attending AACN passed a resolution to move APRN education to a practice doctorate level by 2015. Although a recommendation rather than a mandate, much progress has been made in increasing the number of NPs with doctoral degrees in the past decade. By early 2014, more than 240 DNP programs were under way nationwide (Kirschling, 2014).

There are pros and cons related to the DNP degree. The increased time and cost for students are balanced by the increase in knowledge, skill, and prestige that this doctoral degree confers. Pharmacy, audiology, physical therapy, and psychology have doctoral education as their entry to practice. The practice community has quite quickly embraced the DNP preparation; however, whether employers will compensate DNP graduates at levels commensurate with their education is undecided. Physician reactions to the nursing practice doctorate have been mixed; for example, several states have implemented legislation that reserves the term "doctor" for physicians in clinical arenas. A joint dialogue statement eloquently points out that "Graduate educational programs in colleges and universities in the United States confer academic degrees, which permit graduates to be called 'doctor.' No one discipline owns the title 'doctor' " (Nurse Practitioner Roundtable, 2008, p. 2). The DNP degree continues to be debated; the new degree is propelling APRN roles forward with new knowledge and abilities at a time when healthcare reform is at the forefront of the national conversation. Understanding each of the roles is essential.

Nurse Practitioners

Nurse practitioners (NPs) are registered nurses with master's or doctoral nursing preparation who perform comprehensive assessments, promote health, and treat and prevent illness and injury. In doing so they diagnose, develop differential diagnoses, and order and interpret diagnostic tests. They prescribe pharmacological and nonpharmacological treatments while providing care in primary, acute, and long-term care settings. The population foci for NPs include adult-gerontological, family (across the life span), neonatal, pediatrics, women's health-gender related, and psychiatric mental health. NPs practice autonomously and in collaboration with other healthcare professionals as researchers, consultants, and patient advocates.

The NP role first developed in primary care settings. However, NPs now function in tertiary care, and specific competencies and examinations have been developed for acute and emergency-care NPs (American Academy of Emergency Nurse Practitioners, 2015; NONPF, 2016).

Health promotion and health maintenance are emphasized in all the APRN nursing standards. Nurses have traditionally emphasized health-promotion activities as being a key characteristic of the professional practice of nursing. Health promotion, whether it is for persons who have no specific illness or for persons who have chronic health problems, is critical. Implementation of care that focuses on health promotion has also been shown to be cost-effective (Aleshire, Wheeler, & Prevost, 2012; Mundinger et al., 2000; Safriet, 1998). Horrocks, Anderson, and Salisbury (2002) noted that NPs offered more advice on self-care and management than did physicians, and they seemed to identify physical abnormalities more frequently. However, there was no difference in patient health outcomes between the NP- and physician-managed patient groups. A systematic review by Stanik-Hutt et al. (2013) spanning 18 years of research on the quality and effectiveness of care provided by NPs found that outcomes for NPs were comparable to physicians (MDs). Findings also indicated that patient outcomes on satisfaction with care were similar for NPs and MDs.

The NP movement began at the University of Colorado. Loretta Ford, PhD, RN, and Henry Silver, MD, both full professors, collaborated to launch a postbaccalaureate program to prepare nurses for expanded roles in the care of children and their families. Professors Ford and Silver (Ford, 1979) recognized that nurses had the ability to assess children's health status and define appropriate nursing actions. The purpose of the first NP demonstration project was to implement new roles to improve the safety, efficacy, and quality of healthcare for children and their families (Ford, 1979). Although the project's initial focus was on children and their families, Ford noted that she was confident that nurses could be educated to meet the health needs of community-dwelling persons across the life span. Nurses in the Colorado program received 4 months of intensive didactic education in which assessment skills and growth and development were emphasized. The nurses then completed a 20-month precepted clinical rotation in a community-based setting.

Following Colorado's lead, many schools initiated educational programs, admitting nurses with varying levels of educational preparation. The growth of the NP movement was facilitated by many studies through the years, such as those summarized in a meta-analysis by Brown and Grimes (1995). Over the years, NPs have demonstrated that they safely provide high-quality healthcare, and the NP role has expanded into many new practice areas (Martin, 2000; Mundinger et al., 2000; Newhouse et al., 2011; Stanik-Hutt et al., 2013). Although Dr. Ford's goal initially was to prepare NPs within master's programs, societal demand for NPs led to a proliferation of postbaccalaureate continuing education programs rather than graduate education (Ford, 1979, 2005). Federal funding for NP programs also prompted the initiation of numerous postbaccalaureate and graduate NP programs. The length of these early NP programs varied from a few weeks to 2 years, with many certificate programs being 9 to 12 months in length.

The proliferation of postbaccalaureate programs rather than graduate programs for the education of NPs was partially attributable to the resistance of graduate nursing programs to recognize NPs as being a legitimate part of nursing. A number of nursing leaders termed NPs "physician extenders" and did not view NP practice as "nursing." This lack of enthusiasm for NP education exhibited by numerous nursing leaders in the 1960s and 1970s may also have been fostered by the fact that the NP movement grew out of a collaborative nurse–physician effort rather than being solely initiated by nurses. The early NP curricula were viewed as being based on the medical model rather than a nursing framework, although that was not the focus of Dr. Ford's original NP curriculum, which emphasized child development and health promotion (Ford, 1979).

The NP domains and competencies were based on the work by Brykczynski (1989), Benner (1984), and Fenton (1985). The seven domains are (a) management of client health/illness status, (b) NP–patient relationship, (c) teaching/coaching function, (d) professional role, (e) management and negotiation of healthcare delivery systems, (f) monitoring and ensuring the quality of healthcare practice, and (g) culturally sensitive care (NONPF, 2006). Specific competencies are described for each domain. These domains are detailed and encompassing, indicating that APRN practice requires a broad range of knowledge and expertise. NONPF revised the domains for all NP programs in 2012 and developed nine core competencies: scientific foundation, leadership, quality, practice inquiry, technology and information literacy, policy, health delivery system, ethics, and independent practice. NPs are prepared in a multitude of specialties, including acute care, adult health, family health, gerontology, pediatrics, psychiatry, neonatology, and women's health. Population-specific competencies have been elaborated and defined (NONPF, 2013). In 2017, NONPF released an updated, nationally validated set of NP core competencies and curriculum content to support competencies for entry to practice for all NPs that aligned with the nine competencies released in 2012 (NONPF, 2017).

The ANA, along with other organizations, has developed many types of practice standards, some broadly inclusive and others specialty focused (ANA, National Association of Pediatric Nurse Practitioners [NAPNAP], & Society of Pediatric Nurses [SPN], 2010). For example, the ANA, NAPNAP, and SPN created a joint document that outlines pediatric nursing competencies at both basic and advanced practice levels.

The American Association of Nurse Practitioners (AANP, 2018) estimated that there were more than 248,000 NPs in the United States in 2017, 97.8% of whom were prepared with graduate degrees and that 86.6% of NPs are certified in an area of primary care. Many NPs assume positions that combine clinical practice with employment as educators, administrators, and policy makers or choose other employment.

After completing graduate education, NPs are eligible to sit for national certification examinations (NCE) in their specialty areas. Certification is a mechanism for the nursing profession to attest to the entry-to-practice knowledge of NPs. The certification requirement has been adopted by third-party payers such as the Centers for Medicare and Medicaid Services (CMS) and by most state boards of nursing as a standard that assists in protecting the public from unsafe providers. Certification examinations are offered by a variety of bodies: the American Nurses Credentialing Center (ANCC), the American Academy of Nurse Practitioners Certification Board (AANPCB), the Pediatric Nursing Certification Board (PNCB), the American Association of Critical Nurses Certification Corporation (AACNCC), and the National Certification Corporation (NCC) for the obstetric, gynecologic, and neonatal specialties.

Changes in reimbursement laws, regulations, and policies that allow for direct reimbursement of NPs, the rapid increase in managed care as a mechanism to control healthcare costs, and the growing recognition of the significant contributions of NPs to positive patient outcomes have resulted in a rapid increase in the number of NP programs, particularly DNP programs. The AANP (2018) estimated that 23,000 new NPs graduated in

2015–2016. APRNs who are savvy about ascertaining the gaps in health-care and designing roles for themselves that are not merely physician-replacement roles are likely to be very successful in obtaining satisfactory employment.

Scope of practice is regulated by state laws and describes the legal boundaries of health professional practice. NPs practicing outside the designated scope of practice risk legal sanctions and potential liability (Klein, 2005). Changes in scope of practice reflect the dynamic evolution of NP roles. However, great variability exists regarding the regulation of acute and primary care NPs by individual states.

Relative to CNMs and CRNAs, NPs have a relatively short history in the healthcare delivery system. However, in this short period of time, they have gained the respect of many health professionals and of their patients (Scherer, Bruce, & Runkawatt, 2007). NPs have been featured in the media for their expert opinions on healthcare-related matters and the significant contributions they are making to improving health. New areas of practice and settings for NPs continue to arise and in the next 10 years, the Bureau of Labor Statistics predicts a job growth rate for NPs to be 31%, much greater than the average growth rate of 7% (U.S. Department of Labor, 2017). In many instances, NPs have succeeded in caring for persons in rural areas, in inner cities, and for other vulnerable groups. NPs have established themselves as an integral part of the healthcare system.

Nurse-Midwives

Nurse-midwives are unique among APRNs because they are educated in two different professions. Midwifery is a profession in its own right and in many countries around the world nursing is not a prerequisite. The American College of Nurse-Midwives (ACNM, 2012b) defines "certified nurse-midwives" (CNMs) as individuals educated in the two disciplines of midwifery and nursing who complete a graduate degree program accredited by the Accreditation Commission for Midwifery Education (ACME) and pass the NCE of the American Midwifery Certification Board (AMCB). It is important to understand that there are various certifications for midwives, with CNM being just one. Certified midwives (CMs) receive a background in a health-related field other than nursing and graduate from a graduate midwifery education program accredited by the same organization that accredits CNMs, ACME. In contrast, certified professional midwives (CPMs), registered midwives (RMs), and licensed midwives (LMs) enter midwifery through various accredited and nonaccredited programs that may include required academic courses or an apprenticeship program. According to the ACNM (2012b), midwifery as practiced by CNMs and CMs encompasses a full range of primary healthcare services for women from adolescence beyond menopause. These services include the independent provision of primary care, gynecologic and family planning services, preconception care, care during pregnancy, childbirth and the postpartum period, care of the normal newborn during the first 28 days of life, and treatment of male partners for sexually transmitted infections. CNMs and CMs provide initial and ongoing comprehensive assessment, diagnosis, and treatment. They conduct physical examinations; prescribe medications including controlled substances and contraceptive methods; admit, manage, and discharge patients; order and interpret laboratory and diagnostic tests; and order the use of medical devices. Midwifery care practiced by CNMs and CMs also includes health promotion, disease prevention, and individualized wellness education and counseling. These services are provided in partnership with women and families in diverse settings such as ambulatory care clinics, private offices, community and public health systems, homes, hospitals, and birth centers (ACNM, 2012a, p. 1).

Although the focus of midwifery care has historically been prenatal care and managing labor and birth, nurse-midwives are primary care providers for essentially healthy women, including those with acute and stable chronic conditions. Nurse-midwives strongly believe in supporting natural life processes and not using medical interventions unless there is a clear need. This belief and others are reflected in the 2004 ACNM (2004, p. 1) philosophy statement.

Midwives also believe in:

• Watchful waiting and nonintervention in normal processes
• Appropriate use of interventions and technology for current or potential health problems
• Consultation, collaboration, and referral with other members of the healthcare team as needed to provide optimal health care (ACNM, 2004, para. 1)

Midwifery is a very old profession, mentioned in the Bible. The practice of midwifery declined in the 18th and 19th centuries, and obstetrics developed as a medical specialty. In 1925, Mary Breckinridge established the Frontier Nursing Service (FNS) in Kentucky and was the first nurse to practice as a nurse-midwife in the United States (Breckinridge, 1952). She received her midwifery education in England and returned to the United States with other British nurse-midwives to set up a system of care similar to that which she had observed in Scotland. The FNS was begun to care for women and infants who were without adequate healthcare. The nurse-midwives of the FNS provide quality maternal and infant care with significantly improved outcomes.

The first U.S. nurse-midwifery educational program was started at the Maternity Center Association, Lobenstein Clinic, in New York City in 1932 and the ACNM was incorporated in 1955. Nurse-midwifery practice grew slowly until the late 1960s and early 1970s, when the profession experienced increased acceptance and consumer demand increased for nurse-midwives and the kind of care they provided (King et al., 2015). In 2017, there were 11,826 CNMs and 101 CMs in the United States (ACNM, 2018).

Nurse-midwifery education began with certificate programs and has progressed to graduate education. There are presently 39 ACME-accredited programs in the United States. Most midwifery programs are in schools of nursing, but two are in university-based health-related professional schools. A direct-entry (non-nursing) route to midwifery education, using the same nationally recognized accreditation and certification standards, began in 1997 at the State University of New York (downstate campus). CM students are required to complete certain prerequisite health sciences courses, such as chemistry, biology, nutrition, and psychology, before beginning midwifery education. In addition, certain knowledge and skills common in nursing practice are required before beginning the midwifery clinical courses in the program (ACME, 2005). CMs are currently authorized to practice in five states (ACNM, 2018). CPMs, another category of direct-entry midwives who attend out-of-hospital births, are recognized in approximately half of the states and have a different scope of practice and regulation process than midwives who graduate from ACME-accredited programs.

In the 1970s, national accreditation of nurse-midwifery educational programs and national certification of nurse-midwives was begun by ACNM. The ACME accreditation process is recognized by the U.S. Department of Education, and the certification process now conducted by the AMCB is recognized by the National Commission of Health Certifying Agencies. As a result of national accreditation and certification, CNMs have direct third-party reimbursement and prescriptive authority in all 50 states (ACNM, 2018).

The ACNM document, *Core Competencies for Basic Midwifery Practice* (ACNM, 2012a), describes the skills and knowledge that are fundamental to the practice of a new graduate of an ACME-accredited educational program. These competencies guide curricular development in midwifery programs and are used in the nationally recognized accreditation process. Competencies described in the document include professional responsibilities; the midwifery management process; midwifery care of women, including primary care; preconception care; gynecologic care (including contraceptive methods); perimenopausal and postmenopausal care; prenatal, intrapartum, and postpartum care of the childbearing woman; and care of the newborn. Hallmarks of midwifery practice are also delineated.

Nurse-midwives in the United States have consistently demonstrated that their care results in excellent outcomes and client satisfaction among all women, including the large proportion of underserved, uninsured, low-income, minority, and otherwise vulnerable women for whom CNMs provide care. Births attended by CNMs and CMs occur primarily in hospitals; more than 94% of births in the United States occurred in hospitals in 2014, although the number of home and freestanding birth center births has been rising (ACNM, 2018; MacDorman, Mathews, & Declercq, 2014). Research has demonstrated fewer interventions, including lower cesarean birth rates, among CNM-attended births versus physician-attended births, as well as outcomes at least comparable to physician-attended births (Blanchette, 1995;

Hamlin, 2017; MacDorman & Singh, 1998; Newhouse et al., 2011; Rosenblatt et al., 1997; Thornton, 2017).

The Lancet published a four-paper series advocating for midwifery care in 2014. The four papers examined midwifery globally and advocated for an increased midwife presence worldwide to improve maternal and neonatal outcomes (Homer et al., 2014; Renfrew et al., 2014; ten Hoope-Bender et al., 2014; Van Lerberghe et al., 2014). A systematic review and meta-analysis of midwifery care globally demonstrated that women receiving midwifery-led care experienced equivalent or better outcomes—including fewer episiotomies, less anesthesia use, reduced likelihood of preterm birth, and more spontaneous vaginal births—than those receiving other types of care (Sandall, Soltani, Gates, Shennan, & Devane, 2013). Another systematic review identified exclusively U.S.-based studies and found similar results, with equivalent or superior outcomes in initiating breastfeeding, operative and cesarean births, and perineal lacerations (Newhouse et al., 2011). Additional research since 2011 confirmed Newhouse et al.'s finding (Hamlin, 2017; Thornton, 2017). From a policy perspective, midwifery care can be a cost-effective and sustainable approach to meeting society's women's healthcare needs (Renfrew et al., 2014).

Over the nearly 100-year history of nurse-midwifery/midwifery in the United States, a strong base of support documented by research has been developed and is ongoing. The number of educational programs and practitioners has grown substantially. The passage of the Patient Protection and Affordable Care Act in 2010 resulted in a key provision sought by CNMs for nearly 20 years: the same reimbursement as physicians under Medicaid for providing the same service (Bradford, 2013). During this era of healthcare reform, as healthcare dollars continue to be carefully allocated and specific outcomes measured more closely, CNMs and CMs can be expected to play a more prominent role in providing quality primary healthcare to women.

Clinical Nurse Specialists

Clinical nurse specialists (CNSs) are leaders and experts in evidence-based nursing practice (National Association of Clinical Nurse Specialists [NACNS], 2014). They are registered professional nurses with graduate preparation earned at the master's or doctoral level. They may also be educated in a postmaster's program that prepares graduates to practice in specific specialty areas (Lyon, 2004; Lyon & Minarik, 2001). In 2017, 216 schools offered CNS programs, an increase from 147 programs in 1997 (Dayhoff & Lyon, 2001; NACNS, 2017a). The NACNS has developed curriculum recommendations for CNS education (NACNS, 2011) as well as competencies to reflect the *Essentials of Doctoral Education for Advanced Nursing Practice* (NACNS, n.d.). CNSs have traditionally worked in hospitals, but they now practice in many settings, including nursing homes, schools, home care, and hospice. Essential characteristics and essential core content of NACNS for CNS programs are based on CNSs' spheres of influence: patients/clients and patients, nurses and nursing practice, and organizations/systems.

The CNS role has had a long history in the United States. The CNS role was developed after World War II. Before that time, specialization for nurses was in the functional areas of administration and education. Recognizing the need to have highly qualified nurses directly involved in patient care, the concept of CNSs emerged. Reiter (1966) first used the term "nurse clinician" in 1943 to designate a specialist in nursing practice. The first master's program in a clinical nursing specialty was developed in 1954 by Hildegard E. Peplau at Rutgers University to prepare psychiatric CNSs. That program launched the CNS role that has been an important player in the nursing profession and healthcare arena ever since, although the role has not been without controversy. Healthcare restructuring and cost-cutting initiatives in the 1980s and 1990s resulted in a loss of CNS positions in the United States. However, after increasingly frequent reports of adverse events in hospital settings in the 1990s (IOM Committee on the Quality of Healthcare in America, 2001; Kohn, Corrigan, & Donaldson, 2000), it became apparent that CNSs were critical to obtaining quality patient outcomes (Clark, 2001; Heitkemper & Bond, 2004), with the result that CNSs are again seen as valuable professionals in many U.S. healthcare systems.

As with the NP movement, the availability of federal funds for graduate nursing educational programs and the Professional Traineeship Program through Health Resources and Services Administration (HRSA) that provides stipends for students have played a role in the development of many graduate CNS programs.

The development and use of complex healthcare technology in the management of patients in hospitals and intricate surgical procedures have resulted in increasing acuity and complexity of patient care delivery. Thus, there is a need for nurses with advanced knowledge and expertise to be integrally involved in working with staff to assess, plan, implement, and evaluate care for these patients. Many hospitals have used CNSs as care coordinators and case managers in which they coordinate the care of patients with acute or chronic illnesses during their hospital stays and prepare them for discharge to their homes or other care facilities. CNSs have also been used as discharge planners working with staff to plan posthospital care for patients who have complex health problems (Naylor et al., 1994; Neidlinger, Scroggins, & Kennedy, 1987). Their importance in care coordination over the care continuum is only now being lauded, exemplified in the work of Naylor and colleagues, who reported that use of gerontologic CNSs as discharge planners resulted in fewer readmissions of elderly cardiac patients.

Since its inception, the CNS role has suffered from role ambiguity (Rasch & Frauman, 1996; Redekopp, 1997). Although the initial vision was for CNSs to be integrally involved in patient care for a specific patient population, they have assumed many other roles, such as staff and patient educators, consultants, supervisors, project directors, and more recently, case managers. Redekopp (1997) noted that it is difficult for CNSs to precisely describe their roles to others because their roles are continually evolving to meet the health needs of a changing patient population in an ever-changing healthcare system. Role ambiguity has made it difficult to measure the impact that CNSs have on patient outcomes. Thus, when budgetary crises have occurred in hospitals, CNSs have frequently had to advocate strongly to maintain their positions because outcome data to support the positive impact of their practice have either not been readily available or simply did not exist.

The area of specialization for a CNS may be defined by population, setting, disease or medical subspecialty, type of care, or type of problem. CNS specialties and subspecialties include psychiatric/mental health nursing, adult health, gerontology, oncology, pediatrics, cardiovascular, neuroscience, rehabilitation, pulmonary, renal, diabetes, and palliative care, to name a few. However, certification exists only for the population areas of adult/gerontology, pediatrics, and neonatal. The two certifying organizations include the ANCC and the AACNCC (NACNS, 2017b). Specialty certifications may be obtained through various speciality nursing organizations. However, some organizations do not specify that master's degrees are required for certification in the specialty, causing confusion regarding the regulation and title of CNS. In the past, many CNSs have not sought third-party reimbursement, so they have not taken specialty CNS certification examinations. With changes in state nursing practice acts and the increase in third-party payment and prescriptive privileges for APRNs, the number of certified CNSs is now increasing. A 2016 census of CNSs conducted by NACNS found that almost 68% of the respondants were nationally certified (NACNS, 2017a). The majority of states require national certification; half of all states allow independent practice for CNSs and prescriptive authority has been granted to CNSs by less than one-third of states (NCSBN, 2017a). CNSs are regulated by state boards of nursing although the APRN role for CNSs is not recognized by three states (NCSBN, 2017a).

In the late 1980s and early 1990s, many discussions and debates took place around the merging of the CNS and NP roles (Page & Arena, 1994). Several studies were conducted comparing the knowledge and skills of these two advanced practice roles (Elder & Bullough, 1990; Fenton & Brykczynski, 1993; Forbes, Rafson, Spross, & Kozlowski, 1990; Lindeke, Canedy, & Kay, 1996). Research indicated that there were many similarities in the educational preparation of these two groups of APRNs. Many CNSs viewed the proposed merger as the demise of the CNS role. NPs were concerned that they would need to abandon the title of NP, a title that had become familiar to many patients and healthcare professionals. The NACNS was formed in 1995 to assist CNSs and to provide a vehicle to publicize the many contributions that CNSs have made and continue to make in providing quality patient care. The CNS role today is a dynamic and needed advanced practice nursing role, and many in the nursing profession anticipate that it will continue to exist for years to come.

Certified Registered Nurse Anesthetists

Nurse anesthesia practice traces its origins to the inception of surgical anesthesia, a major innovation that allowed for the development of surgery as a means of treatment for disease. Anesthesia in the late 1800s was hazardous and crude. There was not a good understanding of the pharmacologic and physiologic effects of anesthetic drugs, primarily diethyl ether and chloroform. These anesthetics were often delivered in a "careless manner" by a surgical resident fresh out of medical school who had little or no training in the effects of the anesthetic (Bankert, 1989, p. 22). This led to disastrous results for patients. Thus, some surgeons turned to religious Hospital Sisters who would devote their entire attention to the well-being of the patient during the delivery of the anesthetic. One of the Hospital Sisters, Sister Mary Bernard, was the first identified nurse who delivered anesthesia at St. Vincent's Hospital in Erie, Pennsylvania, in 1877 (Bankert, 1989).

The practice of utilizing nurses to deliver anesthesia spread rapidly through the Catholic and secular hospitals of the late 1800s and early 1900s. In 1912, a formal program of training in the delivery of anesthesia for nurses was developed in Springfield, Illinois, by Mother Magdalene Wiedlocher of the Third Order of the Hospital Sisters of St. Francis. This Order of Hospital Sisters went on to establish St. Mary's Hospital in Rochester, Minnesota, that we now know as the origin of the Mayo Hospitals. These nurse anesthetists at St. Mary's Hospital became known as experts in the delivery of anesthesia who devoted their full attention and skill to the well-being of the patient receiving anesthesia. One nurse anesthetist, in particular, Alice Magaw, stood out as an example of the diligent care delivered by nurse anesthetists. In addition to skillfully delivering anesthetics, Magaw recorded her work and published it in respected medical journals of the time. One such paper published in 1906 documented 14,000 anesthetics at St. Mary's Hospital "without a death directly attributable to anesthesia" (Bankert, 1989, p. 31). Magaw's legacy is honored in the motto of the American Association of Nurse Anesthetists (AANA): Safe and effective anesthesia care (AANA, n.d.).

Certified registered nurse anesthetists (CRNAs) are registered nurses who have become anesthesia specialists by taking a graduate curriculum that focuses on the development of clinical judgment and critical thinking. They are qualified to make independent judgments concerning all aspects of anesthesia care based on their education, licensure, and certification by the National Board of Certification and recertification for nurse anesthetists. CRNAs are legally responsible for the anesthesia care they provide and are recognized in state law in all 50 states, the District of Columbia, Puerto Rico, and the Virgin Islands (AANA, 2013).

Anesthesia care is delivered in collaboration with surgeons, podiatrists, dentists, radiologists, psychiatrists, cardiologists, and anesthesiologists in outpatient, inpatient, and office-based settings.

The CRNA scope of practice includes comprehensive anesthesia and pain care across the life span in many different settings. The scope includes:

1. *Performing* and documenting a preanesthetic assessment and evaluation of the patient, including requesting consultations and diagnostic studies; selecting, obtaining, ordering, and administering preanesthetic medications and fluids; and obtaining informed consent for anesthesia
2. *Developing* and implementing an anesthetic plan
3. *Initiating* the anesthetic technique that may include general, regional, local, and sedation
4. *Selecting,* applying, and inserting appropriate noninvasive and invasive monitoring modalities for continuous evaluation of the patient's physical status
5. *Selecting,* obtaining, and administering the anesthetics, adjuvant and accessory drugs, and fluids necessary to manage the anesthetic
6. *Managing* a patient's airway and pulmonary status using current practice modalities
7. *Facilitating* emergence and recovery from anesthesia by selecting, obtaining, ordering, and administering medications, fluids, and ventilatory support
8. *Discharging* the patient from a postanesthesia care area and providing postanesthesia follow-up evaluation and care
9. *Implementing* acute and chronic pain management modalities
10. *Responding* to emergency situations by providing airway management, administration of emergency fluids and drugs, and using basic or advanced cardiac life support techniques (AANA, 2013)

The CRNA may also have other responsibilities that could include administration and management activities, education, research, quality improvement, interdepartmental liaison, committee appointments, and oversight of other nonanesthesia departments.

Nurse anesthesia educational programs are offered at both the master's level and the clinical doctoral level. The Council on Accreditation (COA) of Nurse Anesthesia Educational Programs is the entity that accredits all nurse anesthesia educational programs regardless of the degree offered. This formal process of accreditation began in 1952 (Bankert, 1989). At this time, nurse anesthesia programs at the master's degree level are a minimum of 24 months in length and at the doctoral level, a minimum of 36 months. All nurse anesthesia educational programs must provide a minimum number of cases and a minimum curriculum that includes pharmacology of anesthetic agents and adjuvant drugs including concepts in chemistry and biochemistry (105 hours); anatomy, physiology, and pathophysiology (135 hours); professional aspects of nurse anesthesia practice (45 hours); basic and advanced principles of anesthesia practice including physics, equipment, technology, and pain management (105 hours); research (30 hours); clinical correlation conferences (45 hours); radiology; and ultrasound. In addition, the curriculum must include three separate comprehensive graduate-level courses in advanced physiology/pathophysiology, advanced health assessment, and advanced pharmacology.

Students must administer a minimum of 550 clinical cases that prepare them for the full scope of practice in a variety of clinical settings (COA, 2004). Completion of the nurse anesthesia educational program and the required cases qualifies the student to sit for the NCE.

Following publication of the AACN's initiative to move education of advanced practice nursing into doctoral frameworks by 2015, the AANA established a task force on doctoral education for nurse anesthetists in 2005. The task force recommended to the board of directors of the AANA that all nurse anesthesia educational programs be offered in a clinical doctoral framework by the year 2025. The COA will not consider any new master's degree programs for accreditation beyond 2015. Students accepted into an accredited program on January 1, 2022, and thereafter must graduate with doctoral degrees (COA, 2004). Unlike other nursing advanced practice specialties, nurse anesthesia programs are not necessarily housed in schools of nursing. Of the 115 programs of nurse anesthesia accredited in the United States, 39 are in a variety of non-nursing academic units (COA, 2017). These programs may offer the Doctorate of Nurse Anesthesia Practice (DNAP) degree. Wherever the educational program is housed, all nurse anesthesia educational programs must be accredited through the COA and the graduates must pass the NCE. Thus, the public is assured that every nurse anesthetist has met a set of predetermined qualifications for entry into practice.

In 1986, the passage of the Omnibus Budget Reconciliation Act marked nurse anesthetists as the first group of advanced practice nursing professionals to be granted direct reimbursement for anesthesia and pain management services to Medicare enrollees. This paved the way for entrepreneurship and innovative practice settings for nurse anesthetists. Furthermore, in 2001, the CMS published its anesthesia care rule granting state governors the ability to opt out of the federal physician supervision requirement, thus allowing nurse anesthetists to work in collaboration with other healthcare providers without physician supervision (AANA, 2018). To date, 17 states have opted out of the CMS requirement for physician supervision of nurse anesthetists. No states have opted out since 2012. In a study completed after states had opted out of the requirement and involving outcomes in states with physician supervision and those opt-out states, no negative outcomes or harm were found when CRNAs delivered anesthesia without physician supervision (Dulisse & Cromwell, 2010).

Nurse anesthesia practice is remarkably varied and flexible. Nurse anesthetists function in fast-paced trauma team settings in urban areas and in highly independent rural settings. Nurse anesthetists provide critically needed surgical and obstetric anesthesia, acute pain management, trauma stabilization, and, in some instances, chronic pain management for the rural communities in which they live. Without the services of nurse anesthetists, many of these small rural hospitals would close (Siebert, Alexander, & Lupien, 2004). Nurse anesthetists have served in the military in peace and on the battlefield in every armed conflict since the World War I, including the most recent conflicts in Iraq and Afghanistan (AANA, 2010). Nurse anesthetists are a crucial part of the modern healthcare system today both in terms of quality of care and access to highly skilled afford-able care. The education and training of nurse anesthetists position these advanced practice nurses to lead healthcare into the future.

International

Although the content in this chapter has focused on APRNs in the United States, it is encouraging to see the continuing development of these roles in other countries. Midwifery, a profession often distinct from nursing, has a longer history internationally than in the United States. The International Confederation of Midwives, so named in 1954, has more than 130 mid-wifery association members representing 112 countries (see www.internationalmidwives.org). The recent *Lancet Series on Midwifery* highlighted midwifery as "a vital solution to the challenges of providing high-quality ma-ternal and newborn care for all women and newborn infants, in all coun-tries" (Renfrew et al., 2014, p. 1). Clinical specialization in nursing has existed in many countries for a long time. In countries such as Australia, Canada, Ireland, the Netherlands, and New Zealand, nurse practitioners have become a major player in the healthcare system (Maier, Barnes, Aiken, & Busse, 2016), while the clinical nurse specialist was one of the first advanced practice nurse (APN) roles to evolve in Asian countries (Pulcini, Jelic, Gul, & Loke, 2010). Many countries have adopted some form of advanced practice nursing.

SUMMARY

APRNs have made significant contributions to quality healthcare, partic-ularly for vulnerable populations. If all Americans are to receive quality, cost-effective healthcare, it is critical that greater use be made of APRNs. Their advanced knowledge and skills, both in nursing and related fields, make valuable contributions to the current and future healthcare system, especially in the task of meaningful healthcare reform. As the United States becomes more diverse, APRNs play key roles in providing culturally com-petent care. They assume leadership in developing new practice sites and innovative systems of care to enhance healthcare outcomes. A bright future awaits nursing and APRNs.

ACKNOWLEDGMENT

The authors acknowledge the contributions of Linda Lindeke, Melissa Avery, and Kathryn White who contributed to this chapter in the previous edition.

REFERENCES

Accreditation Commission for Midwifery Education. (2005). *The knowledge, skills, and behaviors prerequisite to midwifery clinical coursework.* Silver Spring, MD: Author.

Advanced Practice Registered Nurses Consensus Workgroup & APRN Joint Dialogue Group. (2008). Consensus model for APRN regulation: Licensure,

accreditation, certification, and education. Retrieved from https://www
.ncsbn.org/Consensus_Model_for_APRN_Regulation_July_2008.pdf

Aleshire, M. E., Wheeler, K., & Prevost, S. S. (2012). The future of nurse practitioner practice: A world of opportunity. *Nursing Clinics of North America,*
47(2), 181–191. doi:10.1016/j.cnur.2012.04.002

American Academy of Emergency Nurse Practitioners. (2015). Overview of
emergency nurse practitioners (ENP's). Retrieved from http://aaenp-natl
.org/images/AAENP_ENPOverview.pdf

American Association of Colleges of Nursing. (2006). *The essentials of*
doctoral education for advanced nursing practice. Washington, DC: Author.
Retrieved from https://www.aacnnursing.org/Portals/42/Publications/
DNPEssentials.pdf

American Association of Colleges of Nursing. (2011). *The essentials of master's edu-*
cation for advanced practice nursing. Washington, DC: Author.

American Association of Nurse Anesthetists. (n.d.). Who we are. Retrieved from
http://www.aana.com/about-us/who-we-are

American Association of Nurse Anesthetists. (2013). Scope of nurse anesthesia
practice. Retrieved from https://www.aana.com/docs/default-source/
practice-aana-com-web-documents-(all)/scope-of-nurse-anesthesia-practice
.pdf?sfvrsn=250049b1_2

American Association of Nurse Anesthetists. (2018). Fact sheet concerning
state opt-outs and November 13, 2001, CMS rule. Retrieved from https://
www.aana.com/advocacy/state-government-affairs/federal-supervision
-rule-opt-out-information/fact-sheet-concerning-state-opt-outs

American Association of Nurse Practitioners. (2018). NP fact sheet. Retrieved
from https://www.aanp.org/all-about-nps/np-fact-sheet

American College of Nurse-Midwives. (2004). *Philosophy of the American College of*
Nurse-Midwives. Silver Spring, MD: Author.

American College of Nurse-Midwives. (2012a). *Core competencies for basic mid-*
wifery practice. Washington, DC: Author.

American College of Nurse-Midwives. (2012b). *Definition of midwifery and scope*
of practice of certified nurse-midwives and certified midwives. Silver Spring,
MD: Author.

American College of Nurse-Midwives. (2018). Essential facts about midwives.
Silver Spring, MD: Author. Retrieved from http://www.midwife.org/
Essential-Facts-about-Midwives

American Nurses Association. (2015a). *Code of ethics for nurses with interpretive*
statements (2nd ed.). Silver Spring, MD: Author.

American Nurses Association. (2015b). *Nursing: Scope and standards of practice* (3rd
ed.). Silver Spring, MD: Author.

American Nurses Association, National Association of Pediatric Nurses
Practitioners, & Society of Pediatric Nurses. (2010). *Pediatric nursing: Scope and*
standards of practice. Silver Spring, MD: American Nurses Association.

Bankert, M. (1989). *Watchful care: A history of America's nurse anesthetists.* New York,
NY: Continuum.

Benner, P (1984). *From novice to expert: Excellence and power in clinical nursing prac-*
tice. Menlo Park, CA: Addison-Wesley.

Blanchette, H. (1995). Comparison of obstetric outcome of a primary-care access clinic staffed by certified nurse-midwives and a private practice group

of obstetricians in the same community. *American Journal of Obstetrics & Gynecology, 172*(6), 1868–1871. doi:10.1016/0002-9378(95)91424-2

Bradford, H. M. (2013). Women's health and maternity care policies: Current status and recommendations for change. In M. D. Avery (Ed., pp. 301–330), *Supporting a physiologic approach to pregnancy and birth: A practical guide*. Ames, IA: Wiley-Blackwell.

Breckinridge, M. (1952). *Wide neighborhoods, a story of the frontier nursing service*. Lexington: The University Press of Kentucky.

Brown, S., & Grimes, D. (1995). A meta-analysis of nurse practitioners and nurse midwives in primary care. *Nursing Research, 44*, 332–339. doi:10.1097/00006199-199511000-00003

Brykczynski, K. (1989). An interpretive study describing the clinical judgment of nurse practitioners. *Scholarly Inquiry for Nursing Practice: An Interpretive Journal, 3*, 113–120.

Clark, A. (2001). What will it take to reduce errors in health care settings? *Clinical Nurse Specialist, 15*(4), 182–183.

Council on Accreditation of Nurse Anesthesia Educational Programs. (2004). Standards for accreditation of nurse anesthesia educational programs, Revised June 2016. Retrieved from http://home.coa.us.com/accreditation/Documents/2004%20Standards%20for%20Accreditation%20of%20Nurse%20Anesthesia%20Educational%20Programs,%20revised%20June%202016.pdf

Council on Accreditation of Nurse Anesthesia Educational Programs. (2017). *Nurse anesthesia programs summary of 2016 annual report data*. Park Ridge, IL: Author.

Dayhoff, N., & Lyon, B. (2001). Assessing outcomes of clinical nurse specialist practice. In R. Kleinpell (Ed.), *Outcome assessment in advanced nursing* (pp. 103–129). New York, NY: Springer Publishing.

Dulisse, B, & Cromwell, J. (2010). No harm found when nurse anesthetists work without supervision by physicians. *Health Affairs* 29(8), 1469–1475. doi: 10.1377/hlthaff.2008.0966

Edkins, R. E., Cairns, B. A., & Hultman, C. S. (2014). A systematic review of advance practice providers in acute care: Options for a new model in a burn intensive care unit. *Annals of Plastic Surgery, 72*(3), 285–288. doi:10.1097/SAP.0000000000000106

Edwardson, S. (2004). Matching standards and needs in doctoral education in nursing. *Journal of Professional Nursing, 20*, 40–46. doi:10.1016/j.profnurs.2003.12.006

Elder, R., & Bullough, B. (1990). Nurse practitioners and clinical nurse specialists: Are the roles merging? *Clinical Nurse Specialist, 4*, 78–84. doi:10.1097/00002800-199022000-00006

Fenton, M. (1985). Identifying competencies of clinical nurse specialists. *Journal of Nursing Administration, 15*, 31–37. doi:10.1097/00005110-198512000-00008

Fenton, M., & Brykczynski, K. (1993). Qualitative distinctions and similarities in the practice of clinical nurse specialists and nurse practitioners. *Journal of Professional Nursing, 9*, 313–326. doi:10.1016/8755-7223(93)90006-X

Forbes, K., Rafson, J., Spross, J., & Kozlowski, D. (1990). Clinical nurse specialist and nurse practitioner core curricula survey results. *Nurse Practitioners, 15*, 45–48. doi:10.1097/00006205-199004000-00010

Ford, L. (1979). A nurse for all settings: The nurse practitioner. *Nursing Outlook, 27*, 516–521.

Ford, L. (2005). Opinions, ideas and convictions for NPs' founding mother, Dr. Loretta Ford. *The American Journal for Nurse Practitioners, 9*(3), 31–33.

Hamlin, L. (2017). Comparison of births by provider, place, and payer in New Hampshire. *Policy, Politics, & Nursing Practice, 18*(2), 95–104. doi:10.1177/1527154417720680

Heitkemper, M., & Bond, E. (2004). Clinical nurse specialists: State of the profession and challenges ahead. *Clinical Nurse Specialist, 18*(3), 135–140. doi:10.1097/00002800-200405000-00014

Homer, C.S.E., Friberg, I.K., Dias, M.A.B., ten Hoope-Bender, P., Sandall, J., Speciale, A.M., & Bartlett, L.A. (2014). The projected effect of scaling up midwifery. *Lancet, 384*(9948), 1146–1157. doi:10.1016/S0140-6736(14)60790-X

Horrocks, S., Anderson, E., & Salisbury, C. (2002). Systematic review of whether nurse practitioners working in primary care can provide equivalent care to doctors. *British Medical Journal, 324*(7341), 819–823. doi:10.1136/bmj.324.7341.819

Institute of Medicine Committee on the Quality of Healthcare in America. (2001). *Crossing the quality chasm: A new health system for the 21st century.* Washington, DC: National Academies Press.

King, T. L., Brucker, M. C., Kriebs, J. M., Fahey, J. O., Gegor, C. L., & Varney, H. (2015). *Varney's midwifery* (5th ed.). Boston, MA: Jones & Bartlett.

Kirschling, J. M. (2014). *Reflections on the future of doctoral programs in nursing.* Retrieved from http://www.aacnnursing.org/Portals/42/DNP/JK-2014-DNP.pdf

Klein, T. (2005). Scope of practice and the nurse practitioner: Regulation, competency, expansion, and evolution. *Topics in Advanced Practice Nursing eJournal, 7*(3), 1–10.

Kohn, L. T., Corrigan, J. M., & Donaldson, M. S. (Eds.). (2000). *To err is human: Building a safer health system.* Washington, DC: National Academies Press.

Kopanos, T. (2014). Celebrating mile markers. *The Journal for Nurse Practitioners, 10*(7), A13, A14.

Lindeke, L, Canedy, B., & Kay, M. (1996). A comparison of practice domains of clinical nurse specialists and nurse practitioners. *Journal of Professional Nursing, 13,* 281–287. doi:10.1016/S8755-7223(97)80105-6

Lyon, B. (2004). What to look for when analyzing clinical nurse specialist statutes and regulations. *Clinical Nurse Specialist, 16*(1) 33–34. doi:10.1097/00002800-200201000-00013

Lyon, B., & Minarik, P. (2001). Statutory and regulatory issues for clinical nurse specialist (CNS) practice: Ensuring the public's access to CNS services. *Clinical Nurse Specialist, 15*(3), 108–114. doi:10.1097/00002800-200105000-00014

MacDorman, M. F., Mathews, T. J., & Declercq, E. (2014). *Trends in out-of-hospital births in the United States, 1990–2012. NCHS data brief, no. 144.* Hyattsville, MD: National Center for Health Statistics.

MacDorman, M. F., & Singh, G. K. (1998). Midwifery care, social and medical risk factors, and birth outcomes in the USA. *Journal of Epidemiology and Community Health, 52*(5), 310–317. doi:10.1136/jech.52.5.310

Maier, C. B., Barnes, H., Aiken, L. H., & Busse, R. (2016). Descriptive, cross-country analysis of the nurse practitioner workforce in six countries: Size growth, physician substitution potential. *British Medical Journal Open, 6*(9), e011901. doi: 10.1136/bmjopen-2016-011901

Martin, K. (2000). Nurse practitioners: A comparison of rural-urban practice patterns and willingness to serve in underserved areas. *Journal of the*

American Academy of Nurse Practitioners, 12, 491–496. doi:10.1111/j.1745 -7599.2000.tb00163.x

Mundinger, M., Kane, R., Lenz, E., Totten, A., Tsai, W., Cleary, P., . . . , Shelanski, M. L. (2000). Primary care outcomes in patients treated by nurse practitioners or physicians: A randomized trial. *Journal of the American Medical Association, 283,* 59–68. doi:10.1097/00132586-200012000-00026

National Association of Clinical Nurse Specialists. (n.d.). Organizing framework and CNS core competencies. Retrieved from http://www.nacns.org/docs/ CNSCoreCompetencies.pdf

National Association of Clinical Nurse Specialists. (2011). Criteria for the evaluation of clinical nurse specialist master's, practice doctorate, and post-graduate certificate educational programs. Retrieved from http://www.nacns .org/docs/CNSEducationCriteria.pdf

National Association of Clinical Nurse Specialists. (2014). What is a clinical nurse specialist? Retrieved from http://www.nacns.org/html/cns-faqs1.php

National Association of Clinical Nurse Specialists. (2017a). CNS census. Retrieved from http://nacns.org/professional-resources/practice-and-cns -role/cns-census

National Association of Clinical Nurse Specialists. (2017b). What is a CNS? Retrieved from http://nacns.org/about-us/what-is-a-cns

National Council of State Boards of Nursing. (2017a). APRN roles recognized. Retrieved from https://www.ncsbn.org/5399.htm

National Council of State Boards of Nursing. (2017b). Implementation status map. Retrieved from https://www.ncsbn.org/5397.htm

National Organization of Nurse Practitioner Faculties. (2006). *2006 Domains and core competencies of nurse practitioner practice.* Washington, DC: Author. Retrieved from http://www.nonpf.org/NONPF2005/CoreCompsFINAL06.pdf

National Organization of Nurse Practitioner Faculties. (2013). Population-focused nurse practitioner competencies. Retrieved from http://c .ymcdn.com/sites/www.nonpf.org/resource/resmgr/competencies/ populationfocusnpcomps2013.pdf

National Organization of Nurse Practitioner Faculties. (2016). Adult-gerontology, acute care and primary care NP competencies 2016. Washington, DC: Author. Retrieved from https://cdn.ymaws.com/www.nonpf.org/resource/resmgr/ competencies/NP_competencies.pdf

National Organization of Nurse Practitioner Faculties. (2017). *Nurse practitioner core competencies content.* Washington, DC: Author. Retrieved from http:// www.nonpf.org/resource/resmgr/competencies/2017_NPCoreComps_ with_Curric.pdf

Naylor, M., Brooten, D., Jones, R., Lavizzo-Mourey, R., Mezey, M., & Pauly, M. (1994). Comprehensive discharge planning for the hospitalized elderly: A randomized clinical trial. *Annals of Internal Medicine, 120,* 999–106. doi:10.7326/0003-4819-120-12-199406150-00005

Neidlinger, S., Scroggins, K., & Kennedy, L. (1987). Cost evaluation of discharge planning for hospitalized elderly. *Nursing Economic$, 5,* 225–230.

Newhouse, R. P., Stanik-Hutt, J., White, K. M, Johantgen, M., Bass, E. B., Zangaro, G., . . . , Weiner, J. P. (2011). Advanced practice nursing outcomes 1990–2008: A systematic review. *Nursing Economic$, 29,* 230–250.

Nurse Practitioner Roundtable. (2008). *Nurse practitioner DNP education, certification and titling: A unified statement.* Washington, DC: Author.

Page, N., & Arena, D. (1994). Rethinking the merger of the clinical nurse specialist and the nurse practitioner roles. *Image: The Journal of Nursing Scholarship, 26,* 315–318. doi:10.1111/j.1547-5069.1994.tb00341.x

Pulcinic, J., Jelic, M., Gul, R., Loke, A.Y, (2010). An international survey on advanced practice nursing education, practice and regulation. *Journal of Nursing Scholarship, 42*(1) 31–39. doi:10.1111/j.1547-5069.2009.01322.x

Rantz, M. J., Birtley, N. M., Flesner, M., Crecelius, C., & Murray, C. (2017). Call to action: APRNs in U.S. nursing homes to improve care and reduce costs. *Nursing Outlook, 65*(6), 689–696. doi:10.1016/j.outlook.2017.08.011

Rasch, R., & Frauman, A. (1996). Advanced practice in nursing: Conceptual issues. *Journal of Professional Nursing, 12,* 141–146. doi:10.1016/S8755-7223(96)80037-8

Redekopp, J. (1997). Clinical nurse specialist role confusion: The need for identity. *Clinical Nurse Specialist, 11,* 87–91. doi:10.1097/00002800-199703000-00017

Reiter, F. (1966). The nurse clinician. *American Journal of Nursing, 66,* 274–280. doi:10.2307/3419873

Renfrew, M. J., Homer, C. S. E., Downe, S., McFadden, A., Muir, N., Prentice, T., & ten Hoope-Bender, P. (2014). Midwifery: An executive summary for *The Lancet's* series. *The Lancet,,* 1–8. Retreived from https://www.thelancet.com/pb/assets/raw/Lancet/stories/series/midwifery/midwifery_exec_summ.pdf

Rosenblatt, R., Dobie, S., Hart, L., Schneeweiss, R., Gould, D., Raine, T. R., . . . , Perrin, E. B. (1997). Interspecialty differences in the obstetric care of low-risk women. *American Journal of Public Health, 87,* 344–351. doi:10.2105/AJPH.87.3.344

Safriet, B. (1998). Still spending dollars, still searching for sense: Advanced practice nursing in an era of regulatory and economic turmoil. *Advanced Practice Nursing Quarterly, 4,* 24–33.

Sandall, J., Soltani, H., Gates, S., Shennan A., & Devane, D. (2013). Midwife-led continuity models versus other models of care for childbearing women. *Cochrane Database of Systematic Reviews, 2016*(4), CD004667. doi:10.1002/14651858.CD004667.pub5

Scherer, Y. K., Bruce, S. A., & Runkawatt, V. (2007). A comparison of clinical simulation and case study presentation on nurse practitioner students' knowledge and confidence in managing a cardiac event. *International Journal of Nursing Education, 4*(1), 1–14.

Siebert, E., Alexander, J., & Lupien, A. (2004). Rural nurse anesthesia practice: A pilot study. *American Association of Nurse Anesthetists Journal, 72*(3), 181–190. Retrieved from http://www.aana.com/newsandjournal/Documents/181-190.pdf

Stanik-Hutt, J., Newhouse, R. P., White, K. M., Johantgen, M., Bass, E. B., Zangaro, G., . . . Weiner, J. P. (2013). The quality and effectiveness of care provided by nurse practitioners. *The Journal for Nurse Practitioners, 9*(8), 492–500.e13. doi:10.1016/j.nurpra.2013.07.004

ten Hoope-Bender, P., de Bernis, L., Campbell, J., Downe, S., Fauveau, V., Fogstad, H., ...Van Leberghe, W. (2014). Improvement of maternal and newborn health through midwifery. *Lancet, 384*(9949), 1226–1235. doi:10.1016/S0140-6736(14)60930-2

Thornton, P. (2017). Characteristics of spontaneous births attended by midwives and physicians in US hospitals in 2014. *Journal of Midwifery & Women's Health, 62*(5), 531–537. doi:10.1111/jmwh.12638

U.S. Department of Labor, Bureau of Labor Statistics. (2017). Occupational out-look handbook: Nurse anesthetists, nurse midwives, and nurse practitioners. Retrieved from https://www.bls.gov/ooh/healthcare/nurse-anesthetists -nurse-midwives-and-nurse-practitioners.htm

Van Lerberghe, W., Matthews, Z., Achadi, E., Ancona, C., Campbell, J., Channon, A., ...Turkmani, S. (2014). Country experience with strengthening of health systems and deployment of midwives in countries with high maternal mortality. *Lancet, 384*(9949), 1215–1225. doi:10.1016/S0140-6736(14)60919-3

Woo, B. F., Lee, J. X., & Tam, W. W. (2017). The impact of the advanced practice nursing role on quality of care, clinical outcomes, patient satisfaction, and cost in the emergency and critical care settings: A systematic review. *Human Resources for Health, 15*(1), 63. doi:10.1186/s12960-017-0237-9

Patricia A. Ducklow

ADVANCED PRACTICE WITHIN A NURSING PARADIGM

Every nurse's philosophy and beliefs influence his or her daily nursing practice. This philosophy for each nurse reflects the nurse's values and includes paradigms and theories, and overall, is the reference framework and foundation of practice. A paradigm is characterized by the unique constructs, concepts, tenets, and presuppositions on which it is built (Bahramnezhad, Shiri, Asgari, & Afshar, 2015). Some presuppositions for many nursing paradigms include key concepts such as person, health, environment, and nursing. Paradigms provide guidance to the profession and discipline of nursing. Each paradigm also informs the research, development, and implementation of nursing theories that are the bridges connecting nursing theory and nursing practice. An APRN is a registered nurse with expert knowledge built on the competence of the professional nurse and is characterized by the application of a broad range of theoretical- and evidenced-based knowledge (American Nurses Association [ANA], 2010). APRNs are nurses who have earned a master's degree, postmaster's certificate, or Doctor of Nursing Practice degree in one of four specific roles: certified nurse-midwife (CNM), nurse practitioner (NP), clinical nurse specialist (CNS), or certified registered nurse anesthetist (CRNA).

The most important word in the title of APRN is the last one: *nurse*. Advanced education enables nurses to expand their knowledge base and expertise in nursing so that their practices differ not only from those of nurses with an associate's or bachelor's degree but also from those of other health professionals, particularly physicians or physician assistants. Nurses often underestimate the profound positive effect that their care can have on improving individual and population outcomes and the impact on the quality of care. Florence Nightingale, in *Notes on Nursing* (1859/1992), noted that people in her day often thought of nursing as signifying "little more than the administration of medicines and the application of poultices" (p. 6). Efforts are still necessary to convey the full scope of advanced nurse practice to other nurses, professionals, and to the public so that APRNs' contributions to positive health outcomes are understood, respected, valued, and reimbursed. So often the media have focused on the physical assessment skills, tasks, and prescriptive privileges of APRNs rather than on the distinctive and unique knowledge, education, abilities, and expertise that characterize advanced practice nursing.

The impetus for improving healthcare delivery and the need to demonstrate positive healthcare outcomes are consequences of the work undertaken by the Institute of Medicine (IOM). The role of the IOM is not to regulate or create law pertaining to healthcare delivery systems, but to influence policy creation for the delivery of excellent, predictable healthcare (Finkelman, 2013). The IOM publishes detailed reports compiled by expert panels that highlight critical flaws in healthcare delivery that contribute to poor quality healthcare and disparities. Governmental agencies, such as Centers for Medicare and Medicaid (CMS), and regulatory bodies such as The Joint Commission (TJC) utilize these reports that provide the basis for essential improvement strategies such as setting hospital standards, elements of performance, National Patient Safety Goals, and Accreditation Participation Requirements. A necessary component of improving healthcare is the mandatory reporting and benchmarking of safety events, which are accessible to the general public. Poor outcomes, hospital-acquired conditions, and newer events result in the withholding of reimbursement by Medicare and Medicaid, which causes significant financial losses for the organization. Better informed consumers are also demanding high-quality care and are quick to challenge the ever-increasing cost of care. Therefore, demonstrating positive outcome achievement is of paramount importance in healthcare.

One area identified by the IOM requiring significant improvement is the preparation of new graduates entering the healthcare arena. Healthcare professionals should meet five essential core competencies prior to the completion of their educational program: (a) provide patient-centered care, (b) work in interdisciplinary/interprofessional teams, (c) use evidence-based practice (EBP), (d) apply quality improvement (QI), and (e) utilize informatics (Greiner & Knebel, 2003). APRNs expertly demonstrate these five core competencies making their contribution essential in leading improvement strategies. The rigor and experience provided by APRN curricula produce transformational leaders who can serve as the bridge to quality.

APRNs are particularly adept as change agents as they apply theory to practice across the three spheres of influence; patient/client, nurses and nursing practice, and organizations/systems. Working within these three spheres of influence, the APRN is perfectly situated to understand the impact of cumbersome processes at the micro and macro level of an organization (Hanson, 2015). APRNs expertly maneuver through the complexities of healthcare, identifying and removing barriers to advance nursing practice and improve patient outcomes. As change agents, APRNs drive the necessary improvements by integrating new knowledge and guiding nurses to achieve desired outcomes, education, process, and policy (Mayo, Ray, Chamblee, Urden, & Moody, 2017). Consultation and collaboration are inherent to APRNs, making them integral in the success of interdisciplinary teams achieving best quality outcomes and integrating best practices (Fulton, 2011). The unique skill sets of APRNs help to substantiate the value and contribution to healthcare that nurses make, by supporting, conducting, and showcasing nursing research. APRNs encourage nurses to participate in research, which results in new knowledge and ownership of practice. These contributions build on EBP and provide the opportunity for nurses to think independently and to practice autonomously (Morley & Jackson, 2017).

As advanced practice nursing moves rapidly toward the practice doctorate as entry into practice, an excellent opportunity exists to reconceptualize how advanced practice nursing is taught in APRN programs. Burman et al. (2009) challenge educators to focus on health promotion and disease management, incorporating theories from a variety of disciplines to improve health behavior and change their pedagogies as doctorate of nursing practice (DNP) programs and curricula continue to develop. Chism (2013) supports the need for DNP curricula to focus on the leadership of chronic disease management, transformational leadership, population management, and the care of our aging population.

WHAT IS NURSING?

Definitions of Nursing

For many years, the nursing profession has sought to define nursing and to identify its scope of practice. It is critical that APRNs and those aspiring to this role have a clear understanding of what nursing is in order for them to provide a clear understanding of nursing's unique contributions to quality healthcare outcomes in their interprofessional interactions. Therefore, several of the many definitions of nursing that have been put forth over the years are reviewed.

Nightingale (1859/1992) formulated one of the earliest definitions of nursing, which went beyond caring for ill patients. She emphasized the whole person, including diet and environment. The aim of nursing care, according to Nightingale, is to put the individual in the best possible condition so that nature can act on the person. Nightingale's *Notes on Nursing,* although written 150 years ago, speaks to the substantive basis of nursing. Not only does Nightingale elaborate on interventions nurses can employ; she also underscores the necessity of thorough assessments before planning nursing care. Reading *Notes on Nursing* should therefore be a part of every APRN curriculum.

In Henderson's (1966) definition of nursing, emphasis is placed on the nurse collaborating with the individual to enhance the individual's health status. Henderson defined "nursing" as "Assisting the individual, sick or well, in the performance of those activities contributing to health or its recovery (or to a peaceful death) that he would perform unaided if he had the necessary strength, will, or knowledge. And to do this in such a way as to help him gain independence as soon as possible" (p. 15).

Henderson's definition contains many elements that constitute the substantive nature of nursing. Health promotion and caring are key components of her definition. Not all individuals will recover from their diseases or injuries. It is the nurse's role to assist the individual to achieve the goals he or she has established (Jackson, 2015). Henderson stresses helping the individual gain independence. Independence is a Western belief and may not be a value in all cultures. Thus, it is important for the nurse to ascertain the personal values of each individual and realize that independence may not be one of his or her preferences.

Nojima (1989), a Japanese nursing theorist, defined "nursing practice" as a "human activity carried out by nurses to help individuals organize their health conditions so that they are able to live optimally and realize their potential" (pp. 6–7). In her definition, the focus is on a person's quality of life. The partnership between the nurse and the individual is evident in Nojima's definition of nursing. With the advent of globalization, it is important to review the characteristics of nursing outside of Western medicine (Nojima, Tomikana, Makabe, & Snyder, 2003).

The ANA has defined "nursing" as follows: Nursing is the protection, promotion, and optimization of health and abilities; prevention of illness and injury; alleviation of suffering through the diagnosis and treatment of human response; and advocacy in the care of individuals, families, communities, and populations (ANA, 2010, p. 10). Previously, the definition of nursing focused on persons and their responses to health problems, rather than specific illnesses. The aforementioned definition of nursing developed in 2003, which emphasizes health promotion and optimal health, remains unchanged in current discussions of the ANA's *Social Policy Statement* (ANA, 2010). The focus on health differentiates nursing from the practice of medicine.

Despite the frequent reference to the ANA definition of nursing, many APRNs have encountered difficulty practicing from a nursing model. They have been seemingly forced to launch their practice within the medical model in part because of medical diagnoses used for billing and coding and in part because of the medical community's and the public's perception of APRNs. Although it is important to know the cause of a person's pain or stress, much of nursing care remains the same despite the cause. It has been encouraging to see the Agency for Healthcare Research and Quality (AHRQ) consider problems or responses, rather than disease entities, as the focus of practice guidelines. The AHRQ website (www.ahrq.gov) is an excellent resource for EBP and current clinical practices.

Advanced practice nursing builds on the competence of the professional nurse and is characterized by the integration and application of a broad range of theoretical- and evidence-based knowledge (ANA, 2010). An APRN is defined as a "provider that is certified in one of the four roles, educated in health promotion, assessment, diagnosis, management, pharmacotherapeutics, and direct care to individuals, populations, and communities" (J. M. Stanley, 2012, p. 244).

The APRN Consensus Model: licensure, accreditation, certification, and education (LACE) defines advanced registered nurse practice, provides a regulatory model identifying titles, roles, and population foci (APRN Consensus Workgroup & APRN Joint Dialogue Group, 2008). Specialization within advanced practice focuses beyond the six populations (family/individual across life span, adult gerontology, neonatal, pediatrics, women's health/gender-related, psychiatric/mental health) and provides depth within a population. One of the most important aspects of specialization in nursing is that the distinct specialization is always a part of the whole discipline of professional nursing (ANA, 2010).

The APRN consensus model, LACE, has stipulated that APRNs be educated within an accredited program with advanced pathophysiology, advanced health assessment, advanced pharmacology; complete a minimum of 500 clinical hours; and be nationally certified. The licensure of an APRN is "defined as a legal title and credentials to be granted to all advanced practice registered nurses meeting the definitional criteria. Boards of nursing are responsible for granting a second license to APRNs in all four roles" (M. C. Stanley, 2011, p. 248). The LACE model is relevant to improving, standardizing, and regulating the scope of practice; improving the professional transition for APRNs; and highlighting safety as a motivator for national regulation (Rounds, Zych, & Mallary, 2013).

The ANA's *A Social Policy Statement* (2010) emphasizes the characteristics of nursing practice to include human responses, theory application, evidence-based nursing actions, and outcomes. These characteristics build the foundation for professional nursing (ANA, 2010). Within this model, nursing's paradigms, professional scope of practice, code of ethics, specialization, and certification laid the base for professional nursing. Building on this base in a pyramid model are individual state's nurse practice acts, rules, and regulations. From this level, institutional policies and procedures guide nursing practice, with self-determination as the top level of the pyramid model. This model lays the foundation not only for nursing paradigm, professional nursing but for all its expanded roles and specializations.

Scope of Practice

Gaining more knowledge about the substantive basis of the science of nursing is an essential component of APRN education. Scope of practice can be viewed in several ways. In fact, findings from the numerous studies undertaken to identify, describe, and classify the phenomena of concern and compassion of nurses have helped clarify our understanding of scopes of practice.

In *Future of Nursing: Leading Change, Advancing Health*, the IOM report (2011) emphasizes "the need for nurses to practice to the full extent of their education, achieve higher levels of education, be full partners in healthcare systems, and engage in workplace planning and policy making" (Mayo et al., 2017, p. 72). One way to determine scope of practice from a regulatory framework is to focus on population, with each APRN working within his or her specific practice population and his or her actual practice being determined by the APRN regulatory model as discussed previously. Other initiatives such as nursing diagnoses and human responses delineate the substantive basis of nursing.

Nursing Diagnoses

Nursing diagnoses are one strategy nurses have used to describe phenomena for which nurses provide care. Since the First Nursing Diagnosis Conference in 1973, nurses within the North American Nursing Diagnosis Association International (NANDA-I) have worked to identify, describe, and validate individual problems and concerns that fall within the domain of nursing. Currently, there are 235 approved or revised nursing diagnoses (NANDA-I, 2015). Continued efforts are necessary to identify and validate and code new diagnoses and to revise existing diagnoses. APRNs have provided and can continue to provide leadership in the nursing diagnosis movement.

NANDA-I diagnoses are grouped under nine functional patterns: exchanging, communicating, relating, valuing, choosing, moving, perceiving, knowing, and feeling. According to Newman (1984), it is important for nurses to determine changes in an individual's patterns. In approaching assessment in this manner, the focus is on the whole person rather than on specific diagnoses.

Nursing diagnoses have been widely accepted not only in the United States but also internationally (NANDA-I, 2015). As the first effort to develop a common language for nursing phenomena, and despite numerous criticisms, using such diagnoses assists nurses in focusing on those aspects of care for which nursing interventions can be identified and nurse-sensitive outcomes can be determined. In the United States, several projects to identify and classify nursing interventions have been initiated. The National Intervention Classification (NIC) has identified and classified more than 550 research-based nursing interventions (Bulechek, Butcher, Dochterman, & Wagner, 2013; Johnson et al., 2005). To help facilitate the value added by nursing, APRNs need to be familiar with both nursing and medical diagnoses and begin developing new models of reimbursement beyond *International Classification of Diseases*, 10th revision *(ICD-10)* codes.

Human Responses

Human experiences and responses proposed by the ANA (2010) include

> promotion of health and wellness; promotion of safety and quality of care; care and self-care processes, and care coordination; physical, emotional, and spiritual comfort, discomfort, and pain; adaption to physiologic and pathophysiologic processes; emotions related to the experience of birth, growth and development, health, illness, disease, and death; meanings ascribed to health and illness; linguistic and cultural sensitivity; health literacy; decision making and the ability to make

choices; relationships, role performance, and change processes within relationships; social policies and their effects on health; healthcare systems and their relationships to access, cost, and quality of healthcare; and the environment and the prevention of disease and injury.

As with nursing diagnoses, these identified human responses assist APRNs in focusing on the health concerns and needs of the individual, population, or communities. Advanced practice nursing care is of primary importance in producing positive individual outcomes while focusing on health promotion, disease management, education, and wellness. Therapeutics for managing the human responses or assisting the person in managing them may transcend medical care. For example, despite various causes of sleep problems, nursing interventions, such as massage and music therapy, can be used successfully. Viewing nursing in the context of and the perspective of human responses helps all nurses organize the patient-centered plan of care with the nurse's point of view.

THE ART AND SCIENCE OF NURSING
The Art of Nursing

The art of nursing is integrally tied to the caring aspect of nursing. For many years, nursing was defined as both an art and a science. As nurses began to give more attention to establishing a scientific basis for nursing practice, they thereby gained greater acceptance in the scientific community and, yet, the art or caring aspect of nursing received less attention. In practice settings, for example, nurses focused more attention on the high technology used in caring for individuals with complex health problems. Nonetheless, the public has sustained its attachment and desire for APRN-provided caring interventions, such as massage, therapeutic touch, focused listening, guided imagery, and aromatherapy, to name a few. A number of reasons for which people seek nonpharmacological complementary therapies have been proposed: (a) they wish to be treated as whole persons by health professionals; (b) they wish to be active participants in their care; (c) they desire that the treatment not be worse than the disease; and (d) they feel that Western healthcare does not meet all of their needs. Therefore, it is important that APRNs consider how they can integrate the art of nursing, which includes traditional and nontraditional nursing interventions, into their practice.

The essence of the APRN is the caring relationship with the patient. Through sharing knowledge and providing support through communication, caring, and relationship building, the APRN fosters health promotion and disease management with patients, populations, and communities. Caring is a critical element of nursing practice. Leininger (1990), Watson (1988), and Gadow (1980) have each put forth definitions of caring. Watson defined the art of caring as "a human activity consisting of the following: a nurse consciously, by means of certain signs, passes on to others, feelings he or she has lived through, realized or learned; others are united to these feelings and also experience them" (p. 68).

Newman, Sime, and Corcoran-Perry (1991) noted that the focus of nursing is "caring in the human health experience" (p. 3).

Caring requires that a nurse be competent in assessing and intervening. Benner (1998) noted that a caring attitude was not sufficient to make an action a caring practice. The practice must be implemented in an excellent manner in order to be viewed as caring. Caring and the art of nursing convey very similar meanings, but caring nurses also seek the scientific basis for their practice and continue to update their expertise and knowledge. APRNs possess the knowledge and ability to critique research about specific therapies and determine their applicability to specific individual populations.

In 1993, Schoenhoefer and Boykin proposed that the nursing process–based care models, including nursing diagnoses, did not truly address what nurses ought to be doing. Their grand theory of nursing has a framework based on caring that is specific to each nurse, person, and situation, requiring personal individual knowledge of each patient's situation. They acknowledge that all humans care and that nursing is a discipline that requires knowing and developing advanced nursing knowledge. Nursing is also a profession, in which nursing knowledge is applied and used in response to the individual's human needs while still being a dynamic, evolving, creative, and caring process (Schoenhoefer & Boykin, 1993; Zaccagnini & Waud White, 2014). APRNs are well prepared to practice from a theory-driven human-caring basis. A theory-based paradigm-focused advanced nursing practice defines and exemplifies many attributes of the APRN.

Hagedorn and Quinn (2004) proposed a theory of primary caring specific to the APRN that includes five domains: connection, consistency, commitment, community, and change. The domain *connection* describes the APRN's effectiveness based on relationship-centered caring with the patient, family, and community. *Consistency* describes the importance of evidence- and theory-based care in advanced nursing practice. *Commitment* describes how the NP is committed to serve each patient and family to his or her best ability. *Community* illustrates the role of the NP in facilitating full access to healthcare for all persons and strives to meet unmet community health needs. The fifth domain, *change,* explains how APRNs introduce innovative models of healthcare and share decision making with patients.

Basic human needs are to be viewed as those of a whole person and cared for as such. It is the role of the APRN to support and assist the patient in being cared for in a holistic manner. APRNs incorporate the empiric aspects of medicine but practice within a nursing framework. The incorporation of holistic care into practice aids in distinguishing nursing from the medical model. The advantage for patients is that not only are their physical needs met but also there is consideration of their emotional, spiritual, and mental needs (Jasemi, Valizadeh, Zamanzedeh, & Keogh, 2017). The American Holistic Nurses Association/American Association of Nursing (2013, p. 7) identify "compassion, caring trust, and relationships as instruments of healing … and as part of the healing environment." The APRN's qualities and actions of presence, empowerment, reflection, listening, touch, empathy, humor, and knowing the community, as well as the APRN's ability to access care and to directly provide care, ensure patient satisfaction, and provide quality evidence-based outcomes (Hagedorn & Quinn, 2004).

The Science of Nursing

Significant progress has been made in developing the knowledge base that underlies nursing practice, revealing that nursing is characterized by both art and science (ANA, 2004). Although nursing is guided by standards of practice based on clinical evidence and research, additional research is always needed to further develop EBPs so that APRNs will have a sound scientific basis from which to choose specific interventions for individuals or populations (ANA, 2010). The clinical guidelines and evidence-based protocols developed by professional and governmental agencies and available through the National Guideline Clearinghouse exemplify the work that has been done, and that continues to be done, in identifying "best practices" based on research findings. APRNs play a key role in developing, reviewing research, and writing clinical guidelines that integrate the most recent EBP in the literature.

THEORETICAL AND CONCEPTUAL MODELS

During the past 50 years, the nursing profession has given considerable attention to theoretical and conceptual models. This attention has served to differentiate nursing from other disciplines (Marrs & Lowry, 2009; Russell & Fawcett, 2005). However, nursing theories are not new in nursing. Nightingale (1859/1992) elaborated on the relationship of the environment to health and well-being. Numerous theoretical and conceptual models exist.

What relevance do nursing theories have to practice? Cannot nurses merely practice nursing? Meleis (2011) noted that a theory articulates and communicates a mental image of a certain order that exists in the world. This image includes components, and these components inform a model or perspective that guides each nurse's practice. This model may be identical to one of the publicized nursing theories, or it may be based on a theoretical perspective from another discipline. In some instances, eclectic models are used in which nurses combine elements from established nursing theories or theories from other disciplines. New nursing theories continue to be developed. Of particular importance is the delineation of nursing theories that incorporate various cultural perspectives, because the Western philosophical perspective to date has not pervaded many of the existing theories.

There has been much discussion about whether one grand nursing theory is needed. Would the existence of a grand or meta-theory be advantageous to the progression of the profession and discipline? Riehl-Sisca (1989) stated that nursing has benefited from having a multiplicity of theories. The wide range of perspectives elaborated in these theories has helped nurses to more clearly define the nature of the discipline and profession, to evaluate various approaches that can be employed in practice, and to respect diversity as a positive element. Alligood and Marriner-Tomey (2005) identified seven theorists who have developed primary grand theories or conceptual frameworks for nursing: Johnson (1980), King (1971), Levine (1967), Neuman (1974), Orem (1980), Rogers (1970), and Roy (1984). Many other nurses have developed middle-range theories or conceptual frameworks that have served as a basis for research and practice.

More recently, nurses have turned their attention to middle-range theories. Middle-range theories, which focus on a limited number of variables, are more amenable to empirical testing than are grand theories by definition. Examples of middle-range theories include empathy (Olson & Hanchett, 1997), uncertainty in illness (Mishel, 1990), resilience (Polk, 1997), mastery (Younger, 1991), self-transcendence (Reed, 1991), caring (Swanson, 1991), and illness trajectory (Weiner & Dodd, 1993).

Duffy (2009) developed the quality-caring model, providing the APRN with a framework that emphasizes the less visible value of nursing, that is, caring. This is often the less obvious value, but one that guides practice; provides a foundation for quality care, improved outcomes, and patient satisfaction; and supports research. In her model, evidence-based care environment in healthcare today is merged with the caring qualities and attributes of nursing. Caring values, attitudes, knowledge, and behaviors will guide and drive the process of the care plan and interventions, and will establish the foundation for strong relationships. The APRN's patient–nurse relationship is primary and includes all interactions and interventions for which the APRNs are accountable and will implement autonomously. To be a successful APRN leader, collaborative relationships are necessary and include "those activities and responsibilities that nurses share with the members of the interprofessional healthcare team" (Duffy, 2009, p. 82).

Many nurses give little thought to the tenets that guide their practice; however, these philosophical underpinnings have a profound impact on the nature and scope of their practice. When APRNs have a theory-guided practice, they improve the care being provided by offering structure, efficiency in regard to continuity of care, higher quality of care, and improved health outcomes. The discipline of nursing, including professionalism, accountability, and APRN autonomy as a care provider, is supported with a nursing theory–guided practice. Often, an APRN practices and applies clinical decision making within a nursing framework but is not consciously aware of doing so.

Nurses have an ethical and moral responsibility to practice nursing with a consciously defined approach to care. The theoretical or conceptual model used by a nurse provides the basis for making the complex decisions that are crucial in the delivery of high-quality nursing care. In this regard, Smith (1995) stated the following: "The core of advanced practice nursing lies within nursing's disciplinary perspective on human-environment and caring interrelationships that facilitate health and healing. This core is delineated specifically in the philosophic and theoretic foundations of nursing" (p. 3). Thus, nursing theory is an important component of APRN education.

Nursing is a practice discipline, and theories achieve importance in relation to their impact on nursing care. Recently, attempts have been made to relate nursing theories to practice and to begin testing these theories. However, only minimal testing of these theories in practice settings has occurred. The number of theoretical nursing studies, particularly studies examining the efficacy of nursing interventions, is an indication of the apparent separation of theories and practice that has characterized much of nursing practice. As DNP programs continue to mature and develop, it is anticipated that the application gap between theories and practice will narrow.

The theoretical or conceptual framework that an APRN selects and uses has a major impact on the assessments that are made and the nature of the interventions that are chosen to achieve individual outcomes. One's conceptual perspective on clients and on nursing's goals strongly determines what kinds of things one assesses (Gordon, 2007; Johnson, 1959). Everyone has a perspective, whether in conscious awareness or not. Problems can arise if the perspective "in the head" is inconsistent with the actions taken during assessment. Information collection has to be logically related to one's view of nursing. A conceptual model provides the practitioner with a general perspective or a mind-set of what is important to observe, which in turn provides the basis for making nursing diagnoses and selecting nursing interventions.

INCORPORATING NURSING INTO ADVANCED PRACTICE NURSING

Guaranteeing that APRNs view the provision of healthcare from a nursing perspective has implications for graduate curricula. The American Association of Colleges of Nursing (AACN, 2006) includes nursing theory as a component of its document *Essentials of Doctoral Education for Advanced Practice Nursing.* Students also need assistance in utilizing this theoretical content in their practice. Faculty and preceptors who model this approach for advanced practice nursing students are critical for helping them integrate theory into practice and to build bridges over the theory-to-practice gap that currently exists.

APRNs provide healthcare to many individuals and populations in diverse care environments and settings. APRNs have the opportunity to make major contributions to advance the nursing profession. By focusing on the nursing elements of healthcare, APRNs have the opportunity to demonstrate to the public and to policy makers the unique and significant contributions that nursing has on health outcomes. In using nursing frameworks rather than the medical model as the focus of practice, APRNs provide the public with a distinct and adjunctive model of care rather than a substitutive model (i.e., replacing physicians). APRNs may carry out activities that have traditionally been a part of medicine, but the manner, approach, style, and performance of these activities by APRNs need to be translated into the realm of nursing.

SUMMARY

Nursing practice is built on one's philosophy and beliefs. The core of the APRN's practice is the expansion of the professional nursing role. By retaining the fundamental practice of nursing, transitioning from registered nurse to APRN gives the APRN role the "value added" that is separate from other healthcare providers. In order to survive in the current healthcare system, the APRN must not lose sight of the "art of nursing," which transcends the art of medical practice. The art of nursing is built on science, caring, and understanding human experience in health and illness. Regardless of what theoretical framework or constructs are used by APRNs to formulate a model of practice, the key is to remain grounded in nursing. To borrow a phrase from *Hamlet* by William Shakespeare, "This above all: to thine own self be true" (Hamlet Act I, scene 3).

ACKNOWLEDGMENT

The author acknowledges the contributions of Gail B. Katz to this chapter in the previous edition.

REFERENCES

Alligood, M. R., & Marriner-Tomey, A. (2005). *Nursing theory: Utilization and application.* St. Louis, MO: Mosby.

American Association of Colleges of Nursing. (2006). *Essentials of doctoral education for advanced practice nursing.* Washington, DC: Author.

American Holistic Nurses Association/American Association of Nursing. (2013). *Scope and standards of practice: Holistic nursing* (2nd ed.). Silver Spring, MD: American Nurses Association.

American Nurses Association. (2004). *Nursing: Scope and standards of practice.* Silver Spring, MD: Author.

American Nurses Association. (2010) *Nursing's social policy statement: The essence of the profession* (3rd ed.). Silver Spring, MD: Author.

APRN Consensus Workgroup & APRN Joint Dialogue Group. (2008). Consensus model for APRN regulation: Licensure, accreditation, certification & education. Retrieved from http://www.aacn.nche.edu/Education/pdf/APRNReport.pdf

Bahramnezhad, F., Shiri, M., Asgari, P., & Afshar, P. F. (2015). A review of the nursing paradigm. *Open Journal of Nursing, 5,* 17–23. doi:10.4236/ojn.2015.51003

Benner, P. (1998). *Nursing as a caring profession.* Paper presented at the meeting of the American Academy of Nursing, Kansas City, MO.

Bulechek, G. M., Butcher, H. K., Dochterman, J. M., & Wagner, C. (Eds.). (2013). *Nursing interventions classification (NIC)* (6th ed.). St. Louis, MO: Elsevier.

Burman, M. E., Hart, A. M., Conley, V., Brown, J., Sherard, P., & Clarke, P. N. (2009). Reconceptualizing the core of nurse practitioner education and practice. *Journal of the American Academy of Nurse Practitioners, 21,* 11–17. doi:10.1111/j.1745-7599.2008.00365.x

Chism, L. (2013). *The doctor of nursing practice: A guidebook for role development and professional issues* (2nd ed.). Burlington, MA: Jones & Bartlett.

Duffy, J. (2009). *Quality caring in nursing: Applying theory to clinical practice, education and leadership.* New York, NY: Springer Publishing.

Finkelman, A. (2013). Leadership in quality improvement. *Clinical Nurse Specialist, 27*(1), 31–35. doi:10.1097/NUR.0b013e3182776d8f

Fulton, J. S. (2011). Explaining clinical nurse specialist practice to the public. *Clinical Nurse Specialist, 25*(3), 105–106. doi:10.1097/NUR.0b013e31821ada0b

Gadow, S. (1980). Body and self: A dialectic. *The Journal of Medicine and Philosophy, 5*, 172–184. doi:10.1093/jmp/5.3.172

Gordon, M. (2007). *Nursing diagnosis.* (11th ed.). Sudbury, MA: Jones & Bartlett.

Greiner, A. C., & Knebel, E. (Eds.). (2003). *Health professions education: A bridge to quality.* Washington, DC: National Academies Press.

Hagedorn, S., & Quinn, A. (2004). Theory-based nursing practitioner practice: Caring-in-action. *Topics in Advanced Practice Nursing e-Journal, 4*(4), 1–7.

Hanson, M. D. (2015). Role of the clinical nurse specialist in the journey to Magnet recognition. *AANC Advanced Critical Care, 26*(1), 50–57. doi:10.1097/NCI.0000000000000068

Henderson, V. (1966). *Nature of nursing.* New York, NY: Macmillan.

Institute of Medicine. (2011). *The future of nursing: Leading change, advancing health.* Washington, DC: National Academies Press.

Jackson, J. I. (2015). Nursing paradigms and theories: A primer. Virginia Henderson Global Nursing e-Repository. Retrieved from http://www.nursinglibrary.org/vhl/handle/10755/338888

Jasemi, M., Valizadeh, L., Zamanzedeh, V., & Keogh, B. (2017). A concept analysis of holistic care by hybrid model. *Indian Journal of Palliative Care, 23*(1), 71–80. doi:10.4103/0973-1075.197960

Johnson, D. E. (1980). The behavioral system model for nursing. In J. P. Riehl & C. Roy (Eds.), *Conceptual models for nursing practice* (2nd ed., pp. 207–216). New York, NY: Appleton-Century-Crofts.

Johnson, D. E. (1959). The nature of a science of nursing. *Nursing Outlook, 7*(4), 291–294.

Johnson, M., Bulechek, G., Butcher, H., McCloskey Dochterman, J., Maas, M., Moorehead, S. S., & Swanson, E. (2005) *NANDA, NOC and NIC linkages* (2nd ed.). St. Louis, MO: Mosby.

King, I. M. (1971). *Toward a theory of nursing.* New York, NY: John Wiley.

Leininger, M. (1990). Historic and epistemologic dimensions of care and caring with future directions. In J. Stevenson & T. Tripp-Reimer (Eds.), *Knowledge about care and caring* (pp. 19–31). Kansas City, MO: American Academy of Nursing.

Levine, M. (1967). The four conservation principles of nursing. *Nursing Forum, 6*(1), 45–59. doi:10.1111/j.1744-6198.1967.tb01297.x

Marrs, J. A., & Lowry, L. W. (2009). Nursing theory and practice: Connecting the dots. In P. G. Reed & N. C. Shearer (Eds.), *Perspectives on nursing theory* (5th ed., pp. 3–12). Philadelphia, PA: Lippincott Williams & Wilkins.

Mayo, A. M., Ray, M. M., Chamblee, T. B., Urden, L. D., & Moody, R. (2017). The advanced practice clinical nurse specialist. *Nursing Administration Quarterly, 41*(1), 70–76. doi:10.1097/NAQ.0000000000000201

Meleis, A. I. (2011). *Theoretical nursing: Development and progress* (5th ed.). Philadelphia, PA: Lippincott Williams & Wilkins.

Mishel, M. H. (1990). Reconceptualization of the uncertainty in illness theory. *Image: Journal of Nursing Scholarship, 22,* 256–262. doi:10.1111/j.1547-5069.1990.tb00225.x

Morley, G., & Jackson, J. (2017). Is the art of nursing dying? A call for political action. *Journal of Research in Nursing, 22*(5), 342–351. doi:10.1177/1744987117713043

Neuman, B. (1974). The Betty Neuman health care system model: A total person approach to individual problems. In J. P. Riehl & C. Roy (Eds.), *Conceptual approach to individual problems* (pp. 99–114). New York, NY: Appleton-Century-Crofts.

Newman, M. A. (1984). Looking at the whole. *American Journal of Nursing, 84,* 1496–1499. doi:10.1097/00000446-198412000-00068

Newman, M. A., Sime, A. M., & Corcoran-Perry, S. A. (1991). The focus of the discipline of nursing. *Advances in Nursing Science, 14*(1), 1–6. doi:10.1097/00012272-199109000-00002

Nightingale, F. (1992). *Notes on nursing.* Philadelphia, PA: Lippincott. (Originally published 1859.)

Nojima, Y. (1989, May). *The structural formula of nursing practice: A bridge to new nursing.* Paper presented at the 19th Quadrennial Congress of the International Congress of Nurses, Seoul, Korea.

Nojima, Y., Tomikana, T., Makebe, S., & Snyder, M. (2003). Defining characteristics of expertise in Japanese clinical nursing using the Delphi technique. *Nursing Health Science, 5*(1), 3–11. doi:10.1046/j.1442-2018.2003.00129.x

North American Nursing Diagnosis Association International. (2015). *Nursing diagnoses: Definitions and classification 2015-2017* (10th ed.). Ames, IA: Wiley Blackwell.

Olson, J., & Hanchett, E. (1997). Nurse-expressed empathy, individual outcomes, and development of a middle-range theory. *Image-The Journal of Nursing Scholarship, 29,* 71–76.

Orem, D. E. (1980). *Nursing: Concepts of practice.* New York, NY: McGraw-Hill.

Polk, L. V. (1997). Toward a middle-range theory of resilience. *Advances in Nursing Science, 19*(3), 1–13. doi:10.1097/00012272-199703000-00002

Reed, P. G. (1991). Toward a nursing theory of self-transcendence: Deductive reformulation using developmental theories. *Advances in Nursing Science, 13*(4), 64–71.

Riehl-Sisca, J. (1989). *Conceptual models for nursing practice.* Norwalk, CT: Appleton & Lange.

Rogers, M. (1970). *An introduction to the theoretical basis of nursing.* Philadelphia, PA: F. A. Davis.

Rounds, L., Zych, J., & Mallary, L. (2013). The consensus model for regulation of APRNs: Implications for nurse practitioners. *Journal of the American Associate of Nurse Practitioners, 25*(4), 180–185. doi:10.1111/j.1745-7599.2013.00812.x

Roy, C. (1984). *Introduction to nursing: An adaptation model.* Englewood Cliffs, NJ: Prentice Hall.

Russell, G. E., & Fawcett, J. (2005). The conceptual model for nursing and health policy revisited. *Policy, Politics and Nursing Practice, 6*(4), 319–326. doi:10.1177/1527154405283304

Schoenhoefer, S. O., & Boykin, A. (1993). Nursing as caring: An emerging general theory of nursing. In M. E. Parker (Ed.), *Patterns of nursing theories in practice* (pp. 82–92). New York, NY: National League for Nursing.

Smith, M. C. (1995). The core of advanced practice nursing. *Nursing Science Quarterly, 8*(1), 2–3. doi:10.1177/089431849500800102

Stanley, J. M. (2012). Impact of new regulatory standards on advanced practice registered nursing. The APRN consensus model and LACE. *Nursing Clinics of North America, 47*(2), 241–250. doi:10.1016/j.cnur.2012.02.001

Stanley, M. C. (2011). *Advanced practice nursing. Emphasizing common roles* (3rd ed.). Philadelphia, PA: F. A. Davis.

Swanson, K. M. (1991). Empirical development of a middle-range theory of caring. *Nursing Research, 40,* 161–166. doi:10.1097/00006199-199105000-00008

Watson, J. (1988). *Nursing: Human science and human care: A theory of nursing.* New York, NY: National League for Nursing.

Wiener, C. L., & Dodd, M. J. (1993). Coping amid uncertainty: An illness trajectory. *Scholarly Inquiry in Nursing Practice, 7*(1), 17–30.

Younger, J. B. (1991). A theory of mastery. *Advances in Nursing Science, 14*(1), 76–89. doi:10.1097/00012272-199109000-00009

Zaccagnini, M., & Waud White, K. (2014). *The doctor of nursing practice essentials and new model for advanced practice nursing* (2nd ed.). Burlington, MA: Jones & Bartlett.

Jana G. Zwilling

MULTIFACETED ROLES OF THE APRN

Before delving into the various roles of the APRN, the impact of current healthcare reform issues since the inauguration of the Patient Protection and Affordable Care Act (Public Law 111–148, 2010) and the Health Care and Education Affordability Reconciliation Act (Public Law 111–152) on the APRN role is reviewed. These laws are collectively referred to as the Patient Protection and Affordable Care Act (ACA) in this chapter. The ACA was signed into law on March 23, 2010. This comprehensive healthcare legislation is the biggest change in the U.S. healthcare system since the creation of Medicare and Medicaid programs in 1965. The ACA has led to insurance coverage for approximately an additional 20 million previously uninsured Americans (Research AND Development [RAND], 2017). This new regulation has left the U.S. healthcare system in an uproar regarding reimbursement, access to care, and lack of healthcare providers. The country is now waiting, with bated breath, for the possibility of a repeal or adjustment to the ACA. The most recently approved legislation eliminated the individual mandate, thus removing the penalty for an individual having no insurance coverage. There seem to be multiple viewpoints regarding the best way to fund healthcare in the United States; however, there is little discussion about true reform which could potentially decrease costs to start with.

The Centers for Medicare & Medicaid Services (CMS) have been pushing more cost control and quality care by incentivizing healthcare providers and healthcare institutions. The Advanced Alternative Payment Models (APMs) and the Merit-based Incentive Payment System (MIPS) under the CMS Quality Payment Programs are two methods posed to providers to achieve these aims (CMS, 2017). For providers participating in these programs, the Medicare and Medicaid reimbursement rates are based on the provider submission of quality indicators meeting certain standards. Negative incentives are also provided. Unfortunately, for APRNs, only nurse practitioners (NPs), clinical nurse specialists

(CNSs), and certified registered nurse anesthetists (CRNAs) can participate in these programs; certified nurse-midwives (CNMs) were not included. However, participation is not yet mandatory in these programs, so many providers and organizations continue on the fee-for-service models (CMS, 2017).

The vacillation of policy makers can certainly impact APRNs' practice. However, the bottom line is caring for the patient. Regardless of potential future policy changes, the current system needs repair in order to cost-effectively provide care to an increased patient population. APRNs need to look at patient-centered holistic care versus simply federal dictation. Ultimately, the patient is in charge of his or her health and APRNs are the guide. Certainly, disease prevention and health promotion are more cost-effective than chronic disease care. Therefore, APRNs should contribute to a redesign focusing on these factors.

The upheaval of healthcare reform in the United States has created a necessity for the doctorate of nursing practice (DNP)–prepared APRN. The DNP degree focuses on preparing APRNs not only for practice but also to be leaders in practice improvements. The DNP interprets original research into clinical application, health policy changes, and improvement of clinical outcomes with interdisciplinary collaboration (American Association of Colleges of Nursing [AACN], 2006). The ACA includes provisions for strengthening primary care, ensuring quality care, and reducing the costs associated with healthcare. DNP-prepared APRNs can use their practice background and systems thinking to initiate new processes and policies to better serve the potentially increased number of patients. The public has also been enlightened to the role of the APRN in healthcare delivery via the Institute of Medicine's (IOM's) report on the future of nursing (IOM, 2010). Whether it be the certified nurse practitioner (CNP) in an underserved area, the CNM providing access to obstetric care, the CRNA providing a cost-effective solution to anesthetic care, or the CNS maximizing the specialty care provided at the patient bedside, APRNs are poised to be forces of change in the future of healthcare.

Traditionally, the roles of the APRN have been clinically focused, as clinician, patient advocate, case manager, and collaborator, to name a few. Other roles have been underlying for many years, but more recently these have pushed into the limelight. These are the roles of leader, educator, researcher, and independent clinician. Ultimately, the APRN's foundation is that of a clinician—and always will be. With healthcare reform, we need to keep our clinical roots, but must expand to best serve our patients and profession. This chapter examines the various roles, focusing on incorporating them into the whole and consummate professional.

APRN ROLES

Several APRN nursing models have reviewed and researched roles for this growing profession. Hamric's integrative model of advanced nursing practice is a very comprehensive model that includes primary criteria for the APRN as well as central and core competencies (Hamric, Spross, & Hanson, 2013). Primary criteria included in this model are graduate education, certification in the specialty, and a focus on clinical practice. Core competencies referenced by Hamric, Spross, and Hanson (2013) are direct clinical practice, collaboration, guidance and coaching, evidence-based practice, ethical decision making, consultation, and leadership. This model also incorporates outside elements affecting APRN practice. A framework for advanced practice nursing developed by Brown (1998, 2005) looked at the external issues, roles, APRN scope, and competencies, as well as outcomes of the APRN role. The Strong Model of Advanced Practice (Ackerman, Norsen, Martin, Wiedrich, & Kitzman, 1996) is one of the few that has been tested for validity (Mick & Ackerman, 2000). This model has also been supported throughout the literature and used in other research, such as the development of a role-delineation tool by Chang, Gardner, Duffied, and Ramis (2012).

The Strong Model breaks down APRN roles by service parameters. These parameters include direct comprehensive care, support of systems, education, research, and publication and professional leadership. This model, with some modification, is used to further define APRN roles in this chapter.

Direct Care

Patient care is, and should remain, the priority of the APRN. Within this realm, several roles emerge, including patient advocate, educator to the patient and family, case manager, and collaborator. All these roles rely on APRNs using evidence-based practice as a basis for their care and decision-making processes. APRNs need to be staunch supporters of continued research and integrate these findings into practice. The continued advancement of healthcare depends on a culture of support for new and innovative ideas (Ackerman et al., 1996).

Patient Advocate

Advocacy for patients must remain fundamental to the practice of nursing. It is the underpinning of the nurse–patient relationship. "Advocacy" is defined as "the act, or process of pleading for, supporting, or recommending a cause or course of action" (Fowler, 2015, p. 37). Advocacy has progressed to being a guardian of the patient's rights and freedoms of choice. Although several other elements may be included in advocacy, a nurse's advocacy is guided by respect for the individual (Fowler, 2015).

Advocacy can be viewed from a variety of perspectives. Nelson (1998) maintains that advocacy includes legal advocacy, moral–ethical advocacy, substitutive advocacy, political advocacy, and spiritual advocacy. Newer models of patient advocacy are focused on empowering patients to take an active role in their own healthcare, while still maintaining the role of evidence-based healthcare provider. In this sense, the APRN can educate the patient on current practices, yet take a patient-centered approach in assisting the patient with his or her health.

In legal advocacy, the nurse supports the patient's legal rights, such as informed consent or the right to refuse treatment. This may include ensuring that all patients have a copy of the institution's bill of rights. Moral–ethical advocacy requires that the nurse respects the patient's values and supports decisions that are consistent with those values, such as decisions regarding abortion. In substitutive advocacy, if the patient is unable to express an opinion, the nurse should continue to respect the rights of the patient or surrogate and support any wishes that the patient may have previously expressed. In spiritual advocacy, the APRN ensures that the patient has access to spiritual support such as clergy and that the plan of care includes the spiritual aspects of care.

Advocacy must occur for all patients. APRNs should advocate for all patients to complete living wills and advance directives to make sure that healthcare issues are well documented and patient wishes are respected. On occasion, issues of patient competency may arise in areas such as substitutive advocacy and moral–ethical advocacy. When competency is a concern, the APRN must be familiar with laws governing competence, including criteria for the assessment of competence. At the same time, the APRN should be instrumental in establishing policies for direct action when a patient is judged incompetent. In such a case, the APRN must communicate the patient's expectations, if they are known, to the surrogate and/or the patient's family to support any requests and decisions to be made based on the patient's past recommendations. Because there can be confusion and conflict among family, friends, surrogates, and even healthcare professionals during these times, the APRN should have no reservation about convening family–patient conferences and implementing ethics committee evaluations if questions or controversies arise.

Advocacy carries a significant ethical dimension; therefore, principles of ethics can help to evaluate a nurse's effectiveness (ANA, 2015). Pinch (1996) points out that some ethical principles may conflict. For example, the principle of autonomy (self-determination) could clash with distributive justice (fair, equitable distribution of goods or services) if the patient's decisions were to affect the community's greater need or safety. If a patient requested no treatment and is discharged with a dangerous communicable disease that may infect the community, or if a patient demanded resources that jeopardized the financial or medical resources of a community, the patient's autonomy may be at risk of being overshadowed by what is best for the majority. In maintaining advocacy, the APRN would need to be sure that there was, indeed, a conflict in distributive justice and no prejudices existed toward an individual or group.

Concerns, in the past, have existed regarding the ability of a nurse to be an advocate, given our current healthcare systems and associated cost-containment measures (Donagrandi & Eddy, 2000; Kalaitzidis & Jewell, 2015; Nelson, 1998). Is the APRN in a position to maintain advocacy despite the demands of the system? Nelson (1998) contends that the APRN can rise above these constraints. Cost-effectiveness is a strong suit of APRN practice. Payments for Medicare beneficiaries seeing an NP were approximately 29% less than the payments for beneficiaries seeing an MD (Perloff, DesRoches, & Buerhaus, 2016). Multiple other studies have also demonstrated cost savings (Chenoweth, Martin, Pankowski, & Raymond, 2005; Eibner, Hussey, Ridgely, & McGlynn, 2009). On the individual patient level, it has been well established that APRNs provide high-quality care, even in comparison with other provider types (Everett et al., 2013; Kuo, Chen, Baillargeon, Raji, & Goodwin, 2015; Kuo, Goodwin, et al., 2015). The APRN is in a unique position of influence through interaction with other team members, ensuring advocacy through policy formulation that directs patient care and through legislative involvement. Additionally, the APRN should be well versed in the areas of evidence-based practice, standards of care, ethics policies, accreditation criteria, nursing licensure regulations, and professional association standards that can help support an APRN's advocacy position.

Educator to the Patient and Family

Advanced practice nursing education makes the APRN an excellent resource for current knowledge in content areas, supportive resources, research findings, and the implementation of evidence-based practice. This is imperative when educating patients and their families. Today's healthcare consumers are very knowledgeable about their health and medical treatment. Assessment of this knowledge base is essential. Patients are using the Internet as a primary source of information. Some sources have information that is directed to healthcare professionals and is more likely to be reliable. The information that individuals gather is generated from a wide variety of Internet sources, such as chat rooms, blogs, nonevidence-based medical sites, or sites with medical opinions from nonmedical personnel. Information also comes from advertisements, brochures, newspapers, television, health kiosks, nontraditional care providers, and family and friends. This information can be skewed, inaccurate, or incomplete. The APRN should take the time to access and review these sources to appraise the accuracy and reliability of the information that is being provided. Patients may experience fears or preconceived ideas regarding care strategies and inappropriate outcomes. These apprehensions can either motivate them to become very knowledgeable or to remain very uninformed about their health concerns. Just as you might ask students for content references, the APRN should ask patients for their information sources.

The APRN needs to make a point of screening-related health information made available by the healthcare organizations as well. Many patients are overwhelmed simply by their diagnosis, much less their medication, treatment course, or plan of care. Therefore, most printed or electronically distributed educational content should be constructed at a fifth- to eighth-grade reading level. Background, color, and print format are other considerations. Printed or electronic information can be given to a patient to reinforce verbal information, but must be at the patient consumer level, not the medical professional level.

Case Manager

Case management is becoming a more common dimension of the APRN role with the enactment of the ACA. This role is greatly expanding with the implementation of more fixed or bundled reimbursement and inclusion of more patients with preexisting conditions. Healthcare organizations are looking to APRN case managers to coordinate the care of these individuals to reduce costs while providing comprehensive care. Coffman (2001) describes "case management" as a collaborative process promoting quality care and cost-effective outcomes to specific patients and groups. Umbrell (2006) outlines the value of an advanced practice trauma case manager in orchestrating a comprehensive plan to reduce fragmentation of care and better utilization of resources. The key features of the case manager as outlined by Benoit (1996) include (a) standardized resources for a length of stay for selected patient care, caregiver, and system outcomes; (b) collaborative team practice among disciplines; (c) coordinated care over the course of an illness; (d) job enrichment for the caregiver; (e) patient and physician satisfaction with the care; and (f) minimized costs to the institution.

Taylor (1999) initially described the two primary types of case management as (a) the patient-focused model, which supports the patient throughout the continuum of care and helps the patient access healthcare, and (b) the system-focused model, which involves the service environment and is structured for cost containment of a specific group of patients and use of critical pathways for cost-effective outcomes. However, Taylor advanced her model of comprehensive case management that incorporates elements of cultural competency, consumer empowerment, clinical framework, and multidisciplinary practice in addition to other activities of assessment, service, planning, plan implementation, coordination and monitoring, advocacy, and termination. The focus in healthcare is on patient empowerment and quality service based on process improvement, outcome measurements, and performance-based expectations. In the past, case management was associated with the utilization of clinical pathways to drive the plan of care—therefore focusing on process—but the focus since the early 2000s has been on outcome measures. Taylor asserts that this new model is optimal because it incorporates components of both patient and system models to ensure that the patient receives needed services.

Ethical concerns have persisted as to how APRNs who are active in nursing and case management can remain advocates for patients in the new Accountable Care Organizations (ACO) and patient-centered medical home models. The disconnect is maintaining the five principles of ethical behavior while attempting to follow insurance, reimbursement, and other regulations that will come up as a result of this new legislation. The five principles include autonomy, beneficence, nonmaleficence, justice, and fidelity. These are basic principles we, as nurses, learn from the very beginning and need to bring forth despite other overreaching pressures.

The utilization of APRNs as case managers has been advocated (Donagrandi & Eddy, 2000; Taylor, 1999). APRNs have enhanced capabilities in interdisciplinary coordination, advanced clinical decision making, autonomy, synthesis, and critical thinking. The APRN expertise would also be valuable in the development of outcome standards, communication and coordination among disciplines, and analysis of patient care trends. In addition, a focus on complex patient populations requiring extended lengths of stay or long-term care resources is very ably managed by the APRN (Abdellah, Fawcett, Kane, Dick, & Chen, 2005).

Collaborator

Collaboration integrates the individual perspectives and expertise of various team members on behalf of providing quality patient care (Resnick & Bonner, 2003). Interdisciplinary collaboration has become a hot topic in today's healthcare environment. With escalating demands and the prospect of a rise in chronic illness, a cooperative effort among healthcare disciplines will be the most effective means to provide quality care.

One of the key messages in the IOM's report *The Future of Nursing: Leading Change, Advancing Health* (2011) is, "Nurses should be full partners, with physicians and other health professionals, in redesigning healthcare in the United States" (p. 4). The ACA also emphasizes interdisciplinary collaboration as a means to provide cost-effective and comprehensive care. Matthews and Brown (2013) outline a collaborative health management model for effectively managing patients with chronic disease. This model includes the APRN, physician, registered nurse, medical assistant, pharmacist, social worker, mental health provider, and specialty consultants. The authors focus on goals of promoting patient self-management, preventive or proactive care, and close follow-up (Matthews & Brown, 2013).

Unfortunately, there are varied thoughts about the definition of this collaborative process. Influences on these discrepancies include provider gender, level of professionalism, environment, and the traditional push for autonomy in the nursing field. Fast-paced clinical environments and traditional hierarchical roles contribute to poor communication across the disciplines. APRNs will need to lead the way to introduce the collaborative process as a professional behavior and best practice for the care of patients.

Systems Support

Within the paradigm of the healthcare system, the APRN needs to be a leader, a mentor, and a nursing advocate. These three roles ultimately support optimal and innovative patient care practices. The roles are so intertwined that it is difficult to dissect one from the others. This section presents the three as a cumulative role of leader.

The U.S. Army defines "leadership" as "the process of influencing people by providing purpose, direction, and motivation to accomplish the mission and improve the organization" (Army Doctrine Publication, 2012, p. 1). There are many levels of both formal and informal leaders within the military structure. Some of these are by virtue of the position alone, which does not always constitute a good leader. Others, although not necessarily in a leadership position, clearly match the definition of a leader. An effective leader earns respect by setting the example, promoting an open and caring environment, being an inspiration to others, using resources wisely, and creating a strong and supportive team. The role of a leader is relatively new and extremely important for the APRN. With the transition to DNP-prepared APRNs, the career field is now fully equipped to be the "tip of the spear" for change in our healthcare system.

The DNP-prepared APRN, although not a role in itself, contributes significantly to the advancement of APRNs in the leadership role. The AACN DNP essentials specify two key components geared toward leadership. The first is "Organizational and Systems Leadership for Quality Improvement and Systems Thinking." The key here is emphasizing practice while working to improve health outcomes and patient safety on a practice-level or system-wide basis. The second essential relating to leadership is "Health Care Policy for Advocacy in Health Care." The DNP-prepared APRN has the capabilities to broaden the scope of nursing leadership and take on public and nursing profession policy issues (Ehrenreich, 2002).

The National Organization of Nurse Practitioner Faculties (NONPF) outlines NP leadership with seven core competencies: (a) assumes complex and advanced leadership roles to initiate and guide change; (b) provides leadership to foster collaboration with multiple stakeholders to improve healthcare; (c) demonstrates leadership that uses critical and reflective thinking; (d) advocates for improved access, quality, and cost-effective healthcare; (e) advances practice through the development and implementation of innovations incorporating principles of change; (f) communicates practice knowledge effectively, both orally and in writing; (g) participates in professional organizations and activities that influence advanced practice nursing and/or health outcomes of a population focus (NONPF, 2017). The other APRN disciplines have similar competency statements. The CNS Systems Leadership Competency has 13 issues addressed within the leadership scope, including system change, fiscal and budgetary decision making, evaluation of the effect of nursing, dissemination of outcomes of change, provision of clinically competent care by team, assessments performed at the systems level, and interdisciplinary collaboration (National Association of Clinical Nurse Specialists [NACNS], 2010). The American Association of Nurse Anesthetists (AANA,

2013, p. 1) states, "Nurse anesthetists are innovative leaders in anesthesia care delivery, integrating progressive critical thinking and ethical judgment." The American College of Nurse-Midwives (ACNM) delineates leadership competencies as professional responsibilities of the CNM. Some of the outlined responsibilities include knowledge of national and international issues and trends, support of legislation and policy initiatives, and knowledge of issues and trends in healthcare policy and systems (ACNM, 2012).

There are obviously varied levels of leadership. The APRN is well suited for this role at all levels, including clinical, system, community, national, and international. Clinically, the APRN is automatically placed in a leadership role as a result of preparation at the advanced level. The knowledge base of the clinician is the foundation of clinical leadership and ultimately of other echelons as well. As a knowledgeable clinician, the APRN can lead collaborative teams for the improvement of care delivery and outcomes. The healthcare system can also be an important arena for the APRN to lead. APRNs have a unique view of the patient, community, and healthcare system needs and thus can bring needed insight to the administration of hospitals, clinics, and other healthcare delivery formats. On the community, national, and international levels, the APRN can be involved and lead various professional organizations and influence healthcare policy. This is a very important area in which APRNs should be involved. It can be very time-consuming and frustrating, but ultimately very rewarding as APRNs advocate not only for improved healthcare but also for the nursing profession. APRNs make a huge impact not only at the bedside but also by using that clinical knowledge to induce change.

The IOM report *The Future of Nursing: Leading Change, Advancing Health* (2010) emphasizes mentoring as an important part of the leadership role for APRNs. For example, APRNs can take the lead in fostering growth and promoting forward thinking in new or less-experienced nursing staff and APRNs. Some facilities or programs have introduced formal mentoring programs for nurse leaders. In these programs, a senior nursing leader will partner with a newer nursing leader for a period of time to guide the newer nursing leader in his or her role (Bally, 2007). It has also been suggested that APRN educational programs include more of a focus on leadership qualities. Superior leaders require not only a strong clinical background but also formal education on leadership models, behaviors, and communication in interpersonal and large-scale formats (Adeniran, Bhattacharya, & Adeniran, 2012). Bedside mentoring would be the most effective for the majority of APRNs. However, in our fast-paced system, new trends are emerging. Mentoring can take place via email, social networking sites, and blogs. Ultimately, however the relationship is carried out, it is most important to have a good rapport between the individuals and promote an open and caring environment for learning.

Advocacy for nursing directs the APRN to support other nurses in their professional growth and to contribute to the evolution of the nursing profession (Nelson, 1998). Nelson suggests that this is an opportunity for APRNs to facilitate and empower other nurses through leadership, education, and modeling standards for practice. APRNs are in a unique position of influence through interaction with other team members, ensuring advocacy through policy formulation that directs practice and through legislative involvement. In addition, APRNs are versed in the areas of evidence-based practice, standards of care, ethics policies, accreditation criteria, nursing licensure regulations, and professional association standards that can help to support an APRN's advocacy position.

Educator

The APRN has a wealth of experiences for developing standards for practice, strategies for use of equipment and procedures, assessment of patient issues and concerns, and evaluations of nursing staff capabilities and limitations. Advanced practice nursing education makes the APRN a resource for current knowledge in content areas, supportive resources, research findings, and implementation of evidence-based practice. When providing education to students and staff, APRNs can provide sound clinical examples that enhance the application of content. APRNs may find it helpful to seek assistance from their colleagues in academic settings when they are initially developing educational content. It takes considerable knowledge and skill to develop a sound teaching–learning plan.

Although isolated teaching events can be provided, a planned content series is most effective for ensuring learner outcomes and competencies. When planning for the dissemination, an assessment first needs to be completed to determine what knowledge is needed so that the APRN can focus the content. This may be guided through planned curriculum, observed problems in patient care, standards or protocols for practice, or common patient questions, to name a few. The assessment identifies what type of learner outcomes (competencies) are to be achieved.

When the assessment is complete, the APRN needs to develop content objectives to achieve these outcomes. Guidelines for the development of objectives were established by Bloom (1956), who divided objectives into three domains of learning: cognitive, affective, and psychomotor. Content objectives are used to guide the development of the learning tools, whether this be a one-on-one instruction, large live lecture, or online asynchronous format. The format needs to properly fit the learning audience to provide the optimal environment for achieving the prescribed outcomes. Demonstrating outcomes or competencies is consistent in evaluating whether learning has occurred. Identification could be done with a written test, skill demonstration, or return presentation of data. Support content such as handouts or video may also need to be developed. These, too, should reflect the level of learning being addressed. With staff, the APRN has the unique opportunity of continuing to work beside a staff member. In this way, a staff member can continue to pursue clarification and assistance, and the APRN can evaluate the staff member for his or her grasp of the information.

With regard to APRN education, there is a trend toward competency-based programs. This concept began in the 1970s and defines educational goals by precise and measurable descriptions of knowledge, skills, and attitudes the students should have at the culmination of their program (Savage, 1993). Competencies can generally be divided into three cores: APRN, role, and population. Each APRN organization and/or certifying body delineates these a little differently. NONPF approved the DNP as the entry level for NP practice in 2008 (NONPF, 2010b). Within this endorsement is a listing of "core competencies." NONPF states that it is more valuable to have successful achievement of these competencies than to be concerned strictly with the number of clinical hours performed (NONPF, 2010a). There are nine core competency areas for the NP graduate regardless of population focus (NONPF, 2017). These include the topics of leadership, scientific foundation, quality, practice inquiry, technology and information literacy, policy, health delivery system, ethics, and independent practice. Released in 2013 are the specific competencies for each NP population focus area, including family across the life span, neonatal, acute care pediatric, primary care pediatric, psychiatric/mental health, and women's health/gender related.

The NACNS produced a similar document in 2010, listing comprehensive, entry-level competencies expected of graduate-level CNSs (NACNS, 2010). The competencies are reflective of all CNS specialty areas and are divided into three categories: direct patient care, consultation, and systems leadership. The Council on Accreditation of Nurse Anesthesia Educational Programs (CANAEP) has recently approved *Standards for Accreditation of Nurse Anesthesia Programs,* which is a practice doctorate standards document (CANAEP, 2017). The competencies for the CRNA specialty are very skill based. This recent document provides a guideline for minimum numbers of cases and clinical hours, as well as preferred number of cases. The cases are broken down into three categories: patient physical status, special cases, and anatomic categories. The variety of anesthesia methods and skill techniques are also addressed (CANAEP, 2017). CNMs have the *Core Competencies for Basic Midwifery Practice* approved by the ACNM in 2012 (ACNM, 2012). This document outlines the midwifery management process as well as skills and professional responsibilities.

APRN programs are using the competencies outlined by their organizations in developing and monitoring their curricula. The core competencies for each type of APRN can be used as a baseline for new clinician performance. Some programs are even using these competencies as criteria for progression and graduation. The competency measures can include, but are not limited to, clinical portfolios, peer reviews, and examinations.

SUMMARY

For the APRN to fully participate in these aforementioned roles, administration needs to be educated about the many aspects of the APRN's position and the benefits that accrue to patient care and the institution in supporting expanded APRN practice. The APRN should market these capabilities to people and groups at all levels—from patients to legislators. Although providing direct patient care is valuable and rewarding, the APRN can continue to evolve and actually have greater effect in patient care, community and social health, and the development of nursing as a profession by pursuing advanced APRN roles. Whether the APRN works as part of a practice or in a separate position, the opportunity to function in these advanced roles will give the APRN personal satisfaction, enhance the care of patients, and contribute to the profession of nursing.

REFERENCES

Abdellah, L, Fawcett, J., Kane, R., Dick, K., & Chen, J. (2005). The development and psychometric testing of the Evercare Nurse Practitioner Role and Activity Scale (ENPRAS). *Journal of the American Academy of Nurse Practitioners, 17*(1), 21–26. doi:10.1111/j.1041-2972.2005.00006.x

Ackerman, M. H., Norsen, L., Martin, B., Wiedrich, J., & Kitzman, H. J. (1996). Development of a model of advanced practice. *American Journal of Critical Care, 5*(1), 68–73. Retrieved from http://ajcc.aacnjournals.org/content/5/1/68.abstract

Adeniran, R. K., Bhattacharya, A., & Adeniran, A. A. (2012). Professional excellence and career advancement in nursing: A conceptual framework for clinical leadership development. *Nursing Administration Quarterly, 36*(1), 41–51. doi:10.1097/NAQ.0b013e31823b0fec

American Association of Colleges of Nursing. (2006). *The essentials of doctoral education for advanced nursing practice.* Washington, DC: Author.

American Association of Nurse Anesthetists. (2013). Scope of nurse anesthesia practice. Retrieved from http://www.aana.com/resources2/professionalpractice/Documents/PPM%20Scope%20of%20Nurse%20Anesthesia%20Practice.pdf

American College of Nurse-Midwives. (2012). Core competencies for basic midwifery practice. Retrieved from http://www.midwife.org/ACNM/files/ACNMLibraryData/UPLOADFILENAME/000000000050/Core%20Comptencies%20Dec%202012.pdf

Army Doctrine Publication 6-22, Army Leadership. (2012). Retrieved from http://armypubs.army.mil/doctrine/DR_pubs/dr_a/pdf/adp6_22_new.pdf

Bally, J. (2007). The role of nursing leadership in creating a mentoring culture in acute care environments. *Nursing Economic$, 25*(3), 143–149.

Benoit, B. C. (1996). Case management and the advanced practice nurse. In J. Hickey, R. Ouimette, & S. Venegoni (Eds.), *Advanced practice nursing:. Changing roles and clinical application* (pp. 107–125). Philadelphia, PA: Lippincott.

Bloom, B. S. (Ed.). (1956). *Taxonomy of educational objectives.* New York, NY: David McKay.

Brown, S. J. (1998). A framework for advanced practice nursing. *Journal of Professional Nursing, 14*(3), 157–164. doi:10.1016/S8755-7223(98)80091-4

Brown, S. J. (2005). Direct clinical practice. In A. B. Hamric, J. A. Spross, & C. M. Hanson (Eds.), *Advanced practice nursing: An integrative approach* (3rd ed., pp. 143–185). Philadelphia, PA: Elsevier Saunders.

Centers for Medicare & Medicaid Services. (2017). Quality payment program. Retrieved from https://qpp.cms.gov

Chang, A. M., Gardner, G. E., Duffield, C., & Ramis, M. A. (2012). Advanced practice nursing role development: Factor analysis of a modified role delineation tool. *Journal of Advanced Nursing, 68*(6), 1369–1379. doi:10.1111/j.1365-2648.2011.05850.x

Chenoweth, D., Martin, N., Pankowski, J., & Raymond, L.W. (2005). A benefit-cost analysis of a worksite nurse practitioner program: First impressions. *Journal of Occupational and Environmental Medicine, 47*(11), 1110–1116. doi:10.1097/01.jom.0000182093.48440.4c

Coffman, S. (2001). Examining advocacy and care management in managed care. *Pediatric Nursing, 23*(3), 287–289, 304.

Council on Accreditation of Nurse Anesthesia Educational Programs. (2017). Standards for accreditation of nurse anesthesia programs: Practice doctorate. Retrieved from http://home.coa.us.com/accreditation/Documents/Standards%20for%20Accreditation%20of%20Nurse%20Anesthesia%20Programs%20-%20Practice%20Doctorate,%20rev%20May%202017.pdf

Donagrandi, M. A., & Eddy, M. (2000). Ethics of case management: Implications for advanced practice nursing. *Clinical Nurse Specialist: The Journal for Advanced Nursing Practice, 14*(5), 241–249. doi:10.1097/00002800-200009000-00019

Ehrenreich, B. (2002). The emergence of nursing as a political force. In D. Mason, D. Leavitt, & M. Chaffee (Eds.), *Policy & politics in nursing and health care* (4th ed., pp. xxxiii–xxxvii). St. Louis, MO: Saunders.

Eibner, C., Hussey, P. S., Ridgley, M. S., & McGlynn, E. A. (2009). Controlling health care spending in Massachusetts: An analysis of options. Santa Monica, CA: RAND Corporation.

Everett, C., Thorpe, C., Palta, M., Carayon, P., Bartels, C., & Smith, M. (2013). Physician assistants and nurse practitioners perform effective roles on teams caring for Medicare patients with diabetes. *Health Affairs, 32*(11), e1942–e1948. doi:10.1377/hlthaff.2013.0506

Fowler, M. D. M. (2015). *Guide to the code of ethics for nurses with interpretive statements: Development, interpretation, and application.* Silver Spring, MD: American Nurses Association.

Hamric, A. B., Spross, J. A., & Hanson, C. M. (2013). *Advanced practice nursing: An integrative approach* (4th ed.). Philadelphia, PA: W. B. Saunders.

Institute of Medicine. (2010). *The future of nursing: Leading change, advancing health.* Washington, DC: National Academies Press.

Kalaitzidis, E., & Jewell, P. (2015). The concept of advocacy in nursing: A critical analysis. *The Healthcare Manager, 34*(4), 308–315. doi:10.1097/HCM.0000000000000007

Kuo, Y. F., Chen, N. W., Baillargeon, J., Raji, M. A., & Goodwin, J. S. (2015). Potentially preventable hospitalizations in medicare patients with diabetes: A comparison of primary care provided by nurse practitioners versus physicians. *Medical Care, 53*(9), 776e783. doi:10.1097/MLR.0000000000000406

Kuo, Y. F., Goodwin, J. S., Chen, N. W., Lewin, K. K., Baillargeon, J., & Raji, M. A. (2015). Diabetes mellitus care provided by nurse practitioners vs primary care physicians. *Journal of the American Geriatrics Society, 63*(10), e1980–e1988. doi:10.1111/jgs.13662

Matthews, S. W., & Brown, M. A. (2013). APRN expertise: The collaborative health management model. *Nurse Practitioner, 38*(1), 43–48. doi:10.1097/01 .NPR.0000423382.33822.ab

Mick, D., & Ackerman, M. (2000). Advanced practice nursing role delineation in acute and critical care: Application of the Strong model of advanced practice. *Heart & Lung, 29*(3), 210–221. doi:10.1067/mhl.2000.106936

National Association of Clinical Nurse Specialists. (2010). Clinical nurse specialist core competencies. Retrieved from http://www.nacns.org/docs/ CNSCoreCompetenciesBroch.pdf

National Organization of Nurse Practitioner Faculties. (2010b). Clinical hours for nurse practitioner preparation in doctor of nursing practice programs. In: *Clinical education issues in preparing nurse practitioner students for independent practice: An ongoing series of papers.* Retrieved from http://c.ymcdn .com/sites/www.nonpf.org/resource/resmgr/imported/clinicaleducationis suespprfinalapril2010.pdf

National Organization of Nurse Practitioner Faculties. (2010b). Eligibility for NP certification for nurse practitioner students in doctor of nursing practice programs. In: *Clinical education issues in preparing nurse practitioner students for independent practice: An ongoing series of papers.* Retrieved from http://c .ymcdn.com/sites/www.nonpf.org/resource/resmgr/imported/clinicaleduc ationissuespprfinalapril2010.pdf

National Organization of Nurse Practitioner Faculties. (2017). Nurse practitioner core competencies content. Retrieved from http://c.ymcdn.com/sites/www .nonpf.org/resource/resmgr/competencies/2017_NPCoreComps_with_ Curric.pdf

Nelson, M. (1998). Advocacy. In M. Snyder & R. Lundquist (Eds.), *Complementary/ alternative therapies in nursing* (3rd ed., pp. 337–352). New York, NY: Springer Publishing.

Patient Protection and Affordable Care Act of 2010, 42 U.S.C.A. § 18001 *et seq.* Retrieved from https://www.gpo.gov/fdsys/pkg/PLAW-111publ148/pdf/ PLAW-111publ148.pdf

Perloff, J., DesRoches, C. M., & Buerhaus, P. (2016). Comparing the cost of care provided to Medicare beneficiaries assigned to primary care nurse practitioners and physicians. *Health Services Research, 51*(4), 1407–1423. doi:10.1111/1475-6773.12425

Pinch, W. J. (1996). Ethical issues in case management. In D. L. Flarey & S. S. Blancett (Eds.), *Handbook of nursing case management: Health care delivery in world of managed care* (pp. 443–460). Gaithersburg, MD: Aspen Publishers.

Research AND Development. (2017). The future of U.S. healthcare: Replace or revise the Affordable Care Act? Retrieved from https://www.rand.org/ health/key-topics/health-policy/in-depth.html

Resnick, B., & Bonner, A. (2003). Collaboration: Foundation for a successful practice. *Journal of the American Medical Directors Association, 4*(6), 344–349. doi:10.1016/S1525-8610(04)70395-3

Savage, L. (1993). *Literacy through a competency-based education approach.* Washington, DC: Center for Applied Linguistics.

Taylor, P (1999). Comprehensive nursing case management: An advanced practice model. *Nursing Case Management, 4*(1), 2–9.

Umbrell, C. E. (2006). Trauma case management: A role for the advanced practice nurse. *Journal of Trauma Nursing, 13*(2), 70–73. /doi:10.1097/00043860-200604000-00009

Jana G. Zwilling

ADVANCED PRACTICE NURSING WITHIN HEALTHCARE SETTINGS: ORGANIZATIONAL ROLES

The U.S. healthcare system has undergone a huge shift with the implementation of the Patient Protection and Affordable Care Act (ACA) and more potential changes will be forthcoming. These fluctuations have and will continue to require the APRN not only to be clinically competent but also to have an understanding of the organizations in which care is presently delivered. The APRN must have knowledge of and the ability to create the systems of care that will ensure the high-quality and cost-effective care needed in the future.

The economics of healthcare have become increasingly complex. In an attempt to achieve cost efficiencies, merging healthcare organizations have given birth to giant healthcare corporations. However, the goal of cost savings has not necessarily been consistently achieved. This is evidenced by ever-increasing healthcare costs and the percentage of the national budget being spent on healthcare today, with less-than-ideal-outcome for all citizens (Centers of Medicare & Medicaid Services [CMS], 2016; National Center for Health Statistics, 2017).

THE U.S. HEALTHCARE SYSTEM

Healthcare delivery systems in the United States are unlike those of any other country in the world. Most other developed countries have national health insurance programs run by governments and financed through general taxes, so almost all citizens are entitled to receive healthcare. The United States has recently taken steps toward a national health insurance program. The ACA was signed into law in March 2010. As all laws do, it takes time to put processes in place and see the effects and outcomes of the new legislation. The initial year for individuals and their families to sign up for health insurance as mandated by the ACA was 2014. As with many laws, new leadership has different opinions than previous leadership. As recently as November 2017, the individual insurance mandate holds the potential for repeal. If passed, this would remove the penalty individuals must pay if they have no insurance coverage.

There are varying opinions regarding healthcare reform laws. Enabling insurance coverage regardless of preexisting conditions or the ability to pay the insurance premiums is a benefit for many. Other benefits of new laws can include tax credits for small businesses to offer employee health coverage and the mandate that all coverage must include preventive services. There are some perceived drawbacks to new healthcare legislation. Every individual is mandated to have some form of health insurance or will have to pay a fine. This can be perceived as taking away an individual's choice; however, it could also decrease the number of uninsured. Also, the increasing costs of premiums need to be considered, because insurance companies can no longer deny coverage and companies will need to raise rates to ensure coverage for everyone. Unfortunately, despite the increased premium costs, insurance reimbursement to healthcare providers has also decreased. This has created an environment of strategic healthcare implementation.

There is traditionally strong evidence that health insurance coverage improves access and quality of health and medical care, contributing to the overall health of individuals and their families. According to 2014–2015 data from the National Hospital Ambulatory Medical Care Survey (NHAMCS, 2014; National Ambulatory Medical Care Survey, [NAMCS], 2015):

- In emergency departments, the percentage of visits by patients who had some form of insurance coverage was seven times higher than that of uninsured visits.
- The number of patient visits to physicians' offices was more than 15 times higher for individuals with private health insurance or Medicaid/ Children's Health Insurance Program (CHIP) compared with those with no insurance.

An increasing number of Americans are gaining access to insurance coverage with the implementation of the ACA. In 2012, 45.5 million Americans, or 14.7% of the U.S. population, were underinsured or uninsured, including working-age adults (those aged 18–64 years; Cohen & Martinez, 2012; Kaiser Commission on Medicaid and the Uninsured, 2012). A Gallup poll showed percentages of uninsured as low as 10.9% in the third quarter of 2016. However, the fourth quarter of 2017 revealed the rate of the uninsured had been increased to 12.2% (Auter, 2018). These reports also show a narrowing in the inequity of coverage based on race and ethnicity, gender, and age. Uninsured persons are defined as persons without private health insurance, Medicare, Medicaid, State Children's Health Insurance Program (SCHIP) coverage, a state-sponsored or other government-sponsored health plan, or a military plan. Also included among the underinsured and uninsured are persons who have only Indian Health Service coverage or a private plan that pays for only one type of service, such as accidents or dental care (National Health Interview Survey, 2012). It remains to be seen how the passing of the Republican tax bill in late 2017, which includes a repeal of the individual insurance mandate effective in 2019, will affect numbers of uninsured.

The complexities of the various systems of care—which include nonprofit and proprietary organizations; large and small corporations; local, regional, and worldwide conglomerates; small and multisystem plans; multistate healthcare systems and payment mechanisms; and regulatory requirements—can be overwhelming to the new APRN. Few nurses have a strong background or experience in the organizational influences of healthcare. Content on the complexity of healthcare coverage has historically been minimal in nursing undergraduate education. This knowledge deficit is compounded by the fact that most nurses have neither experience with the organizational dimensions of healthcare nor access to quality leadership mentoring (Ramseur, Fuchs, Edwards, & Humphreys, 2018).

What remains to be seen is the impact on the healthcare system of increasing access. Many believe this will cause a huge influx of patients needing care, thus overburdening an already short supply of primary care providers. Rationing of care has been discussed as a potential and negative outcome of this increased patient load (Robinson, Williams, Dickinson, Freeman, & Rumbold, 2012). This could mean long waits for nonemergent care and nonexistent elective services. A formal priority-setting approach has yet to be implemented on a large scale. Preventive care will become the focus, and nontraditional forms of healthcare delivery will need to be implemented (Cornelissen et al., 2014). The shortage of primary care physicians and the emphasis on preventive services create an opportunity for APRNs to have an impact on the healthcare delivery systems.

Organizational Influences

How does an understanding of these organizational influences affect the APRN's roles and functions? Many factors are involved, and these influences can clearly change during the tenure of the APRN's career. A beginning APRN needs to understand these organizations when selecting future employment and providing care to clients. As APRNs become more confident in their role as care providers, they can expand their roles as leaders and change agents to influence their organizations. To do so requires enhanced knowledge and skills in organizational design, systems, function, and complexity. Therefore, advanced knowledge in such fields as organizational behavior, cost analysis, risk management, patient satisfaction, safety, and quality is necessary to fully implement the role of the APRN. To ensure that the APRN is on the forefront of new and innovative care delivery practices, an understanding of the healthcare systems and organizations that are and should be in place where the APRN practices is a needed prerequisite.

Even though these rapidly changing healthcare system settings are ripe for innovation, the APRN may find it a daunting task to understand and negotiate them. Traditionally educated to provide advanced nursing care more closely aligned to a specific system or setting of care, the APRN is now faced with the challenge of a multisystem arena for care delivery. Understanding system issues has been identified as a necessary component of graduate education for nurse administrators and APRNs for many years, but the recommendation has not been fully embraced. As early as 1998, Lynn, Layman, and Englebardt (1998) identified the importance of incorporating such topics as leadership, financial management policies, health policy, and organizational culture and structure into course content in advanced practice educational programs.

The American Association of Colleges of Nursing (AACN) *Essentials of Doctoral Education for Advanced Nursing Practice* (AACN, 2006) identifies that advanced nursing practice includes an organizational and systems leadership component. This requires political skills, systems thinking, and business and financial expertise. In this environment of ongoing changes in the organization and financing of healthcare, this document asserts that it is imperative that all graduates of practice doctorate degree nursing programs have a keen understanding of healthcare policy, organization, and financing of healthcare. The purpose of this content is to prepare a graduate to provide quality cost-effective care, to participate in the design and implementation of care in a variety of healthcare systems, and to assume a leadership role in managing human, fiscal, and physical healthcare resources.

Analysis of Organizations

For the new APRN, understanding healthcare organizations is vital in determining the most appropriate place or setting for employment. The ability to understand an organization is based on several factors. Examples of questions APRNs should ask include:

- What is the organizational structure of the organization?
- What is the philosophical underpinning of the organization?
- What are the directions and goals of the organization?
- What are the culture and climate of the organization?

Organizational structure is one dimension that is important to understand. Historically, healthcare organizations have been structured in the more traditional hierarchical and bureaucratic organizational models. Many experts in organizational functioning believe that these traditional models will no longer work in the emerging healthcare arena. They have proposed that the new models need to be flat, innovative, nimble, and responsive to change. The healthcare organizations that will survive in the frenetic pace of today's world will promote greater flexibility and have the ability to deal with ambiguity and uncertainty. The healthcare systems of the future will be driven by a free market system and need to push the envelope on quality and affordability in order to sustain business from the more informed patient (Wesslund, 2017).

The APRN should evaluate the structure of the organization and how it will influence his or her ability to provide care and perform the various aspects of the APRN role. For instance, organizational structure clearly affects communication in a healthcare system and influences how and by whom decisions are made. The APRN should identify how many layers of the organization lie between the APRN and the person or persons who are responsible for making decisions that will affect the APRN's clinical decisions, the latitude of the APRN's daily practice, and the costs of care related to patient care. The APRN should understand the "official" organizational structure and recognize the "informal" lines of communication and decision-making networks.

Every organization has different philosophical underpinnings that frame the organization's direction for the future and give the APRN insight into how decisions will be made. An organization's mission, vision, values, philosophy, and organizational objectives are important. The mission of the organization describes the purpose for which that organization exists. The mission statement provides valuable information about the organization's direction and goals for the future. Mission statements allow the reader to understand what is meaningful to the organization, how that meaning may be measured, and clearly define the organization's reason for existing. They can also lead to an enhanced understanding of the ethics, principles, and standards for which the employees will be held accountable (Danna, 2011).

Mission statements should provide vision for the organization. The vision should be an image of the future, whereas value statements should bond people and set behavioral standards in the organization. The philosophy of the organization outlines values, concepts, and beliefs that establish the organization's care practices. Mission and vision statements can help a prospective employee understand the value placed on the clients and workers in an organization. Having a clear understanding of these foundational aspects of an organization can help inform the APRN about an agency's present and future goals and expected outcomes. For instance, an APRN who has a strong belief in providing care to all people regardless of their ability to pay or who has a strong belief in a certain ethical orientation is wise to identify that the organization being considered has values that are consistent with that person's belief system. Simply hoping that an organization promotes the same level of quality care that the individual APRN aspires to give or believing that all organizations are the same is naive and will affect whether the APRN will survive or strive in the practice setting.

A common method of analyzing healthcare organizations is to use a systems theory approach. The healthcare organization is considered an open system; it has permeable boundaries that are affected by the society in which it operates. Change in society forces internal change in the operation of an organization. The rapidity with which these changes have occurred recently is responsible for the chaotic situations in which many health-care practitioners and administrators operate today (Lee & Mongan, 2009). Given the extraordinary complexity of these healthcare systems, an emerging field of science has been suggested as an alternative approach to understanding them. This emerging field, termed "complexity science," offers alternative leadership and management strategies for the chaotic, complex healthcare environment (Miles, 2009).

One method to evaluate an organization is to examine an organization's outcomes or its "organizational effectiveness." Danna (2011) provides a helpful listing of indicators to monitor organizational effectiveness. Those indicators include patient satisfaction with care; family satisfaction with care; staff satisfaction with work; staff satisfaction with rewards, intrinsic and extrinsic; staff satisfaction with professional development; staff satisfaction with organization; and management's satisfaction with staff, community relationships, and organizational health. A malfunctioning organization would be reflected by such elements as focusing on the wrong elements of the operation, having too many meetings attended by too many people accomplishing little work, and having too many levels of administration, to name a few.

Healthy environments support meaningful work and provide an environment in which the APRN can excel and feel an important part of the team. The American Organization of Nurse Executives (AONE, 2009) has identified six critical factors to improve workplace initiatives, extracted from a study of workplace implementation and innovation. These factors are leadership development, empowered collaborative decision making, work design and service delivery innovation, a values-focused organizational culture, recognition and rewards systems, and professional growth and accountability.

Organizational Climate and Culture

All healthcare organizations have a climate and culture. "Climate" is described as the emotional states, feelings, and perceptions shared by the members of the organization. Climate can be described by such terms as positive or negative, hopeful or negative, trusting or suspicious, and competitive or nurturing. The APRN can influence the climate or be influenced by it. Climate can influence interactions and responses by patients and coworkers alike. It is a component of job satisfaction and enjoyment in one's work life. An organizational climate that is inconsistent with an APRN's preferred orientation can cause dissatisfaction and limit the ability to excel. However, the seasoned APRN can be pivotal in establishing the day-to-day climate in the practice setting.

An organization's social system, including its beliefs, norms, mission, philosophies, traditions, and values, makes up its "culture." It represents the perspectives, values, assumptions, language, and behaviors that have been effectively used by the members of the organization. Culture influences the formal and informal methods and styles of communication. When considering employment in an organization, an APRN should assess the culture and climate of an organization to determine whether it is an appropriate fit. The APRN may wish to practice with a specific population or within a specialty area. However, without an appreciation of the organization's climate and culture, the APRN may be unable to implement the changes and level of care he or she hopes to provide. Finding an organization that is consistent with the APRN's preferred culture and climate can provide a solid and more comfortable practice arena for an individual practitioner.

The Culture of Safety and Quality

Beginning in the 1980s and continuing with increased emphasis during the past decade, there has been a nationwide agenda to address the culture of safety and quality in healthcare organizations. National healthcare quality accreditation and regulatory agencies have taken major steps to enhance quality and safety by identifying evidence-based best practices and encouraging measurement and monitoring of these practices and care outcomes. The Joint Commission (formerly known as the Joint Commission on the Accreditation of Healthcare Organizations [JCAHO]), the Institute of Medicine (IOM), the Agency of Healthcare Research and Quality (AHRQ), and the CMS of the U.S. Department of Health and Human Services (HHS) are just a few of the many organizations and agencies focused on enhancing healthcare quality and safety.

The IOM (now the Health and Medicine Division of the National Academies of Science, Engineering, and Medicine) has identified safety concerns and problems with quality of care. In the IOM's *Crossing the Quality Chasm: A New Health System for the 21st Century* (2001), six dimensions of healthcare performance were deemed to be in need of improvement: safety, effectiveness, patient-centeredness, timeliness, efficiency, and equity. The IOM defines "healthcare quality" as "the degree to which health services for individuals and populations increase the likelihood of desired health outcomes and are consistent with current professional knowledge" (pp. 128–129). The care should be based on evidence-based practice and provided in a technically and culturally competent manner with good communication and shared decision making (Pelletier & Beaudin, 2018, p. 3).

A series of IOM reports help illustrate how wide the quality chasm is and how important it is to close the gulf between our standards of high-quality care and the prevailing norm in practice. Two landmark reports released by the IOM, *To Err Is Human: Building a Safer Health System* (Kohn, Corrigan, & Donaldson, 2000) and *Crossing the Quality Chasm: A New Health System for the 21st Century* (2001), moved the national dialogue, asserting that reform is not accomplished by simply addressing the issues around its margins. The third phase of the IOM's *Quality Initiative* focuses on setting the vision outlined in *Quality Chasm* into operation. This implementation is on three levels: environmental, healthcare organization, and interaction between clinicians and patients. Thus far, focus has been on the redesign of care delivery, reform of health professions' education, technology implementation, safety, and quality care that is accessible and cost-effective. Details of these foci are addressed in multiple IOM reports from 2003 to 2006 including: *Health Professions Education: A Bridge to Quality* (Greiner & Knebel, 2003), *Key Capabilities of an Electronic Medical Record* (IOM, 2003), *Patient Safety: Achieving a New Standard for Care* (Aspden, Corrigan, Wolcott, & Erickson, 2004), *Performance Measurement: Accelerating Improvement* (IOM, 2005), and *Medicare's Quality Improvement Organization Program: Maximizing Potential* (IOM, 2006).

The overall goal for the Quality and Safety Education for Nurses (QSEN) project (Cronenwett et al., 2007) is to meet the challenge of preparing future nurses who will have the knowledge, skills, and attitudes (KSAs) necessary to continuously improve the quality and safety of the healthcare systems in which they work. Using the IOM *Health Professions Education: A Bridge to Quality* (Greiner & Knebel, 2003) competencies, QSEN faculty and a national advisory board have defined quality and safety competencies for graduate-level nursing and proposed targets for the KSAs to be developed in APRN programs for each competency (AACN, 2012). These competencies serve as a guide to curricular development for formal academic programs, transition to practice, and continuing education programs (Cronenwett et al., 2009).

CMS finalized its initiatives to develop quality measures of healthcare providers following the institution of the ACA in 2011. One of these initiatives is the "Pay for Reporting and Pay for Performance" standard. This standard outlines four quality measures that will be tracked, and provider reimbursement will be affected by the outcomes. These measures are tracked with a variety of methods, including patient surveys, claims calculation, electronic health record (EHR) review, and group practice reporting option (CMS, 2012). The APRN should be aware of these outcome measures when considering a place of employment and use them as a mechanism to monitor the quality of services provided by his or her organization. There are now innumerable quality and safety initiatives nationwide, and astute APRNs will understand what is occurring in their place of employment and will help shape its practices to enhance quality. Several studies show APRNs' practices are already demonstrating high-level outcomes for patient satisfaction and chronic disease management (Dinh, Walker, Parameswaran, & Enright, 2012; Newhouse et al., 2011). Continued positive outcomes will propel APRNs to be exemplary models of quality healthcare.

SUMMARY

The APRN of today and tomorrow will need to address organizational and system issues. Although it may seem daunting in our changing healthcare landscape, APRNs must develop the knowledge to analyze organizational variables and the skills and abilities to enhance quality and safety. The APRN must be a leader and change agent instrumental in creating the care delivery systems that will be needed in the future.

REFERENCES

American Association of Colleges of Nursing. (2006). Essentials of doctoral education for advanced practice nursing. Retrieved from http://www.aacnnursing .org/Portals/42/Publications/DNPEssentials.pdf

American Association of Colleges of Nursing. (2012). QSEN education consortium. Graduate-level QSEN competencies: Knowledge, skills, and attitudes. Retrieved from http://www.aacnnursing.org/Portals/42/AcademicNursing/ CurriculumGuidelines/Graduate-QSEN-Competencies.pdf

American Organization of Nurse Executives. (2009). Retrieved from http://www .aone.org

Aspden, P., Corrigan, J. M., Wolcott, J., & Erickson, S. M. (Eds.). (2004). *Patient safety: Achieving a new standard for care.* Washington, DC: National Academies Press.

Auter, Z. (2018). U.S. uninsured rate steady at 12.2% in fourth quarter of 2017. Gallup-Sharecare Well-Being Index. Retrieved from http://news.gallup .com/poll/225383/uninsured-rate-steady-fourth-quarter-2017.aspx

Centers for Medicare & Medicaid Services. (2012). Guide to quality performance standards for accountable care. Retrieved from http://www.cms .gov/Medicare/Medicare-Fee-for-Service-Payment/sharedsavingsprogram/ Downloads/ACO-Guide-Quality-Performance-2012.PDF

Centers for Medicare & Medicaid Services. (2016). National health expenditures by type of service and source of funds, CY 1960-2016. Retrieved from http:// www.cms.gov/Research-Statistics-Data-and-Systems/Statistics-Trends-and -Reports/NationalHealthExpendData/NationalHealthAccountsHistorical .html

Cohen, R. A., & Martinez, M. E. (2012). Health insurance coverage: Early release of estimates from the National Health Interview Survey, 2012. Retrieved from http://www.cdc.gov/nchs/data/nhis/earlyrelease/insur201306.pdf

Cornelissen, E., Mitton, C., Davidson, A., Reid, C., Hole, R., Visockas, A., & Smith, N. (2014). Determining and broadening the definition of impact from implementing a rational priority setting approach in a healthcare organization. *Social Science & Medicine, 114,* 1–9. doi:10.1016/j.socscimed.2014.05.027

Cronenwett, L., Sherwood, G., Barnsteiner J., Disch, J., Johnson, J., Mitchell, P., ... Warren, J. (2007). Quality and safety education for nurses. *Nursing Outlook, 55*(3), 122–131. doi:10.1016/j.outlook.2007.02.006

Cronenwett, L., Sherwood G., Pohl, J., Barnsteiner, J., Moore, S., Sullivan, D., . . . Warren, J. (2009). Quality and safety education for advanced nursing practice. *Nursing Outlook, 57,* 338–348. doi:10.1016/j.outlook.2009.07.009

Danna, D. (2011). Organizational structure and analysis. In L. Roussel (Ed.), *Management leadership for nurse administrators* (6th ed.). Boston, MA: Jones & Bartlett.

Dinh, M., Walker, A., Parameswaran, A., & Enright, N. (2012). Evaluating the quality of care delivered by an emergency department fast track unit with both nurse practitioners and doctors. *Australasian Emergency Nursing Journal, 15*(4), 188–194. doi:10.1016/j.aenj.2012.09.001

Greiner, A. C., & Knebel, E. (Eds.). (2003). *Health professions education: A bridge to quality.* Washington, DC: National Academies Press.

Institute of Medicine. (2001). *Crossing the quality chasm: A new health system for the 21st century.* Washington, DC: National Academies Press.

Institute of Medicine. (2003). *Key capabilities of an electronic medical record.* Washington, DC: National Academies Press.

Institute of Medicine. (2005). *Performance measurement: Accelerating improvement.* Washington, DC: National Academies Press.

Institute of Medicine. (2006). *Medicare's quality improvement organization program: Maximizing potential.* Washington, DC: National Academies Press.

Kaiser Commission on Medicaid and the Uninsured. (2012). The uninsured and the difference health insurance makes. *Kaiser Family Foundation.* Retrieved from http://www.kff.org/uninsured/upload/1420-14.pdf

Kohn, L. T., Corrigan, J. M., & Donaldson, M. S. (Eds.). (2000). *To err is human: Building a safer health system.* Washington, DC: National Academies Press.

Lee, T., & Mongan, J. (2009). *Chaos and organization in health care.* Cambridge: Massachusetts Institute of Technology Press.

Lynn, M., Layman, E., & Englebardt, S. (1998). Nursing administration research priorities: A national Delphi study. *Journal of Nursing Administration, 15,* 7–11.

Miles, A. (2009). Complexity in medicine and healthcare: People and systems, theory and practice. *Journal of Evaluation in Clinical Practice, 15,* 409–410. doi:10.1111/j.1365-2753.2009.01204.x

National Ambulatory Medical Care Survey. (2015). 2015 Outpatient department summary tables. Retrieved from https://www.cdc.gov/nchs/data/ahcd/namcs_summary/2015_namcs_web_tables.pdf

National Center for Health Statistics. (2017). *Health, United States, 2016: With chartbook on trends in the health of Americans.* Hyattsville, MD: Department of Health and Human Services. Retrieved from https://www.cdc.gov/nchs/data/hus/hus16.pdf

National Health Interview Survey. (2012). Early release of selected estimates based on data from the January–June 2012 national health interview survey. Retrieved from http://www.cdc.gov/nchs/data/nhis/earlyrelease/earlyrelease201212_01.pdf

National Hospital Ambulatory Medical Care Survey. (2014). 2014 Emergency department summary tables. Retrieved from https://www.cdc.gov/nchs/data/nhamcs/web_tables/2014_ed_web_tables.pdf

Newhouse, R. P., Stanik-Hutt, J., White, K. M., Johantgen, M., Bass, E. B., Zangaro, G., . . . Weiner, J. P. (2011). Advanced practice nurse outcomes 1990–2008: A systematic review. *Nursing Economics, 29*(5), 1–22. doi:10.1234/12345678

Pelletier, L. R., & Beaudin, C. L. (2018). *HQ solutions: Resource for the healthcare quality professional* (4th ed.). Glenview, IL: National Association for Healthcare Quality.

Ramseur, P., Fuchs, M. A., Edwards, P., & Humphreys, J. (2018). The implementation of a structured nursing leadership development program for succession planning in a health system. *The Journal of Nursing Administration, 48*(1), 25–30. doi:10.1097/NNA.0000000000000566

Robinson, S., Williams, I., Dickinson, H., Freeman, T., & Rumbold, B. (2012). Priority-setting and rationing in healthcare: Evidence from the English experience. *Social Science & Medicine, 75*(12), 2386–2393. doi:10.1016/j.socscimed.2012.09.014

Wesslund, R. E. (2017). Reform is a market issue. Retrieved from http://www.bdcadvisors.com/wp-content/uploads/2015/08/bdc_2011_reformisamarketissue.pdf

Kathryn A. Blair

INTERPROFESSIONAL COLLABORATIVE TEAMS AND EDUCATION: ROLES FOR THE APRN

With the Patient Protection and Affordable Care Act (ACA), a forced transformation of healthcare that promoted access to care and affordability began to evolve. However, the progress has been slow and the current system remains reactive.

The old reactive model of care does not involve a variety of healthcare professionals in coordinated care but rather results in a lack of continuity of care (Nuño, Coleman, Bengoa, & Sauto, 2012). Mitchell et al. (2012) reported that Medicare patients may see multiple physicians yearly (at least two primary care providers and five specialists). This number does not include other professionals involved in the patient's care, such as pharmacists, nurses, physician assistants, APRNs, social workers, dietitians, and chiropractors. Most of these professionals are working in isolation, addressing a specific problem. If a provider engages other professionals in patient care, the typical pattern is parallel or consultative and not integrated or collaborative. This model of care encourages duplications of services and fragmented care.

As early as 2003, the Institute of Medicine's (IOM) *Health Professions Education: A Bridge to Quality* identified that the present-day system of healthcare fails to translate research into practice, apply technology to enhance care and reduce errors, and fully utilize the available resources (Greiner & Knebel, 2003). The failure to use nurses to their full capacity was repeated in the IOM's *The Future of Nursing: Leading Change, Advancing Health* (2010) document. This report recommended that nurses be full partners, with physicians and other health professionals, in redesigning healthcare in the United States. Unfortunately, the current system continues to fail to use nurses, especially APRNs, to their full capabilities, and the present-day model of care encourages underuse and/or overuse of resources, subop-timal care, inefficiencies, rising expenditures, and provider and patient dissatisfaction.

In addition to transforming the healthcare system, the ACA created a significant shortage of providers and uneven geographical distribution of providers (Busen, 2014; Washko & Fennel, 2017). Predictions from the Bureau of Labor Statistics suggest the current employment of 203,800 nurse anesthetists, nurse-midwives, and nurse practitioners will increase to 267,000 by 2026, a 31% increase (Bureau of Labor Statistics, U.S. Department of Labor, 2017). The growing demand for healthcare providers, specifically APRNs, places the APRNs in pivotal roles to change the current healthcare delivery system and promote and participate in team-based care.

One proposed solution to address the shortage of healthcare providers, rising healthcare costs, errors, and suboptimal/fragmented care is the utili-zation of "teams." Team-based healthcare has been defined as care provided by two or more healthcare professionals who have different skills and ex-pertise and who work together on common goals to provide quality patient-centered care (Mitchell et al., 2012). This definition could be expanded beyond healthcare providers to include non–healthcare professionals, such as administrators, community leaders, and others.

If team care is important, then what kind of team? There exist several forms of teams: disaster teams; teams in the acute care setting caring for critically ill patients; community-based teams that care for people in their homes; office-based care teams; and teams that include the patient, family members, and supporting healthcare providers (Mitchell et al., 2012). Other teams are defined by their structure: multidisciplinary, transdis-ciplinary and interprofessional, or interdisciplinary. "Interdisciplinary" and "interprofessional" are interchangeable terms. Given the recent trend for promoting interprofessional collaboration, the term "interpro-fessional" will be used in place of "interdisciplinary." Multidisciplinary team members assume a hierarchical role that is governed by profes-sional identities. Transdisciplinary team members cross disciplines, and individual expertise blurs roles of team members. This team model is not often seen in healthcare, in part because medical education continues to marginalize other healthcare professionals such as "nondoctors," and healthcare systems continue to legitimize medical dominance (Paradis, Pipher, Cartmell, Rangel, & Whitehead, 2017). Interprofessional team member roles are synergistic and interdependent, characterized by open communication, collaboration, and leadership that is task driven. When there is effective communication and collaboration in an interprofessional team, then members are empowered to take a leadership role based on their expertise for the patient's problem. One key element of the team-based care that is interprofessional is *collaboration*. In essence, interprofes-sional collaboration requires a partnership, including patient, family, and healthcare providers who engage in a unified, coordinated approach with shared decision making regarding health and social issues (Canadian Interprofessional Health Collaborative, 2010). The interprofessional collaborative team (ICT) model promotes active engagement and joint decision making (Lapkin, Levett-Jones, & Gilligan, 2013).

In 2001, the authors of the IOM report *Crossing the Quality Chasm: A New Health System for the 21st Century* argued that patient safety, quality care, and cost containment are bundled in ICTs. If ICTs are necessary for improving healthcare, what are the fundamental principles guiding these teams? The Interprofessional Education Collaborative Expert Panel (2011; updated 2016) classified four competency domains: values and ethics, roles and responsibilities, interprofessional communication, and team and teamwork and argues that these domains must be incorporated into professional identity for ICTs to function. Other researchers examining ICTs have identified six core elements necessary for interprofessional collaborative practice that is patient-centered: (a) knowledge and skills for team functions, (b) communication, (c) leadership, (d) cooperation and negotiation for conflict resolution, (e) understanding and strength in one's professional role, and (f) appreciation of the professional roles of others (Patrician et al., 2012; Templeton, Robinson, & McKenna, 2016).

Composition of the ICT is another topic for exploration. Although the primary members of a healthcare team are identified as a physician and primary care nurse, other healthcare professionals such as pharmacists, social workers, psychologists, and dietitians are included depending on the needs and goals of the patient (Sayah, Szafran, Robertson, Bell, & Williams, 2014). The question to be addressed is whether physician participation is necessary in all teams. As the APRN role continues to evolve, the answer may be no. This is not to be construed as marginalizing the physician's role, but rather to highlight that there may be instances where the APRN is the primary provider of care or directly responsible for the care of a particular patient independent of a physician.

What remains elusive is when and where the ICTs are necessary. The day-to-day care for minor acute illnesses does not require an ICT—or does it? When conceptualizing an ICT on a macro level, then ICTs are necessary for all aspects of care. This might encompass system operations, population-based models of care, standards of practice, evidence-based practice models, and quality improvement projects. On a micro level, or the process of delivering care to the individual patient, the ICTs may be indicated for patients with chronic, complex healthcare issues, when minor illnesses are later defined as more complex than originally thought, or when instituting preventive services.

BARRIERS FOR ICTs

Professional barriers for ICTs include the classic physician-driven model with the physician as the leader of the team. The introduction of medical homes by the Accountable Care Organization promotes this concept of a physician-driven team model. This model dissuades the integration of ICTs into the healthcare system. Other barriers to collaboration are related to differences in each discipline's professional orientation (Paradis et al., 2017), lack of clarity of roles, or liability and competence (Schadewaldt, Mcinnes, Hiller, & Gardner, 2013). Traditional hierarchical roles, ownership of specific knowledge, technical skills, and clinical territory between professions produce interdisciplinary conflict and subsequent disruption of ICTs (Brooten, Youngblut, Hannan, & Guido-Sanz, 2012; Munro, Kornelsen, & Grzybowsk, 2013).

Systems factors such as regulatory issues and billing practices have been cited as barriers for ICTs (Munro et al., 2013; Weinstein, Brandt, Gilbert, & Schmitt, 2014). Yet another confounding variable is the current reimbursement system. Although team care is reimbursed in the form of care management and pay-for-performance benchmark payments (Roett & Coleman, 2013), the work of the team behind the scenes is not reimbursed resulting in a disincentive to form teams.

Role confusion has been recognized as a common barrier for effective ICTs. The ambiguity between roles is particularly troublesome for those professions with overlapping roles (e.g., APRNs and physicians).

Professional Socialization

The greatest barrier for ICTs is *professional socialization*. "Professional socialization" is the developmental stage when a student learns about the profession from historical and social perspectives and incorporates the values and attitudes of that profession.

Although many healthcare professionals are members of the healthcare team, nurses and physicians play a central role, given the status of medicine and the number of nurses. "Given the centrality of the nurse–physician relationship within healthcare, and the importance of collegiality to professional and organizational outcomes, promoting interprofessional respect and collaboration between nursing and medicine is of critical importance" (Price, Doucet, & McGillis-Hall, 2014, p. 106).

Traditionally, medicine remains at the top of the healthcare hierarchy, with all other healthcare professions deemed as second best (Price et al., 2014). Physicians assume a superior role in patient care decision making based on medical education and socialization. Historically, physician education prepares physicians for independence and autonomy. Ultimately, this socialization discourages cooperation and interdependence.

Nurses are viewed as relying on physicians for direction; however, with the advent of academic degrees and training, increasing technology, and increasing healthcare complexity, nurses have expanded their scope of practice. The failure to educate the public and other healthcare providers has resulted in the APRN appearing second rate to the physician. "True collaboration between the two professions will remain elusive until nurses cease to attribute their knowledge to physicians, recognizing collective decision making and authority, effectively ending this historical game" (Price et al., 2014, p. 105).

With closer examination of the historical perspective of both professions, the roles of physicians were reflective of the roles of women and men. Several social changes have occurred over the past 50 years, such as the improved status of women and the advanced practice nursing options, and have contributed to a more collegial relationship between physicians and nurses. Unfortunately, "nurses are subordinate to not only medicine, but organizational structures as well" (Price et al., 2014, p. 106).

APRNs' expansion of practice and the development of doctorally pre-pared clinical nurses can and will challenge preconceived notions of pro-fessional practice. Without regulatory support through legislation and regulatory policies, the notion of APRNs being second best will persist. In addition to regulatory changes, healthcare organizations, communities, and educational institutions need to embrace interprofessional collabora-tion as the norm rather than the exception to providing the best patient care.

ICT: Role for APRNs

To address the professional barriers, APRNs must begin to unravel the con-fusion around nursing knowledge, skills, and roles. Nurse educators and nurses, including APRNs, need to clearly articulate what they know and do to increase nurses' visibility and participation in the design of an interpro-fessional healthcare system. Unifying the conflicting views among nurse scholars and educators regarding the relationship of nursing knowledge to practice will add additional clarity (Sommerfeldt, 2013).

With the expansion of the nursing role, the pervasive notion that medicine is superior to nursing is beginning to change. The belief that only nurses function within a caring, nurturing, and holistic model while physicians function within a scientific-based model is no longer true. The time has come to recognize that the practices of medicine and nursing (specifically the APRN role) have a great deal of overlap and the roles complement one another rather than compete against each other. With the continued evolu-tion of the APRN role and the doctorate of nursing practice (DNP), these old viewpoints and models of practice are being challenged (Price et al., 2014).

APRNs need to challenge the early professional socialization by edu-cating the public about the role and functions of the APRN. The school system can be one venue. When local schools have career days, the APRN can articulate the uniqueness of nursing and advanced practice nursing so that when students think about healthcare careers, nursing will be the first choice and not the second choice if they cannot get into medical school.

Using the media to foster public education is critical. In 2002, the Johnson & Johnson Corporation sponsored commercials about nursing. Although these commercials increased public awareness about the profession, they did little to emphasize the depth of nursing education, skills, and scope of practice. The commercials focused on "Dare to care" or nursing historical roots of being a "caring" profession.

Becoming involved in local health policies is another way to reach the public. The key is to become visible. APRNs need to engage legislators, in-surance companies, industry stakeholders, and other stakeholders in facil-itating the change in attitudes about nursing. If APRNs sit at the sidelines and wait for someone else to do the work, they will remain "second best."

To address systems barriers, the APRN is in a pivotal position to facilitate the changes necessary to redesign the healthcare system such that ICTs can work. APRNs can foster partnerships among stakeholders (patients, families, and community leaders) to foster support for ICT healthcare initiatives; can become involved in legislative activities to change federal and state regulations regarding reimbursement and scope of practice issues; can work with technology experts to design information systems that support ICTs; and can develop a better understanding of how to encourage teamwork through asynchronous healthcare delivery (Djukic, Fulmer, Adams, Lee, & Triola, 2012; Kuziemskya & Varpiob, 2011; Nuño et al., 2012).

With the increased use of health information systems (HISs) as a tool in providing care, APRNs can collaborate with information technology experts in the development and design of HISs to support collaborative care delivery (Kuziemskya & Varpiob, 2011). The redesign of HISs needs to incorporate communication mechanisms that interface with patients and families, communities, and other healthcare providers. This can facilitate asynchronous collaborative team efforts.

Reconceptualizing the APRN role as the liaison between and among team members (Légaré et al., 2011) and as the coordinator of care will clarify one function of the APRN within the team. The APRN is the glue that holds the team together. This does not mean always assuming the leadership role, but rather keeping the patient/family connected with the entire team.

APRNs can participate in or conduct research examining team factors that promote optimal performance in applied clinical practice (Andreatta & Marzano, 2012). With this information, APRNs can work with educators to design interprofessional collaborative team education (ICTE) programs as well as role model behaviors that contribute toward a functioning ICT that meets the needs of the patient without increasing cost by decreasing duplication of services and improving patient outcomes.

An overlooked dimension of ICT is "team science," which "entails team members with training and expertise in different health profession fields working together to combine and integrate their knowledge, skills, and perspectives into single research projects that are clinically focused" (Little et al., 2017, p. 17). Using team science may be an avenue to promote the ICT model in the future.

ICT Education: Role of the APRN

A variety of organizations have argued that fostering ICTs begins with ICTE. As articulated earlier, most healthcare professionals are educated in silos, interfacing little with other professions. The incorporation of ICTE into curricula challenges the status quo, blurs professional boundaries, and requires involvement of individual stakeholders (Lawlis, Anson, & Greenfield, 2014). In other words, to implement ICTE, there must be support from the top down. Unless the leadership, academicians, and regulatory authorities are willing to support the initiative, ICTE will not be initiated or sustained as part of the curricula and clinical learning environment (Missen, Jacob, Barnett, Walker, & Cross, 2012; Schmitt, Gilbert, Brandt, & Weinstein, 2013).

The components of ICTE programs are many. Some of the elements, such as professional and personal responsibility and accountability, are already embedded in existing curricula. Others, such as mutual trust and respect, interprofessional communication, and coordination, are key for a successful ICTE program (Bridges, Davidson, Odegard, Maki, & Tomkowiak, 2011) and may need expansion in existing curricula. Although the didactic portion is important, the actual operationalizing of these behaviors is critical.

Aligning medical, nursing, and other professional schools' curricula (didactic and/or clinical experiences) is a daunting task, nevertheless using simulations and other technology to facilitate the ICT learning and experience has been used with some success (Djukic et al., 2012; Liaw, Zhou, Ching Lau, Siau, & Wai-chi Chan, 2014). Most students' attitudes about ICTE were positive, whether they participated face-to-face or via asynchronous web-based activities. Most students believed the experience was useful in helping them understand the roles of various professions and in improving their communications skills. The evidence of these learning experiences translating into sustainable practice is inconclusive (Lapkin et al., 2013).

For ICTE to be implemented and sustained in academic centers, leadership among educators, healthcare professionals, and regulatory authorities must be incorporated into the planning as well as the implementation. From a student perspective, the ICTE must not be perceived as an "add-on" to curricula that are already full. Threads of communication, collaboration, joint decision making, conflict resolution, and role realignment from profession-centered care to patient-centered care (Veerapen & Purkis, 2014) should be woven into the existing courses and should have didactic experiences that enable the student to operationalize these concepts. The clinical setting is a great opportunity to apply these concepts into practice. This can be done in the direct clinical experiences or through simulation.

The APRN can play a role in designing the threads as an academician, practicing clinician, or team member (role-modeling). Research suggests that role-modeling behaviors are as important as knowledge (Pollard, Miers, & Rickaby, 2012).

Introducing the concept of ICTE begins in school but continues in the workplace. Incorporating ICTE in the workplace is an example of "learning by doing" (Brennan, Olds, Dolansky, Estrada, & Patrician, 2014; Kuipers, Ehrlich, & Brownie, 2014). Novice practitioners (whether physicians or APRNs) struggle with roles and skills after graduation; however, continued work in this area will indirectly facilitate sustainability. When systems adopt ICTs as a mode of operation, the players will practice in ICTs.

For decades, healthcare scholars have discussed the role of ICTs in healthcare delivery systems, while educational researchers examined the processes of ICTE. Although the literature is filled with research in both domains, little has been done to institute ICTs in clinical practice or to incorporate ICTE in curricula.

Today's APRNs and those in the future will be responsible for determining the role of ICTs in the future healthcare system. If nurses and APRNs fail to become engaged in the discussion about healthcare reform and the structure and function of ICTs, they run the risk of being overlooked and irrelevant (Sommerfeldt, 2013). The future of nursing's contributions to ICTE and ICTs will depend on the participation of current and future nurses, especially APRNs, in the discussions about healthcare reform. The time is right for the development of new models of care through creating ICTs, remodeling academic nursing education curricula, and incorporating ICTE as a thread or theme; it is time for nursing as a profession to assume a major role in reconstructing healthcare.

SUMMARY

With an aging population and the complexity of chronic disease management, the days of a solo primary care are vanishing. With outcome-based reimbursement, providers from various disciplines need to work together in teams to coordinate care, reduce healthcare costs, ensure patient safety, and enhance quality care. ICTs are the future in healthcare delivery systems. APRNs will play a critical role in establishing ICTs through the role of a change agent. APRNs will have to break down the barriers of traditional hierarchical roles through professional socialization, modifying regulatory and reimbursement systems through political activism, and change the current notion that APRNs are "midlevel providers." When the APRN establishes "value added" to healthcare, then new models of ICTs can evolve.

REFERENCES

Brennan, C. W., Olds, D. M., Dolansky, M., Estrada, C. A., & Patrician, P. A. (2014). Learning by doing: Observing an interprofessional process as an interprofessional team. *Journal of Interprofessional Care, 28*(3), 249–251. doi:10.3109/135 61820.2013.838750

Bridges, D. R., Davidson, R. A., Odegard, P. S., Maki, I. V., & Tomkowiak, J. (2011). Interprofessional collaboration: Three best practice models of interprofessional education. *Medical Education Online.* doi:10.3402/meo.v16i0.6035

Brooten, D., Youngblut, J. M., Hannan, J., & Guido-Sanz, F. (2012). The impact of interprofessional collaboration on the effectiveness, significance, and future of advanced practice registered nurses. *Nursing Clinics of North America, 47,* 283–294. doi:10.1016/j.cnur.2012.02.005

Bureau of Labor Statistics, U.S. Department of Labor. (2017). Nurse anesthetists, nurse midwives, and nurse practitioners. *Occupational Outlook Handbook.* Retrieved from https://www.bls.gov/ooh/healthcare/nurse-anesthetists -nurse-midwives-and-nurse-practitioners.htm

Busen, N. H. (2014). An interprofessional education project to address the health care needs of women transitioning from prison to community reentry. *Journal of Professional Nursing, 30*(4), 357–366. doi:10.1016/j.profnurs.2014.01.002

Canadian Interprofessional Health Collaborative. (2010). A national interprofessional competency framework. Retrieved from http://www.cihc.ca/files/ CIHC_IPCompetencies_Feb1210.pdf

Djukic, M., Fulmer, T., Adams, J. G., Lee, S., & Triola, M. M. (2012). NYU3T: Teaching, technology, teamwork: A model for interprofessional education scalability and sustainability. *Nursing Clinics of North America, 47,* 333–346. doi:10.1016/j .cnur.2012.05.003

Greiner, A. C., & Knebel, E. (Eds.). (2003). *Health professions education: A bridge to quality.* Washington, DC: National Academies Press.

Institute of Medicine. (2001). *Crossing the quality chasm: A new health system for the 21st century.* Washington, DC: National Academies Press.

Institute of Medicine. (2010). *The future of nursing: Leading change, advancing health.* Washington, DC: National Academies Press.

Interprofessional Education Collaborative Expert Panel. (2011). *Core competencies for interprofessional collaborative practice: Report of an expert panel.* Washington, DC: Interprofessional Education Collaborative. Retrieved from https://www.aacom.org/docs/default-source/insideome/ccrpt05-10-11 .pdf?sfvrsn=77937f97_2

Interprofessional Education Collaborative. (2016). *Core competencies for interprofessional collaborative practice: 2016 update.* Washington, DC: Interprofessional Education Collaborative. Retrieved from https://nebula.wsimg.com/2f68a39 520b03336b41038c370497473?AccessKeyId=DC06780E69ED19E2B3A5&dispos ition=0&alloworigin=1

Kuipers, P., Ehrlich, C., & Brownie, S. (2014). Responding to health care complexity: Suggestions for integrated and interprofessional workplace learning. *Journal of Interprofessional Care, 28*(3), 246–248. doi:10.3109/1356182 0.2013.821601

Kuziemskya, C. E., & Varpiob, L. (2011). A model of awareness to enhance our understanding of interprofessional collaborative care delivery and health information system design to support it. *International Journal of Medical Informatics, 8,* 150–160. doi:10.1016/j.ijmedinf.2011.01.009

Lapkin, S., Levett-Jones, T., & Gilligan, C. (2013). A systematic review of the effectiveness of interprofessional education in health professional programs. *Nurse Education Today, 33,* 90–102. doi:10.1016/j.nedt.2011.11.006

Lawlis, T. R., Anson, J., & Greenfield, D. (2014). Barriers and enablers that influence sustainable interprofessional education: A literature review. *Journal of Interprofessional Care, 28*(4), 305–310. doi:10.3109/13561820.2014.895977

Légaré, F., Stacey, D., Pouliot, S., Gauvin, F.-P., Desroches, S., Kryworuchko, J., Dunn, S., . . . (2011). Interprofessionalism and shared decision-making in primary care: A stepwise approach towards a new model. *Journal of Interprofessional Care, 25*(11), 18–25. doi:10.3109/13561820.2010.490502

Liaw, S. Y., Zhou, W. T., Ching Lau, T. C., Siau, C., & Wai-chi Chan, S. (2014). An interprofessional communication training using simulation to enhance safe care for a deteriorating patient. *Nurse Education Today, 34,* 259–264. doi:10.1016/j.nedt.2013.02.019

Little, M. M., St Hill, C. A., Ware, K. B., Swanoski, M. T., Chapman, S. A., Lutfiyya, M. N., & Cerra, F. B. (2017). Team science as interprofessional collaborative research practice: A systematic review of the science of team science literature. *Journal of Investigative Medicine, 65*(1), 15. doi:10.1136/ jim-2016-000216

Missen, K., Jacob, E. R., Barnett, T., Walker, L., & Cross, M. (2012). Interprofessional clinical education: Clinicians' views on the importance of leadership. *Collegian, 19,* 189–195. doi:10.1016/j.colegn.2011.10.002

Mitchell, P., Wynia, M., Golden, R., McNellis, B., Okun, S., Webb, C. E., . . . Von Kohorn, I. (2012). *Core principles and values of effective team-based health care.* Discussion Paper. Washington, DC: Institute of Medicine. Retrieved from http://www.academia.edu/14373686/Core_principles_and_values_of_ effective_team-based_health_care._Institute_of_Medicine

Munro, S., Kornelsen, J., & Grzybowsk, S. (2013). Models of maternity care in rural environments: Barriers and attributes of interprofessional collaboration with midwives. *Midwifery, 29,* 646–652. doi:10.1016/j.midw.2012.06.004

Nuño, R., Coleman, K., Bengoa, R., & Sauto, R. (2012). Integrated care for chronic conditions: The contribution of the ICCC framework. *Health Policy, 105,* 55–64. doi:10.1016/j.healthpol.2011.10.006

Paradis, E., Pipher, M., Cartmill, C., Rangel, J. C., & Whitehead, C. R. (2017). Articulating the ideal: 50 years of interprofessional collaboration in medical education. *Medical Education, 51,* 861–872. doi:10.1111/medu.13331

Patrician, P. A., Dolansky, M., Estrada, C., Brennan, C., Miltner, R., Newsom, J., . . . Moore, S. (2012). Interprofessional education in action: The VA Quality Scholars Fellowship Program. *Nursing Clinics of North America, 47,* 347–354. doi:10.1016/j.cnur.2012.05.006

Pollard, K. C., Miers, M. E., & Rickaby, C. (2012). "Oh why didn't I take more notice?" Professionals' views and perceptions of pre-qualifying preparation for interprofessional working in practice. *Journal of Interprofessional Care, 26,* 355–361. doi:10.3109/13561820.2012.689785

Price, S., Doucet, S., & McGillis-Hall, L. (2014). The historical social positioning of nursing and medicine: Implications for career choice, early socialization and interprofessional collaboration. *Journal of Interprofessional Care, 28*(2), 103–109. doi:10.3109/13561820.2013.867839

Roett, M. A., & Coleman M. T. (2013). Practice improvement, part II: Collaborative practice and team based–care. *Family Practice Essentials, 414,* 11–18.

Sayah, F. A., Szafran, O., Robertson, S., Bell, N. R., & Williams, B. (2014). Nursing perspectives on factors influencing interdisciplinary teamwork in the Canadian primary care setting. *Journal of Clinical Nursing, 23*(19–20), 2968–2979. doi:10.1111/jocn.12547

Schadewaldt, V., Mcinnes, E., Hiller, J., & Gardner, A. (2013). Views and experiences of nurse practitioners and medical practitioners with collaborative practice in primary care: An integrative review. *BioMedCentral Family Practice, 14,* 132. doi:10.1186/1471-2296-14-132

Schmitt, M. H., Gilbert, J. H., Brandt, B. F., & Weinstein, R. S. (2013). The coming of age for interprofessional education and practice. *The American Journal of Medicine, 126*(4), 284–288. doi:10.1016/j.amjmed.2012.10.015

Sommerfeldt, S. C. (2013). Articulating nursing in an interprofessional world. *Nurse Education in Practice, 13,* 519–523. doi:10.1016/j.nepr.2013.02.014

Templeton, K., Robinson, A., & McKenna, L. (2016). Advancing medical education: Connecting interprofessional collaboration and education opportunities with integrative medicine initiatives to build shared learning. *Journal of Complementary and Integrative Medicine, 13*(4), 347–355. doi:10.1515/jcim-2016-0002

Veerapen, K., & Purkis M. E. (2014). Implications of early workplace experiences on continuing interprofessional education for physicians and nurses. *Journal of Interprofessional Care, 28*(3), 218–225. doi:10.3109/13561820.2014.884552

Washko, M. M., & Fennell, M. L. (2017). The epicenter of effectiveness and efficacy in health care delivery: The evolving U.S. workforce. *Health Services Research, 53*(1), 353–359. doi:10.1111/1475-6773.12662

Weinstein, R. S., Brandt, B. F., Gilbert, J. H., & Schmitt, M. H. (2014). Bridging the quality chasm: Interprofessional teams to the rescue? [Editorial] *American Journal of Medicine, 126*(4), 276–277. doi:10.1016/j.amjmed.2012.10.014

Kathy J. Wheeler and Lorna L. Schumann

6

GLOBAL HEALTH: DYNAMIC ROLES FOR THE APRN/ ADVANCED PRACTICE NURSE

Never doubt that a small group of thoughtful, committed citizens can change the world. Indeed, it is the only thing that ever has.

—Margaret Mead

Advanced practice nursing is on a rapidly unfolding evolutionary path globally, dictated by need, vision, and opportunity. The need for cost-effective quality healthcare providers is universal. Technology, communications, and new educational methods have allowed global connections, thus effectively making the world seem smaller. Individuals and organizations involved in healthcare delivery have seen and learned from each other at a pace not seen before. Patients, people, and providers have continued and, in some instances, accelerated transitory movements, relocating regionally and internationally. These factors have resulted in several occurrences regarding the role of the APRN or advanced practice nurse (APN): (a) the advanced practice role is emerging and evolving in many countries; (b) those in the advanced practice role need to understand the global community in order to serve, educate, and treat that community; and (c) the migration of people has created global communities that can be served by APRNs/ APNs.

GLOBAL APRN/APN ROLES AND TRENDS

One of the most confusing aspects of advanced practice nursing pertains to the titling, definitions, and interpretations of the various APRN/APN roles throughout the world. For this chapter, the authors have chosen to use the terms "APRN" and/or "APN" according to whatever seemed more appropriate to the text.

Only recently has the United States settled on consistent terms and definitions through the *Consensus Model for APRN Regulation: Licensure, Accreditation, Certification, and Education* (APRN Consensus Work Group & National Council of State Boards of Nursing APRN Advisory Committee, 2008). The APRN Advisory Committee, through the consensus model, settled on the global term "APRN." The consensus model further delineated four roles: certified registered nurse anesthetist (CRNA), certified nurse-midwife (CNM), clinical nurse specialist (CNS), and certified nurse practitioner (CNP). APRNs in the United States are to be educated in one of these four roles, but must also be educated in one or more of six population foci: the family/individual across the life span; adult-gerontology; pediatrics; neonatology; women's health/gender related; or psychiatric/mental health. The consensus model is broader than merely setting titles—its underlying purpose was to create a document that "defines APRN practice, describes the APRN regulatory model, identifies the titles to be used, defines specialty, describes the emergence of new roles and population foci, and presents strategies for implementation" (p. 4).

Just as the United States has struggled over titles, terms, and role interpretations, the same can be said of advanced practice nursing outside the United States. Many countries have chosen to recognize and encourage expanded roles for nurses beyond that of registered nurse, having done so uniquely and with great variety. The International Council of Nurses (ICN) reports that 70 countries have or are developing advanced practice roles for nurses (ICN Nurse Practitioner/Advanced Practice Nursing Network [ICN NP/APNN], 2018). The ICN NP/APNN (2018, para. 1) goes on to define an APN as "a registered nurse who has acquired the expert knowledge base, complex decision-making skills, and clinical competencies for expanded practice, the characteristics of which are shaped by the context and/or country in which he or she is credentialed to practice. A master's degree is recommended for entry level." The term "advanced practice nurse" (APN) is the commonly accepted international term. Despite the definition, cited characteristics, competencies, and scopes of practice specified by ICN, there is tremendous variation in titles, education, credentialing, policies, recognition, and support worldwide. A 2008 web-based survey identified 13 different titles for APNs in countries recognizing advanced practice. The same survey also showed the following in respondent countries: 71% had some sort of APN education, 50% cited the master's degree as the primary credential, 72% had formal recognition of the role, and 48% had licensure or renewal requirements (Pulcini, Jelic, Gul, & Loke, 2009).

More recent research shows similar variation. A meeting was convened in 2014 in Philadelphia, Pennsylvania, to discuss APN practice around the globe, specifically for the purpose of improving access to cost-effective, quality care in parts of the world where the APN role is absent or underutilized. According to Tine Hansen-Turton (personal communication, September 17, 2014), the meeting brought together 30 health leaders from around the world. Attendees included representatives from the ICN, multiple universities, multiple ministries of health, the Organization for Economic Co-operation and Development (OECD), the Commission on Graduates of Foreign Nursing Schools (CGFNS), and other health organizations. The first recommendation of the report focused on removing the barriers to practice for APNs. These barriers are identified by the Global APN Nursing Symposium as follows:

• Lack of defined role for APNs
• Inconsistent educational and training standards
• Inconsistent or unnecessary regulation
• Unstable healthcare funding from government or third-party payers

Key findings were summarized as follows:

• APNs have the potential to play a much larger role in improving the health of people worldwide.
• Different nations are in different stages of developing their nursing workforce, and opportunities for advanced nursing practice vary significantly from country to country.
• Countries where APNs have a well-defined role and greater practice authority have increasingly used nurses to improve access to primary and preventive healthcare.
• APNs have been successfully deployed in both developed and developing countries to improve health.
• APNs around the globe have worked with governments, consumer groups, funders, investors, and business leaders to create innovative programs and interventions that improve people's health.
• APNs can be a cost-effective solution to existing healthcare access and quality problems, but additional data are needed to fully evaluate and capture the value of their services.

Based on these issues, the group recommended the following:

• Standardize the definition of the APN role.
• Improve the educational curricula for APNs while respecting each country's unique cultural and political context.
• Increase access to primary and preventive healthcare services by removing policy barriers that prevent APNs from practicing to the full extent of their education and training.
• Reform healthcare funding mechanisms to allow for APN-based practice models.
• Collect data and share information on APN quality and outcomes in a variety of countries/settings.

The results of this meeting are detailed in a video of the Global Advanced Practice Nursing Symposium (Philadelphia, 2014), available from: https://vimeo.com/11059.3150

Although the role will evolve according to unique regional issues, there are commonalities, such as the universal need for cost-effective quality healthcare. APRNs/APNs can meet the need, and support for APRNs/APNs will happen through the development and maintenance of policies that provide for APRN/APN education, practice, and research frameworks.

BROADER GLOBAL TRENDS AND NEEDS

To prepare for a global experience, the APRN/APN should understand political, social, economic, and healthcare trends and, more broadly, megatrends. "Megatrends" are defined as high-level trends that generally operate largely outside of industry and geography. Futurists offer unique predictions on megatrends according to perspective. However, in terms of healthcare, most agree the following are megatrends APRNs/APNs need to anticipate: urbanization to cities and towns (Bolwell, 2016; Lancefield & Sviokla, 2018), globalization (Hay Group, 2018), climate change and scarcity of resources (Lancefield & Sviokla, 2018; Weller, 2018), population growth and changing demographics (Hay Group, 2018; Lancefield & Sviokla, 2018; Weller, 2018), workforce shortages (ICN, 2017), increase in chronic disease (World Health Organization [WHO], 2018), rise in infectious disease outbreaks (Ordway & Sokol, 2016), shift to primary care (WHO, 2008), distance learning (Digital Learning Compass, 2017), and increased technology and innovation in communication and healthcare delivery (Lancefield & Sviokla, 2018).

The United Nations (2013) estimates the world's population will reach 9.6 billion by 2050. The prediction suggests populations in developed countries will remain largely unchanged; however, in 49 of the least developed regions, population growth is expected to double. More than half of these countries will be in Africa. This is significant because these areas struggle with limited resources and healthcare delivery. Most of the predicted population explosion will be explained by increased life expectancy. A variety of improved conditions in the world have led to a steady increase in life expectancy in high resource and low resource countries. By 2045 to 2050, the global life expectancy will likely be 76 years, and by the end of the century, it is thought life expectancy will be 89 years in high resource countries and 81 years in low resource countries (United Nations, 2013). Increased life expectancy will have significant repercussions. For example, there will be more wheelchairs and walkers than baby carriages in portions of Europe, there will be fewer family caretakers and income-earning adults to support the aging populace, and people will expect better health than their parents and grandparents (Massachusetts Institute of Technology, 2014).

However, despite the expectation of improved health, the reality will likely be more individuals with chronic disease. With ever-increasing diseases, such as obesity, diabetes, hypertension, and cardiovascular disease, this issue becomes even more significant as low resource countries attempt to deal with increasing numbers of people with these noncommunicable diseases (NCDs), while still struggling with significant communicable disease (Anjana et al., 2011). Although NCDs are the primary cause of morbidity and mortality globally, the rise in outbreaks of infectious disease is another concern. The 2014 Ebola outbreak and the 2016 declaration of Zika as an international public health emergency by the WHO are only two recent examples of how infectious disease can grip the world, create a destructive path, and challenge healthcare systems (Ordway & Sokol, 2016).

Another predicted trend is the potential shortage of healthcare workers, estimated at 18 million by 2030, of which half will be registered nurses (ICN, 2017). In 2006, the WHO issued the *The World Health Report 2006—Working Together for Health* (WHO, 2006), which was devoted to an assessment of the global health workforce in order to offer solutions. The report discussed recruitment, education, pay, resources, worker input, lifelong learning, and technology. The report also discussed the problems of migration of healthcare workers and the importance of balancing choice of individuals to pursue work as needed against the backdrop of healthcare need, putting retention strategies in place, and working with wealthier countries to adopt responsible recruitment. This last issue is a particular responsibility of the United States, United Kingdom, Canada, and Australia, as they are the primary recipients of medical migration workers (Zackowitz, 2014). To assist with this issue, O'Brien and Gostin (2011) recommend the following:

• Address the health worker shortage in the United States
• Develop a plan to address the global health worker shortage
• Provide global leadership in addressing the global health worker shortage
• Reform United States–global health assistance programs in partner countries
• Increase financial assistance for global workforce capacity development
• Increase the number of health workers being trained in the United States
• Empower an appropriate agency to regulate recruiters of foreign-trained health workers (pp. 4–7)

Nichols, Davis, and Richardson (2011), in the the Institute of Medicine's (IOM's) *The Future of Nursing: Leading Change, Advancing Health,* reiterate many of these same points:

• Promote targeted educational investment in foreign-educated nurses in the U.S. nursing force
• Promote baccalaureate education for entry into practice in the United States
• Harmonize nursing curricula
• Add global health as a subject matter to undergraduate and graduate nursing curricula
• Establish a national system that monitors and tracks the inflow of foreign nurses, their countries of origin, the settings in which they work, and their education and licensure
• Create an international body to coordinate and recommend national and international workforce policies

TABLE 6.1 Millennium Development Goals

1. Eradicate extreme poverty and hunger
2. Achieve universal primary education
3. Promote gender equality and empower women
4. Reduce child mortality
5. Improve maternal health
6. Combat HIV/AIDS, malaria, and other diseases
7. Ensure environmental sustainability
8. Develop a global partnership for development

Source: United Nations. (2018). From MDGs to SDGs. Retrieved from http://www.sdgfund.org/mdgs-sdgs

In 2000, world leaders from 189 countries met at the United Nations (2018) and agreed on eight Millennium Development Goals (MDGs), listed in Table 6.1 (United Nations, 2018). The MDGs specified multiple measurable targets aimed at solving the most demanding problems of the time. Significant progress has been made toward goal achievement, particularly poverty reduction, improved access to water, reduction in infectious disease, reduction in disparities of education, and increased participation of women in policy. However, not all goals were fully met. In 2012, the United Nations Conference on Sustainable Development met in Rio de Janeiro to create new goals, sustainable development goals (SDGs). After extensive involvement with stakeholders, the United Nations General Assembly Working Group proposed 17 new goals for global development from 2015 to 2030. These goals are listed in Table 6.2 (United Nations, 2018), and measurable targets can be accessed at www.sdgfund.org/mdgs-sdgs.

Agencies Involved in the Global APRN/APN Experience

The ICN has been guiding global nursing since 1899 with a mission "to represent nursing worldwide, advancing the profession and influencing health policy" (ICN NP/APNN, 2018, para. 1). In 2000, the ICN and the American Association of Nurse Practitioners (AANP; formerly the American Academy of Nurse Practitioners) created the NP/APNN. This network is considered a primary global resource for APRNs/APNs and those interested in advancing the role (AANP, 2018). The organization is composed of a core steering committee and multiple subgroups, monitors global trends in advanced practice, and disseminates information about advanced practice nursing (AANP, 2018). Membership is free and can be accessed at the network website, at www.icn-apnetwork.org.

Other nursing organizations known for supporting nursing around the world are Sigma Theta Tau International (STTI), and the National Organization of Nurse Practitioner Faculties (NONPF). Currently, STTI is working with world health leaders on the Global Advisory Panel on the Future of Nursing (GAPFON), which has been tasked to create a global

TABLE 6.2	Sustainable Development Goals

1. End poverty in all forms everywhere.
2. End hunger, achieve food security and improved nutrition, and promote sustainable agriculture.
3. Ensure healthy lives and promote well-being for all at all ages.
4. Ensure inclusive and equitable quality education and promote lifelong learning opportunities for all.
5. Achieve gender equality and empower all women and girls.
6. Ensure availability and sustainable management of water and sanitation for all.
7. Ensure access to affordable, reliable, sustainable, and modern energy for all.
8. Promote sustained, inclusive, and sustainable economic growth, full and productive employment and decent work for all.
9. Build resilient infrastructure, promote inclusive and sustainable industrialization and foster innovation.
10. Reduce inequality within and among countries.
11. Make cities and human settlements inclusive, safe, resilient, and sustainable.
12. Ensure sustainable consumption and production patterns.
13. Take urgent action to combat climate change and its impacts.
14. Conserve and sustainably use the oceans, seas, and marine resources for sustainable development.
15. Protect, restore, and promote sustainable use of terrestrial ecosystems, sustainably manage forests, combat desertification, and halt reverse land degradation and halt biodiversity loss.
16. Promote peaceful and inclusive societies for sustainable development, provide access to justice for all and build effective, accountable, and inclusive institutions at all levels.
17. Strengthen the means of implementation and revitalize the global partnership for sustainable development.

Source: United Nations. (2018). From MDGs to SDGs. Retrieved from http://www.sdgfund.org/mdgs-sdgs

nursing voice that will improve global health. STTI (2014) has been supportive to APRNs/APNs through grants, support of research initiatives, continuing education, conferences, and numerous publications. AANP and NONPF have assisted APRNs/APNs through leadership on practice, policy, and education. The WHO has also worked on nursing issues such as education, governance, retention, and migration of nurses, but has not been as involved with advanced nursing.

Several organizations have influenced the standards of APRN/APN practice and education in the United States. Although nations choose to self-determine if or how the APRN/APN role develops, many use the same documents. Table 6.3 provides a partial listing of influential documents.

Certification organizations are beginning to examine educational programs and to certify some APRNs/APNs who attend schools outside the United States. Given the variability of roles and education of international APRNs/APNs, there is little migration of APRNs/APNs across borders. Currently, the CGFNS is working on an APRN/APN education comparability tool to address the underlying issues. At some point, the process of accrediting APRN/APN schools outside the United States may become desirable.

TABLE 6.3 Documents With Potential International Influence

American Association of Nurse Practitioners	• Clinical Outcomes: The Yardstick of Educational Effectiveness • Nurse Practitioner Cost-Effectiveness • Nurse Practitioner Curriculum • Quality of Nurse Practitioner Practice • Scope of Practice for Nurse Practitioners • Standards of Practice for Nurse Practitioners
American Association of Colleges of Nursing	• The Essentials of Baccalaureate Education for Professional Nursing Practice (2008) • The Essentials of Doctoral Education for Advanced Nursing Practice (2006) • The Essentials of Master's Education in Nursing (2011)
NONPF	• Multiple examples of competencies for nurse practitioners available on the NONPF website. Intended for entry into practice, the competencies are numerous, population-specific, and separately include those for both master's and doctoral levels.
American College of Nurse-Midwives	• Certified Midwifery and Nurse-Midwifery Education and Certification • Competencies for Master's Level Midwifery Education • Degree Requirements for Midwifery Faculty • Midwifery Education and DNP • The Practice Doctorate in Midwifery
American Association of Nurse Anesthetists	• Scope of Nurse Anesthesia Practice (2013) • Standards of Nurse Anesthesia Practice (2013) • Quality of Care in Anesthesia (2009)
National Association of Clinical Nurse Specialists	• Clinical Nurse Specialist Core Competencies (2010) • Position Statement on the Importance of the CNS Role in Care Coordination (2013) • Revised CNS Core Competencies (2017)

CNS, clinical nurse specialist; DNP, doctor of nursing practice; NONPF, National Organization of Nurse Practitioner Faculties.

Preparing the APRN/APN for Global Experiences

International advanced practice nursing partnerships have become a popular method of exchanging nursing knowledge in that they provide a forum for access to international practice experiences and a forum for research in international healthcare issues. In today's global healthcare environment, APRNs/APNs educated in global health are prepared to network with international multidisciplinary healthcare providers to develop and deliver quality care. These partnerships have included long-term work assignments and medical brigades (previously called "missions") of varied lengths, most with the goal of developing sustainable healthcare access. How this goal is carried out depends on the needs and plans of the supporting partners and may vary by time of year, current needs of the partner, and the political climate.

Aside from international experiences that occur in the United States, many healthcare providers are willing to volunteer on both short- and long-term undertakings outside the United States. World disasters like the 2010 Haiti earthquake that created catastrophic damage have prompted the need for increasing emergency medical relief and continuing sustainable medical work. Nongovernmental organizations (NGOs) have teams that arrive regularly to provide sustainable help for this nation.

Ethics and Responsibilities: Approach to Care

Any international experience should involve the development of appropriate ethical and cultural approaches by those involved in healthcare delivery. Ethical practice involves respectfully approaching those in need, treating them fairly and equitably, and thoughtfully approaching human rights (Hunter & Crabtree, 2010). A culturally competent health system is "one that acknowledges and incorporates—at all levels—the importance of culture, assessment of cross-cultural relations, vigilance towards dynamics that result from cultural differences, expansion of cultural knowledge, and adaptation of services to meet culturally unique needs" (Batancourt, Green, Carrillo, & Owusu, 2003, p. 294). Chase and Hunter (2002) describe "cultural competence" as a skill that can be learned and emphasize that the APRN/APN should be not only culturally competent but culturally responsive, defining that as someone capable of relating in an ethnorelativistic, not ethnocentric, fashion. With an ethnorelativistic approach, the APRN/APN provides care centered on the values and perspectives of the patient and the community. Resources to educate and assess those skills can be obtained through the National Center for Cultural Competence (n.d.), accessible at https://nccc.georgetown.edu. The Center also emphasizes that the APRN/APN be not only culturally competent, but culturally responsive, providing care centered on the values and perspectives of the patient and the community.

A related issue pertains to the ethics and cultural sensitivity surrounding the level of participation in global experiences—short term (1 day to 1 month) versus long term (1 month to 2 years) versus permanent (2 years or more). APRNs/APNs have participated at all levels. The controversy stems from concerns that any effort without proven benefits to the patient or community is not ethical. Although patients who receive corrective lenses, are cured of an infection, or have a completely decayed tooth pulled may value the intervention, some want the measure of value to be based on level of sustainability. Martiniuk, Manouchehrian, Negin, and Zwi (2012) cited that benefits of short- and long-term medical brigades included transferring medical knowledge, helping communities convey their plight, and giving communities hope that problems might be solved. Negatives included problems of sustainability (unless that was specifically countered), limited relations with nearby healthcare systems, and lack of data analysis. The authors recommended the following to optimize global efforts: cross-cultural dialogue and efforts, determined efforts toward efficacy, transparency, and coordination with existing organizational programming. These are clear messages to any APRN/APN considering such work or evaluating a program before joining.

Fulbright Programs

One organization with a long history of providing high-quality opportunities for international experiences for APRNs/APNs is the Fulbright Program (U.S. Department of State [USDS], 2018). The Fulbright Program offers U.S. nursing professionals, educators, and scholars the opportunity to study, teach, and/or conduct research abroad through the Fulbright Scholar Program and the Fulbright Specialist Program. These are competitive programs that are open to most academic disciplines. The Fulbright initiative was spearheaded by Senator William J. Fulbright as a way to promote peace and mutual understanding at the close of World War II. Funding began in 1946, and now its programs are active in more than 155 countries. The Fulbright Scholar Program publishes the grant opportunities each spring with an application deadline of August 1. Many grant applications require a letter of invitation, so it is helpful to review the online catalog early, speak with the Fulbright staff about the grant specifics, and communicate with the host institution about obtaining an invitation letter. The Scholar Program funds travel and a generous living stipend. These grants may be for teaching, research, or a teaching–research combination, and the time commitment (3–12 months) is specified in the grant opportunity. In contrast, the Fulbright Specialist Program offers an opportunity for experienced professionals and academics to collaborate on projects defined by the host institution for 2 to 6 weeks. Travel and in-country costs are covered. However, the Fulbright Specialist Program does not fund activities, such as direct patient care requiring a license. See www.eca.state.gov/fulbright/about-fulbright for more details on the Fulbright programs.

Healthcare Medical Brigades

Emerging healthcare needs, such as Ebola, severe acute respiratory syndrome (SARS), and Middle East respiratory syndrome (MERS) require global partners working together to develop strategies to treat and prevent the spread of these diseases. The term "healthcare" is used to designate an interdisciplinary approach to deliver care internationally. An interdisciplinary team of healthcare individuals is needed to improve overall healthcare. A well-rounded team is composed of physicians, nurses, APRNs/APNs, dentists, health educators, nutritionists, social workers, pharmacists, physical therapists, occupational therapists, counselors, and students from all disciplines.

Countries such as the United States, Canada, Switzerland, Germany, England, and Australia have large numbers of NGOs and universities that send out healthcare teams regularly for the purposes of providing direct patient care, supervised experiences for students, and opportunities to network on research and education. Table 6.4 lists volunteer international healthcare websites and information to assist in planning a medical brigade.

Pretravel Preparations

Pretravel preparation should begin at least a year in advance. In preparing for a trip, the team leader should review online information about the host country/sponsor, especially data related to finances and bringing medications and supplies. If the brigade is outside the United States, the State Department warnings specific to the country should be reviewed. Networking and developing a relationship with the host country/sponsor may require an initial visit to determine the needs. Issues such as requirements of the host country/sponsor for current provider licenses, medications, and supplies that are approved by the country/sponsor should be determined early in the pretravel period. Transportation and lodging will also need to be worked out with the host. One country (Burundi) requires visa applications be submitted with a letter of invitation from the people with whom the volunteer is staying or documentation of hotel reservations.

There are a variety of ways team members may fund their trip expenses. Some pay the total amount out of pocket. Others will rely on fund-raisers to support all or part of the team's expenses. Some organizations do a one-third method, when the individual pays a third, the organization pays a third, and the last third is from donations or fund-raiser activities (Samaritans Now, 2014).

Funding needs to be discussed at one of the early team meetings—finances can become a source of friction in the group. Airline tickets are the most costly budget item. Some airline companies will provide group rates and allow extra baggage for free. Some airlines request contact at least 60 days in advance of travel.

Team members frequently ask how much cash they should bring. In many cases, it depends on the economy of the host country. For example, costs in Thailand are higher than those in Guatemala. The exchange rates are also higher for larger bills. Many governments require crisp new bills for exchange.

Many countries (e.g., Ecuador, Guatemala) require preapproval for medications, and the expiration date on medications must be at least 6 months into the future. The preapproval requires listing expiration dates, names of the pharmaceutical companies that produced the medications, and quantities of the medications. All documents must be notarized. Table 6.5 lists pharmaceutical organizations that will provide medications to healthcare teams. Table 6.6 provides recommended medications for International Medical Brigades. Some organizations require a physician's signature. If ordering medications outside the United States (e.g., from Action Medeor in Germany), U.S. Customs and Border Protection will need to be contacted for a list of brokerage firms that will support bringing

TABLE 6.4 Volunteer International Websites/Information to Assist in Planning

U.S. State Department Travel Warnings and Consular Information Sheets—provides country-by-country information relevant to health, safety, visa, and entry requirements (travelers may be unable to board planes if they do not have the necessary visa), medical facilities, consular contact information, drug penalties, etc.; www.travel.state.gov/content/passports/en/country.html

Central Intelligence Agency (CIA) Publications and Factbooks—includes among its sections World Factbook (provides a wealth of information on virtually all countries), *Handbook of International Economic Statistics*, CIA Maps and Publications released to the public. www.cia.gov/cia/publications; www.cia.gov/redirects/ciaredirect.html

Center for Disease Control (CDC)—provides information for foreign travel and recommended immunizations. www.cdc.gov

Ford Foundation—is one of the largest U.S. foundations active in national and international health. www.fordfound.org

Hesperian Foundation—publishes low-cost, practical books for use in all aspects of international health practice at the community level. www.hesperian.org

Library of Congress Country Studies—provides detailed information on many of the countries of the world prepared by the Federal Research Division of the Library of Congress. The site has an impressive search engine that can search across the database for any combination of words, ranks the hits in order of closeness to your search terms, and then provides links to the desired text. www.lcweb2.loc.gov/frd/cs/cshome.html#toc, www.loc.gov/collections/country-studies/about-this-collection/#toc

Teaching Aids at Low Cost—lists and distributes many health-related teaching aids that are provided in low-cost format and often in multiple languages for use by healthcare providers and patients in developing countries. www.talcuk.org or healthbooksinternational.org/

World Health Organization—www.who.int/topics/travel/en/

American Council for Voluntary International Action—is a consortium of more than 150 nonprofit organizations working worldwide in health, educational development, and other related fields. It is a source of jobs and volunteer resources. The site includes hotlinks to all of its members. www.interaction.org

Doctors Without Borders USA—is the French-originated organization (Medecins Sans Frontieres) that sends fully qualified health professionals into some of the most challenging parts of the world. Because they do not have job descriptions contracted for nurse practitioners, nurse practitioners function in the role of nurses. www.msf.org

FUNEDESIN—is a clinical rotation program that provides clinical experiences in the Amazon region of Ecuador. It is open to all levels of students and health professionals in the fields of medicine and nursing. Further information can be found on the website. (www.orgs.tigweb.org/funedesin-foundation-for-integrated-education-and-development). The application pack can be requested by emailing clinic@funedesin.org.

Global Health: Making Contacts—contains a gold mine of international health resources and projects, including job opportunities. It provides links with a long list of governmental and nongovernmental agencies and organizations, people, academic institutions, and organizational directories relevant to health. The sections are conveniently grouped according to major mission, affiliation, type, etc.; www.globalhealth.pitt.edu

(continued)

TABLE 6.4	Volunteer International Websites/Information to Assist in Planning *(continued)*

Global Service Corps—provides short- and long-term opportunities to volunteer in health, education, and environment projects in Kenya, Costa Rica, and Thailand. www.globalservicecorps.org

IFESH—provides assistance and opportunities for service much in the fashion of the U.S. Peace Corps. The primary focus is sub-Saharan Africa. Through its IFP, the Foundation has provided 9-month overseas internships for Americans who are graduate students or recent college and university graduates. Fellows are placed with development-focused organizations working overseas. www.payson.tulane.edu/funding-agent/international-foundation-education-and-self-help-ifesh

International Healthcare Opportunities Clearinghouse—provides listings of organizations with Internet links of online resources, courses, and books on international health, as well as information about how to get funding. It has a search engine that can locate organizations according to diverse search criteria and provides links to home pages of organizations where available. www.library.umassmed.edu/ihoc/

IHMEC—provides information about courses, curricula, annotated websites, foreign language study courses, and other materials useful for faculty and students interested in international health. Go to the Resources section of the IHMEC home page. www.globalhealtheducation.org

IMC—is a private, nonsectarian, nonpolitical, humanitarian relief organization established in 1984 by volunteer U.S. physicians and nurses. The home page lists IMC's programs and job openings for doctors, nurses, and other health professionals. www.internationalmedicalcorps.org

MPA International—is a nonprofit Christian relief and development organization, promoting the total health of people living in the world's poorest communities. www.map.org

Medical Missions Foundations—has multiple opportunities for providing surgical and medical care in underserved communities. www.medicalmissionsfoundation.org/

Direct Relief—has many opportunities in the United States and abroad to improve health and lives of people affected by poverty and emergencies. www.directrelief.org

Humanitarian Medical Relief—has more than 60 possibilities for volunteer service and includes a link to Flights for Humanity, a nonprofit Christian organization that flies patients to medical centers for treatment. www.humanitarianmedical.org (in Spanish)

International Health Database Under the American Medical Association—has numerous opportunities. www.ama-assn.org//ama/pub/about-ama/our-people/member-groups-sections/medical-student-section/opportunities/internation-health-opportunities.page

Volunteer Humanitarian Opportunities—has numerous project opportunities for volunteer service. They send more than 10,000 people abroad each year. www.projects-abroad.org

Heal the Nations Christian Medical Missions—focuses on India and Uganda to work with children and families improve their health. www.healthenations.com/

American Medical Resources Foundation—donates used, but fully functional, medical equipment to hospitals serving the poor worldwide. www.amrf.com

HIM—is a nonprofit, nondenominational agency that focuses on the needs of less fortunate children and families. They have served in Guatemala for 35 years. Each trip runs about 10 days and costs about $1,000 for airfare and lodging. www.heartsinmotion.org/index.php

(continued)

| TABLE 6.4 | Volunteer International Websites/Information to Assist in Planning *(continued)* |

International Volunteer Work in India–Delhi—as Mark Twain recounted in *Following the Equator,* India is "the land of dreams and romance, of splendor and rags, of palaces and hovels, the country of a hundred nations and a hundred tongues." www.crossculturalsolutions.org

Monitoring Freedom—Human Rights Around the World—includes expatriate resources and resources for Americans fleeing America. Allows users to search the largest expatriate database of embassies, international jobs, and offshore financial services websites. www.escapeartist.com/jobs/overseas1.htm

International Grants and Funders—provides international grants and funders. www.grantspace .org

Global Volunteer Network—is a resource for those interested in volunteering. www. globalvolunteers.org/

Doctors of the World, USA: Volunteer/Recruitment—offers a wide array of opportunities for health professionals to contribute to ongoing efforts to alleviate suffering and help improve human rights around the world. www.doctorsoftheworld.org/

Healing Touch International: Clinics—is a listing of Healing Touch Clinics that are open to the public. Some clinics are by appointment only, and payment is by donation. Clinic choice can be made on the website. www.healingtouch.net/hti.html https://www.youtube.com/watch?v=ViViitW2f5w

The Medical Foundation, About Us—History—discusses the work of the Medical Foundation for the Care of Victims of Torture, which began more than 25 years ago under the auspices of the Medical Group of Amnesty International. www.freedomfromtorture.org

Mercy & Truth Medical Missions—desires to serve the public, as much as possible. Mercy & Truth Medical Missions is a fee-for-service clinic. www.mercyandtruth.com

Global Health Outreach—organizes short-term medical group missions. Christian Medical & Dental Association, under Medical Missions tab. www.cmda.org/missions/detail/global-health-outreach

Medical Education International—medical education teams with Christian Medical & Dental Association, under Medical Missions tab. www.cmda.org/missions/detail/mei

Northwest Medical Teams International—Their organization's focus is bringing healing to people in crisis. www.medicalteams.org/

Heal the Nations—provides Christian Medical Missions links, a list of volunteer healthcare organizations, both Christian and secular. www.healthenations.com/links.html

USAID—provides economic and humanitarian assistance. www.usaid.gov

Christian Connections for International Health—promotes international health. Has a job search section. www.ccih.org

"Nuestra Senora de Guadalupe"—based in Ecuador, organizes short-term medical missions into the remote areas of the Amazon basin. The Mission at Guadalupe also has a clinic that is looking for providers for longer terms. www.guadalupe-ec.org

(continued)

TABLE 6.4	Volunteer International Websites/Information to Assist in Planning *(continued)*

American Baptist Churches in the U.S.A International Ministries (ABC)—goals are theological education, evangelism, economic development, education, and health. www.internationalministries. org

International Medical Volunteer Association—provides information about volunteering and links to various international organizations. www.imva.org

Doctors for Global Health—a private, not-for-profit organization promoting health, education, art, and other human rights throughout the world. www.dghonline.org

University of Washington—provides information on overseas medical opportunities. www.globalhealth.washington.edu

University of Kentucky—offers weeklong medical brigades four times yearly at permanent UK clinic in Santo Domingo, Ecuador. www.uky.edu/international/shoulder_to_shoulder

American Medical Student Association—strives to extend the scope of members' medical education through institutes, international exchanges and career development opportunities. www. amsa.org/

MAP/Reader's Digest International Fellowships—a global Christian health organization that partners with people living in conditions of poverty to save lives and develop healthier families and communities. www.map.org

Save the Children—focuses on outreach efforts related to maternal, newborn, and child health. www.everybeatmatters.org

ABC, American Baptist Churches; CDC, Centers for Disease Control and Prevention; CIA, Central Intelligence Agency; FUNEDESIN, Foundation of Integrated Education and Development; HIM, Hearts in Motion; IFESH, International Foundation for Education and Self-Help; IFP, International Fellows Program; IHMEC, International Health Medical Education Consortium; IMC, International Medical Corps; USAID, United States Agency for International Development.

the medications into the United States for transport to the host country. Some companies allow APRNs/APNs to purchase low-cost medications, and others require a physician or pharmacist to do the purchasing. This requirement is based on state regulation of the involved APRNs/APNs. Another source to review is www.who.int/medicines/areas/access/sources_prices/international_medicine_price_guidesprice_lists.pdf.

Some university pharmacy departments compound medications for interdisciplinary faculty/student medical brigades or assist in purchasing and packaging of medications. Some hospitals donate at cost medications and supplies. Some pharmaceutical companies will donate over-the-counter medications. Good sources of over-the-counter medications are APRN/APN conferences. At the end of the healthcare conference, companies are willing to donate their remaining products. Table 6.7 provides a list of recommended medications for a trip. Occasionally, there is a request from the host administrator for a specific medication—for example, something to treat hyperthyroidism.

TABLE 6.5 Medical Brigade Pharmaceutical Resources

Agency	Website	Phone or Email/ Contact Person	Application	Pharmaceutical Supplier	Comments
Cross Link International	www.idealist.org/en/nonprofi t/8f628780a11a4fcc8d7910a460 fc4fce-crosslink-international- falls-church?	(703) 534-5465	www.crosslinkinternational.net/ App.shtml		Receiving agency must be a Christian faith–based organization.
Brother's Brother Foundation	www.brothersbrother.org	(412) 321-3160 Mail.@ brothersbrother.org		Yes, and small trays of basic surgical instruments	Most medications are good for 4–6 months. No cost for medications and shipment in the United States.
Catholic Medical Mission Board	www.cmmb.org/programs/ medical-donations/	ktebbett@cmmb.org	www.cmmb.org/pdfs/ HealingHelpMedicalMissionsApp. pdf		Requires submission of an online application.
MAP	www.map.org/medicines	(800) 225-8550	www.map.org/site/DocServer/ MAP_Travel_Pack_Program-		Requires submission of an online application.
Kingsway Charities	www.kingswaycharities.org	(800) 321-9234			Receiving organization must be Christian faith–based.

Organization	Website	Contact	Application	Medications/Supplies	Notes
Vitamin Angels	www.vitaminangels.org	(805) 564-8400			Not for short-term medical teams.
Globus Relief	www.globusrelief.org	(801) 977-0444		Yes, and medical equipment	They try to make pharmaceuticals below cost.
medWish International	www.medwish.org	(216) 692-1685 or info@medwish.org	www.medwish.org/handcarryinfo-app.html	No, only medical supplies	
Project Cure	www.projectcure.org/get-assistance	(303) 792-0729	www.projectcure.org/get-assistance/medical-kits#application	Yes	Most medications provided will have only 3 months remaining on their dating.
FAME	www.fameworld.org	(317) 358-2480 or medicalmissions@FAMEworld.org			Must be a faith-based organization.
International Aid	www.internationalaid.org	healthproduct@internationalaid.org (800) 968-7490		Yes, and lab-in-a-suitcase (www.internat-ionalaid.org/Lab-In-A-Suitcase_files/LIS%20Brochure%20New.pdf)	Need to complete online application.

(continued)

TABLE 6.5 Medical Brigade Pharmaceutical Resources *(continued)*

Agency	Website	Phone or Email/ Contact Person	Application	Pharmaceutical Supplier	Comments
Action Medeor	www.medeor.org	+49 2156 9788-0 or info@medeor.de	info@medeor.de	Yes	Product catalogue: www.medeor.de/en/medeor-market-en/price-indicator.html
World Medical Relief	www.worldmedicalrelief.org/	info@ worldmedicalrelief.org, (313) 866-5333	www.worldmedicalrelief.org	Yes	Accommodates medical brigade teams with pharmaceuticals. Medications do not usually have a year before expiring but such medications can be purchased at lower cost. Need to fill out an online application.
Americares	www.americares.org/ whatwedo/mop/	cmarion@americares. org, (203) 658-9500	www.americares.org/whatwedo/ mop/mopapplication.pdf	Yes	Most medications are short-dated (3–6 months out), but they do have a few longer-dated medications. Suggest a $200 donation.

Blessings International	www.blessing.org	(918) 250-8101; Fax (918) 250-1281	www.blessing.org/wp-content/uploads/2012/09/Blessings-Instructions.pdf	Yes	First-time users must fax a copy of their check for the estimated amount of the order with their application form.
Direct Relief International	www.directrelief.org	(805) 964-4767	www.directrelief.org/wp-content/uploads/VolunteerApplication2013.pdf	Has medication and supplies for volunteers on disaster relief.	Participates in disaster relief worldwide.
Heart-to-Heart International	www.hearttoheart.org	(913) 764-5200	www.hearttoheartinternational.wufoo.com/forms/heart-to-heart-international/	Yes	Physicians, optometrists, dentists, podiatrists, and pharmacists can apply for a standard Ready Relief pack of medications or a custom order.

(continued)

TABLE 6.5 Medical Brigade Pharmaceutical Resources *(continued)*

Agency	Website	Phone or Email/ Contact Person	Application	Pharmaceutical Supplier	Comments
Interchurch Medical Assistance WorldHealth	www.imaworldhealth.org/	(877) 241-7952 or (410) 635-8720	imainfo@imaworldhealth.org	They have medicines and supplies for their own projects. They run their own programs in Haiti, South Sudan, Dominican Republic, Congo, Tanzania, and Indonesia.	They deliver prepacked medicine and supply boxes to treat up to 1,000 patients.
Project HOPE	www.projecthope.org	(800) 544-HOPE	Application to be a volunteer for Project HOPE can be found at www.projecthope.csod.com/ats/careersite/JobDetails.aspx?id=35	They have medication and supplies for their own country.	Project HOPE has worked in more than 120 countries.

Source: Developed by Colleen Strand; modified by Lorna Schumann; reproduced with permission.

TABLE 6.6   Recommended Medications for International Medical Brigades

Analgesics, antipyretics, NSAIDs	Anti-inflammatory drugs
Anesthetics	Antimalarial drugs
Antiallergics	Cardiovascular drugs
Antiamoebic drugs	Dermatologic preparations, disinfectants
Antiasthmatic drugs, antitussives	Diuretics
Antibacterials, antifungals, antiviral drugs	Gastrointestinal drugs
Antidiabetics	Laxatives
Antidiarrheal drugs	Ophthalmologic preparations
Antiepileptics	Psychotherapeutic agents
Antihelminthics, antifilarial drugs	Vitamins and food supplements

NSAIDs, nonsteroidal anti-inflammatory drugs.

Team Meetings

Team meetings are essential to building a strong cohesive team. The meetings should include discussion of cultural traditions and behaviors; boundary setting; cultural differences and cultural sensitivity; and issues of dealing with extreme poverty, serious illnesses, abuse, and starvation. Illicit drug use and drunkenness are not acceptable behaviors on a medical brigade trip. Other issues to address are flights and lodging, itinerary, work schedules, local regional health issues, and practical tips for the trip. See Tables 6.6 to 6.12 for trip preparation materials.

The team should plan at least one or two tourist activities, such as sightseeing to the Taj Mahal and the Red Fort in the Delhi area. Shopping is also a fun experience for most team members, so selecting a hotel close to a shopping area is recommended.

Setting Up a Medical Camp

The host country/sponsor organization selects the sites for the camps and arranges the overall setup. For example, when working in the slum areas of New Delhi, the host rents tents that can be used in areas for slums that do not have school buildings. In some countries, established clinics, schools, or churches/temples can be used for the camp. Occasionally, setup may be under a tree or out in the open.

Setup needs to include a patient check-in station (a triage nurse and interpreter) as the gatekeeper area for the flow of patients. Table 6.13 provides a list of common diseases seen in Central and South America.

TABLE 6.7 Short-Term Healthcare Mission Team Leader Responsibilities

1. Begin planning the trip a year in advance. Decide on the type of project, dates, and location. Work with host country/sponsor team members to plan the medical brigade and determine the needs of the people.
2. Solicit application for team members and select a team. Interview and select team members about 6 months or earlier in advance so that they can request time off work.
3. Develop a budget that includes air flights, all transportation, housing, and food. Share the information with the team. Develop a plan for financing the trip.
4. Set up a schedule for team meetings and post-trip debriefing. The first meeting should cover issues such as waivers, trip insurance, cultural sensitivity, appropriate behaviors for the trip, what to do in case of illness, how to obtain passports (if needed), how to obtain visas (if needed), needed immunizations, the approximate cost of the trip, and any issues the team members may have.
5. The team leader is responsible for coordinating medications and supplies to be taken on the trip. Each team member should pack the medications and supplies he or she is taking and make a list to give to the team leader. The number of bags allowed and the weight of the bags are determined by individual airlines. Some airlines allow only one checked bag free; others will allow up to three. Other luggage will need to be paid for, usually $25 to $75 per bag. A third bag may cost as much as $200. Most airlines are willing to work with medical teams to take three bags for free.
6. The team leader and host country/sponsor leader are responsible for the daily activities and debriefing activities. Should a team problem occur, the team leader and host country/sponsor leader should work together to resolve the issue.
7. Plan an in-country post-trip debriefing meeting to discuss issues that occurred on the trip. This meeting may need to take place on the last evening the team is together—some teams are composed of team members from other countries.

A similar analysis can be made for any region or country in order to prepare, appropriately.

Many organizations have developed forms for recording patient identification information, vital signs, allergies, current medications, significant medical history, and a list of problems the patient wants treated. Teams will need to consider limiting the number of problems they can deal with per patient, because there are often many people waiting to be seen. Occasionally, providers are faced with unknown diagnoses.

Although individuals usually queue up on the basis of first come, first serve, or the sickest first, there is often crowding and claiming rank and status. On a medical mission in a Delhi slum, a Mercedes pulled up, and an elegantly dressed woman went to the front of the line. No one seemed to be bothered by this, except the team members.

Referrals/Transfer to the Hospital

Before opening the clinic, organizers need to check with hosts about referrals and transferring patients to the hospital. In some countries, individuals refuse to go to the hospital because of bad care and high mortality rates, where one-third of patients admitted die. These individuals may also

TABLE 6.8	Recommendations of What to Take for Medical Brigades to Developing Countries
Lightweight (silk, cotton) sleeping bag for warm climates—spray with N,N-diethyl-meta-toluamide (DEET; insect repellent) and put in zip lock bag for penetration of the DEET into the material Miranda@nznature.co.nz ($2 NZ = $1 US)	Learn to adapt and do without for a short time—think: patience, perseverance, and stamina
Aluminum foil blanket for warmth, if needed	Clothespins and roll of heavy string or lightweight rope
Mosquito net and repellent containing DEET (not in pressurized spray can)—recommend spraying suitcase and clothing with DEET before travel	Duct tape, colored (can help visualize bags or brigade team items)
Citron wrist/ankle band to ward off mosquitos (effective for 400 hours)	Otoscope/ophthalmoscope (battery powered for places where there is no electricity) A ready-to-go bag that has stethoscope, blood pressure cuff, otoscope, ophthalmoscope, pens, urine dip sticks, scissors, duct tape, O_2 saturation monitor (inexpensive from www.Amazon.com), Doppler (relatively inexpensive from www.Amazon.com), reliable thermometer, etc.
Sunscreen	Flashlight or headlight (frees hands to fight off the elements), backpack (one that will carry water bottles)
Toiletries (inexpensive shampoo or conditioners, if expensive products are brought Customs may inspect and keep)	Belly pack—keep passport (in a ziplock bag) and money in your pack
Camera, extra camera batteries if battery dependent	Passport must be in a safe place at all times!!!
Towel, washcloth, and soap; hand wipes	Hat and lightweight rain poncho
Toilet paper, one roll—others may be purchased in country	Lightweight clothing that dries fast or scrubs—works well for seeing patients. What is worn depends on the culture. In India, females on the team wear the traditional dress of shalwar, kameez, and dupatta. Avoid wearing shorts and tank tops.
Nutritious snacks	Tennis shoes, closed toe shoes, or boots with socks—recommended to protect from insect bites
Chocolate that will not melt	Colored photocopy of passport to give to the team leader
Flip-flops or Chacos for the shower	Lightweight long-sleeve and long-leg pajamas with tight cuffs— keep the mosquitoes and other insects off the skin

(continued)

TABLE 6.8 Recommendations of What to Take for Medical Brigades to Developing Countries *(continued)*

Language dictionary and medical language dictionary	Leatherman or other knife in *checked bag*
Gifts for people who help and children (stickers, blow-bubbles, inexpensive toys—chosen according to age and safety)	Country-specific electrical adapter plugs and voltage converters, if needed. For information: www.rei.com/learn/expert-advice/world-electricity-guide.html
Water bottle—bottled water usually can be bought in country	Extra batteries of standard sizes—in-country batteries may not be reliable
Locks for suitcase—not for use on flight, to use when working or away from them for the day	Personal medicines
Imodium AD	NSAID of choice (carry on the plane)—helps with jet-lag and high altitudes.
Ciprofloxacin (enough for 3 days), for diarrhea, or use when starting to run a fever—is not effective in all countries	
Azithromycin 500 mg daily for 3 days is the treatment of choice for South East Asia and India	

NSAID, nonsteroidal anti-inflammatory drug.

TABLE 6.9 Pretravel Safety Precautions

Review online travel recommendations:
- From the host country's embassy and other reliable resources
- Immunizations and medications (available at www.cdc.gov)
- Review State Department travel warnings (available at www.travel.state.gov/travel).

Review WHO website for information on travel.
- Notify the State Department of trip purpose/travel itinerary (www.travel.state.gov or 888-407-4748)
- Collect team member licenses and colored copies of team member's signed passports/visas
- Prepare a team emergency kit
- Set up two or three team meetings; a conference call may be helpful using www.freeconferencecall.com

WHO, World Health Organization.

become angry that the team is unable to resolve their problems. The host country/sponsor administrator is the best person to deal with these issues.

Home Visits

Team members may be asked to do a home visit on an individual who cannot come to the clinic or who is dying. For safety, it is best that several

TABLE 6.10	Travel Preparations	
Documents	Passport	Application is available at www.travel.state.gov/passport Cost: $140 (adult first-time passport book and card) + $25 execution fee. Expedited services are an additional $60. Should not expire within 6 months after return to United States.
	Visa(s)	May be required by individual country; check www.travel.state.gov/visa/ to determine visa requirements. Cost: Varies, but often around $150 to $200, when added to cost of FedEx, new photos, and the visa itself.
	Immunization record	Some countries require verification of specific immunizations (especially yellow fever) to enter the country. Immunizations can be expensive for first-time trip members. The receiving country may require a photocopy of the yellow fever immunization when applying for a visa. Information is available at www.nc.cdc.gov/travel/default.aspx.
Travel arrangements	Flights	Flights can be arranged online, but commonly used travel sites (e.g., Travelocity, Cheap Flights, Expedia) are often unable to book international travel to more remote settings. Help may be obtained from a travel agent or the airline. Consider choosing airlines that add frequent flyer miles based on connecting flights with partner airlines. An example is Delta/KLM/Kenya airlines to Nairobi. An excellent site for host country maps is www.WHO.int/maps.
	Lodging	Hotels or other lodging facilities may not accept credit cards; other hotels may not accept *all* credit cards. If going to a malaria-endemic country, a bed net or net sleeping bag and mosquito repellant may be recommended. Recommendations of prophylactic medications can be reviewed at www.cdc.gov/travel. If air-conditioning is available, sleeping quarters need to be kept as cold as possible.
	Food/water	Familiarity of types of food that will be available is helpful; if food security is a potential problem, bringing protein bars, trail mix, and water purification tablets may be necessary. A quality water filter is the Pre-Mac travel well "Trekker" (www.shop.eri-online.com).
Healthcare	Medications	The Yellow Book 2014 from the CDC (www.cdc.gov/features/yellowbook/index.html) is a comprehensive resource for health risks and recommendations for every country, including medications. The Yellow Book is also available for Android and iOS mobile devices. The iTunes store has a Yellow Book app for iPads and iPhones. In-country medications, if available, may not be correctly formulated or may be contaminated. They may also be expensive. One Zofran ODT is $5 in Ecuador.

(continued)

TABLE 6.10 Travel Preparations *(continued)*

		When possible, enough medication (regularly taken medications and any prophylactic medications) to last the entire trip should be brought; some countries may require copies of prescribed medications, especially controlled substances; consider over-the-counter medications for pain, fever, nausea/vomiting, diarrhea, constipation, cuts/scrapes, and insect bites. The team leader should obtain an emergency kit.
	Bed nets	These provide protection in malaria-endemic countries.
	Insurance coverage	Health insurance out-of-network coverage needs to be checked; evacuation insurance (e.g., www.travelinsurancereview.net/plans/evacuation/) needs to be considered. Medicare/Medicaid does not provide coverage outside the United States.
Communication	Itinerary	All participants should carry a paper copy of the itinerary. An additional copy of the travel itinerary (flight, hotel, ground transportation) should be left with someone at home. Flight departures should be confirmed the day before traveling back to the United States.
	In-country contacts	The names and numbers of in-country contacts should be left with someone at home; include country codes as part of the phone number.
	Cell phones	Cell phone and data access can be expensive when used internationally; coverage and charges should be checked before departure to avoid huge bills on return; purchase of an in-country cell phone is another option, with a SIM card to which more airtime can be added, as needed. Downloading WhatsApp to a smartphone for free text messaging when WiFi is available may be useful. Phone providers should be notified of travel outside the United States and may need details of the trip itinerary. Most cell phone plans contain an international plan that can be added to your phone. Verizon charges $10.00 per day, but there are data limits.
Money	ATM cards	Money exchange should be done before leaving the country, if possible. Banks can help with this process. ATM machines are becoming more available in low resource countries, but it cannot be assumed one will be available in all locations; PIN number should be four numbers (many foreign ATM machines do not have letters, just numbers). Use of debit cards can be a problem; it is often safer to use credit cards. Your credit card company may recommend that you do not ask for a receipt from the machine. The card provider needs to be contacted before leaving; otherwise, the card may be terminated or useless. Special debit cards can be purchased for travel (e.g., Contour card). These can be thrown away when the balance is gone. Use outside the United States needs to be verified.

(continued)

TABLE 6.10	Travel Preparations *(continued)*
Traveler's cheques	Although fairly obsolete in many developed countries, traveler's cheques may still be used in some countries
Credit cards	In low resource countries, many businesses (hotels, restaurants, shops) do not accept credit cards. If intending to use credit cards, the credit card company will need to be notified of travel plans prior to the trip.
Cash	All participants need to bring a certain amount of cash, exchanged as described earlier. In addition to personal expenses, there are always opportunities to help others (e.g., obtaining an oxygen tank for a young adult with tetralogy of Fallot). A working understanding of local currency is important to avoid overpaying or underpaying or being short-changed; there are smartphone apps that will help clarify currency exchanges. Cash should be carried in a money belt or belly pack. Some countries (e.g., Thailand) have a better exchange rate for larger bills.

CDC, Centers for Disease Control and Prevention.

members of the team accompany the interpreter. Culturally, this is often a very positive experience for the team members because they have the opportunity to experience what the individual deals with on a daily basis. Wound care may require daily visits.

Team Member Injuries/Serious Illnesses

Typically, most team member illnesses can be treated by the team. However, if a team member is seriously injured, evacuation may be required. Evacuation may also be required for serious illnesses. Contact information for the in-country U.S. embassy can be obtained at www.travel.state.gov. The emergency number for the U.S. embassy is (888) 403-4747. Trip insurance is highly recommended because evacuation can cost more than $50,000 and in-country treatment can also be very expensive. Most U.S. medical insurances and Medicare/Medicaid do not provide coverage outside the United States. Trip health insurance information can be obtained at www.travel.state.gov/travel/tips/brouchures/brochures_1215.html.

The online brochure from the Smart Traveler Enrollment Program (STEP) contains excellent information on safety and preparedness. The link is www.travel.state.gov/tips_1232.html.

In-Country Debriefing

Ideally, debriefing should occur each evening in an informal setting. Discussion includes listing what activities went well and what activities

TABLE 6.11   Packing Suggestions

Checked luggage	Airline luggage limits need to be reviewed. Frequent flyer programs may allow three free bags for Elite members.
	Unnecessary personal items (e.g., expensive jewelry/equipment) need to be left at home. Personal medical equipment without batteries may be checked. Expensive personal or other medical equipment with batteries will need to be in carry-on bags. Do not take items that you cannot afford to lose.
	Pack:
	Water filter, if bottled water will not be available (www.eri-online.com/ERI_ Equipment.html)
	Clothing appropriate for the weather and culture
	N,N-diethyl-meta-toluamide (DEET; insect repellent)
	Itemized list of medications and supplies
	Gifts for hosts and children
	Towel and washcloth for remote areas (Wash clothes are rare in many countries.)
Carry-on luggage	Lightly packed, there may be limits of 10 kg.
	Include:
	Extra change of clothes (in case luggage gets lost or delayed)
	Toiletries
	Travel documents
	Personal medications and medical equipment
	Belly pack
	Cell phone

TABLE 6.12   Airline, Hotel, and Transportation Safety

Airline safety	If there are unusual items being transported, the airline needs to be checked with in advance.
	Unruly passengers need to be avoided.
	Passport *must* be carried on the body.
Hotel safety	Rooms between the second and sixth floors are recommended.
	Hotel business card should be carried in a wallet/belly pack, with the wallet in a front pocket.
	The hotel escape plan should be reviewed.
	Clothes, wallet, and shoes should be kept in the same place for emergency exiting.
	Participants should be observant and avoid crowds.
	Room safes are *not* safe.
Transportation safety	Gasoline shortages are not uncommon in resource-poor settings; it is important to verify that your transport has enough gasoline to complete journeys.
	Some modes of transportation are relatively unsafe (e.g., minibuses). In some countries (e.g., Guatemala), public buses are not safe.
	Some cities have very high rates of traffic accidents, particularly after dark.

TABLE 6.13 Common Diseases/Disorders Exemplar—Central and South America

Burns/trauma/work injuries Shoulder, neck, back, and leg pain	**Eye** Conjunctivitis Cataracts Glaucoma Blindness Pterygium Pinguecula Styes
Cardiac Hypertension (severe)	**Fungal infections** Vaginal: vulvar candidiasis Feet Oral Skin Tinea versicolor
ENT Cerumen impaction Otitis media Otitis externa	**Gastrointestinal conditions** Parasites: pinworms, amoebas, *Giardia* Gastritis Gastroesophageal Reflux Peptic ulcers Diarrhea/constipation
Endocrine Type 2 diabetes Hypothyroidism	**Genitourinary** Urinary tract infections Benign prostatic hyperplasia Prostatitis Bacterial vaginosis Irregular menstrual cycles Pregnancy Chloasma
Musculoskeletal problems Arthritis: osteoarthritis and rheumatoid Post-trauma pain Back pain Myalgias	**Other infectious diseases/mosquito-borne diseases** Sexually transmitted infections Dengue fever Malaria Chikungunya (Africa/India/Caribbean)
Neuropsychologic conditions Depression Headaches Seizures Peripheral neuropathy	**Respiratory diseases** Colds Chronic cough Bronchitis Asthma Pneumonia Environmental allergies

(continued)

TABLE 6.13 Common Diseases/Disorders Exemplar— Central and South America *(continued)*

Nutritional disorders	Skin
Malnutrition	Rashes
Dehydration	Scabies
Anemia	Infections
Hyperhidrosis resulting from lack of B vitamins	
Burning feet	

ENT, ear, nose, throat.

need improvement. As problems arise, it is best to deal with them immediately. Should team conflicts occur, the team leader and the host deal with the issues.

A list of needed medicines/supplies that are to be purchased while in the country should be compiled and then shared with the host to facilitate purchase at a discount. Medication purchases may be required daily. A running list of recommendations for the next trip is another task for the team leader.

Post-Trip Debriefing

Team members need to be given the opportunity to process life-changing experiences, air feelings and reactions, and discuss what worked and what needs to be changed for the future medical brigades. The team leader may need to talk to individuals who had traumatic experiences in caring for patients. Team members may need to receive parasite medications. View Table 6.14 for recommendations on parasite treatments.

ROLE OF THE APRN/APN IN GLOBAL RESEARCH

From a global perspective, the role of the APRN/APN researcher is dynamic and vital to informing and articulating the APRN/APN role, shedding light on the healthcare needs of disadvantaged populations internationally, and establishing a body of evidence of advanced practice nursing knowledge. The scope and perspectives of APRN/APN research are broad and may encompass epistemology; ethnography; role definition, justification, and expansion; exploration of the notion of competence and role-specific competencies; scope of practice and role potential; and disease- and intervention-specific research within APRN/APN roles from an evidence-based practice perspective.

This research reflects both the practice perspectives of the involved APRNs/APNs and the national and international healthcare environments and jurisdictions in which APRNs/APNs work. This research is not confined to APRNs/APNs themselves, though the APRN/APN role may be the subject of much of the international research. For example, taking an international perspective and supported by the WHO, Lassi, Cometto, Huicho, and Bhutta (2013) published a systematic review and

TABLE 6.14 Parasitic Treatments

Parasite	Treatment (Not Recommended During Pregnancy or Lactation)
Worm (roundworm, hookworm, pinworm, whipworm, etc.) Common local beliefs about symptoms: excess salivation, itchy nose/throat, grinding teeth, craves sweets Roundworm: asymptomatic, but while in lungs produces a nonproductive cough Hookworm: mainly asymptomatic, but early manifestations may be epigastric pain or diarrhea, chronic iron-deficiency anemia Whipworm: chronic abdominal pain, anorexia, bloody or mucoid diarrhea, rectal prolapse Pinworm: chronic anal itching (worse at night), rarely abdominal discomfort, weight loss	**Adults and children 2 years and up:** Mebendazole 100 mg twice daily × 3 days or Albendazole 400 mg × 1 dose **Children younger than 2 years**: For ascaris, piperazine 50–75 mg/kg daily × 2 days or For pinworms, piperazine 40 mg/kg daily × 7 days
Giardia Often asymptomatic, early: diarrhea, abdominal pain, bloating, belching, flatus, nausea and vomiting; diarrhea is common, but upper abdominal discomfort predominant Chronic: occasionally diarrhea, most common flatus, loose stools, and sulfurous burping; can cause weight loss	**Adult:** Albendazole 400 mg once daily × 5 days or Metronidazole 250 mg three times daily × 5 days or Metronidazole 2 g daily × 3 days or Tinidazole 2 g × 1 dose **Children:** Albendazole 400 mg once daily × 5 days or Tinidazole 50 mg/kg once daily × 5 days or Metronidazole 5 mg/kg three times daily × 5–7 days
Amebiasis Lower abdominal pain, little diarrhea, malaise, weight loss, abdominal or back pain; can mimic acute appendicitis; small amount of stool but lots of mucus and/or blood; few have fever	**Adult:** Metronidazole 500–700 mg three times daily × 10 days or Tinidazole 2 g × 2 days (liver abscess × 3 days) **Children:** Metronidazole 15 mg/kg three times daily × 10 days or Tinidazole 50–60 mg/kg/day × 3 days (liver abscess × 5 days)

meta-analysis of 53 studies from the scientific literature comparing the quality of care provided by providers such as APRNs/APNs and that by what may be considered higher level providers within developed and developing countries, such as Africa. The review concluded there was no difference between the quality, effectiveness, and outcomes of care provided by the two groups of practitioners. Although the APRN/APN role is well established in North America, the role continues to evolve internationally in both high resource and low resource countries, giving rise to a body of research literature with an evidential and exploratory focus that is rich and evolving.

CONDUCTING GLOBAL RESEARCH

Conducting international nursing research requires an overarching commitment to caring in the context of the local culture. Globally, respect for persons, beneficence, and justice are the foundation for responsible community engagement in the research process. This aligns with the ICN's *Code of Ethics for Nurses*, which states that the universal mandates for nursing practice, and therefore, nursing research, are respect for human rights—the right to life and choice, to dignity, and to be treated with respect. Practically, this requires that APRNs/APNs follow the ethical mandates of the professional practice of nursing as they plan and conduct research. Furthermore, all nurse researchers are expected to know the rules and regulations governing human subject's research where the study will be conducted. Yearly, the U.S. Department of Health and Human Services (DHHS) Office for Human Research Protections provides an updated international compilation of human research standards (www.hhs.gov/ohrp/international/index.html) and the Office of Research Integrity of DHHS provides a primer on the responsible conduct of research (www.ori.hhs.gov/ori-introduction-responsible-conduct-research). In short, all researchers should know international as well as local professional codes, governmental regulations, and institutional policies.

All research codes and policies address the issue of informed consent. However, specific cultural factors, such as decision-making processes and issues of literacy, need to be addressed in the research process (Krogstad et al., 2010). In areas where there is a tradition of communal decision making, community leaders may need to be engaged before potential participants are asked to consent. Also, where there is low literacy and consent is obtained verbally, the researcher must recognize the risk of inconsistent information being shared. To minimize the risk of uninformed consent, an adaptation of "teach back" can be employed whereby the participant's level of understanding is evaluated before consent is confirmed (Krogstad et al., 2010).

Often, APRNs/APNs may be planning to conduct research as they are providing clinical care. This sets up special concerns. Four particular issues have been identified (Laman, Pomat, Siba, & Betuela, 2013). They include the risk of putting a priority on accomplishing the research activity over patient care, confusing the patient's expectation for clinical care with his or her participation consent, setting up inappropriate inducements, and providing "one-time" clinical services that are not sustainable by the host area. According to international nursing ethical standards, patient care must always take precedence over research. As

TABLE 6.15	Journals Known to Publish International APRN/APN Research

- *American Journal of Nursing*
- *Biological Research for Nursing*
- *BMC Nursing*
- *Canadian Journal of Nursing Research*
- *Clinical Nursing Research*
- *Evidence-Based Nursing*
- *International Journal of Evidence-Based Healthcare*
- *International Journal of Nursing Practice*
- *International Journal of Nursing Studies*
- *International Nursing Review*
- *Journal of Advanced Nursing*
- *Journal of the American Association of Nurse Practitioners*
- *Journal of Nursing & Care*
- *Journal for Nurse Practitioners*
- *Journal of Research in Nursing*
- *Nursing Science Quarterly*
- *Western Journal of Nursing Research*

BMC, BioMed Central.

well, local ethics committees can provide important perspectives to minimize patient confusion, counterproposals for what may be considered "inappropriate inducements," and partnership with the researcher to work toward creating sustainable clinical services. Overall, nurses engaged in conducting international research must think globally about gaining new scientific knowledge, but act wisely at the local level, always moving in accordance with nursing's consistent commitment to ethical practice.

Researchers use the traditional available resources, but also enjoy the use of Google Scholar or access to the Joanna Briggs Institute (JBI) and the JBI Library of Systematic Reviews, available at www.connect.jbiconnectplus.org/JBIReviewsLibrary.aspx. Table 6.15 lists journals known to publish international APRN/ANP research.

ROLE OF THE APRN/APN IN EDUCATION DELIVERY AND CONSULTATION

The global nursing shortage of both professional nurses providing care and of nursing faculty creates an environment where the pooling of professional resources is critical (Appiagyei et al., 2014; Bell, Rominski, Bam, Donkor, & Lori, 2013; Nardi & Gyurko, 2013). Nursing providers and faculty are increasingly able to come together to increase the capacity and quality of professional nurses through educational consultation. Technology use, communication that seems to make the world *smaller,* various iterations of distance education, and the ease and improvement of global transportation may profoundly change the landscape of APRN/APN education globally. Currently, most examples of U.S. participation in APRN/APN or other healthcare education and consultation has involved face-to-face work, with students coming to the United States or U.S. faculty going to the host country. The selection of clinical sites for APRNs/APNs requires particular vigilance—some distance programs expect students to come to the United States for this part of the program or work out experiences at U.S. facilities outside the United States (e.g., military bases, embassies). In all instances, the preceptor must be scrupulously reviewed.

Educational consultation falls generally into three categories of professional focus:

- **Individuals:** At this level, educational consultation occurs within the context of medical brigades.
- **Communities:** Educational consultation at this level can occur within the context of medical brigades, but also within broader regional or national populations with health consultation similar to train-the-trainer scenarios (Lasater, Upvall, Nielsen, Prak, & Ptachcinski, 2012).
- **Professional:** Consultation regarding education at this level provides professional infrastructure enrichment, support, or capacity building. Areas for consultation include academic preparation and professional development (Hatzichristou & Rosenfield, 2017).

This professional consultation can occur in a country where a small group of visiting providers comes to receive specialized training/experiences or can occur when a visiting professional can come into a country to provide training or program development. Both areas hold great promise for expanding capacity and quality, yet both raise concerns. Visiting consultors who leave their home for individualized or small group training may not use the training or may not return to their home country at all (Sherwood & Liu, 2005). Visiting single consultants may provide "train-the-trainer" types of experiences within the host country, but they may do so through a cultural lens that is not the same as the host consultant (Palmer & Heaston, 2009).

Process

A similar process undergirds the three categories of educational consultation. At its core, consultation is a process by which people or systems problem solve. This process involves two-way problem solving and is a dynamic method of seeking, giving, and receiving help. Sometimes those receiving the consultation have most of the answers and just need help reaching the goal or solution. The process has three phases: initiation, progression, and culmination.

Initiation

In starting an international educational consultation, there are several questions that need to be answered clearly for all parties involved:

- What are the purpose and outcomes of the consultation?
- What questions/topics need to be addressed?
- What resources are available?
- What resources need to be developed?

Clear answers to these questions provide the basis for the interactions and focus of the consultation.

The first point on which to seek agreement is in regard to the purpose and desired outcome(s). All parties should be specific as to the joint purpose: developing curriculum or programs, addressing specific organizational issues, and/or building infrastructure. That specific purpose will then define the objectives, and they should be concrete and defined and should reflect the consultor's culture, values, state of science, and resources. Each of the parties may have additional purposes that may be served by the consultation, but the primary purpose to be served and goals to be met should be those agreed on by the consultant and consultor (Memmott et al., 2010). For example, building the consultation within the framework of a service-learning program emphasizes the centrality of the agreed-on purpose of the partnership, while acknowledging the benefits of the partnership for all involved (McKinnon & Fealy, 2011).

In defining that purpose, the expected role of the consultant should also be clearly expressed. That definition should include expectations of performance (e.g., conducting classes, designing curricula, delivering continuing education) and time (in preparation, while on site, and on departure) along with workspace (formal academic or in the field) and payment. Forms and amount of communication expected throughout the consultation should also be clarified. Finally, the shared nature of any intellectual property produced as a result of the consultation should be negotiated up front (George & Meadows-Oliver, 2013).

Building on that shared and defined purpose, the next point of agreement is that of the specific questions and topics to be addressed. Does the consultor desire specific subject matter expertise? Who is the intended audience/target learner? Are there programs for professional growth and development to be built or adapted locally or regionally? Are there national, regional, or local implications for practice, licensure, and credentialing that need to be considered and addressed? Awareness of cultural mores and expectations alongside the current practice ecology of the host country is critical for designing and refining content (Scanlan & Abdul Hernandéz, 2014).

Finally, both consultant and consultor need to discuss the resources available. Will translation of materials be needed? What (and, in some cases, if any) is the access to Internet and library resources? What are the resources necessary for sustaining achievement or reproduction of the final goal? Pioneering work in Somalia and China demonstrates that building capacity with no or minimal indigenous resources can begin by identifying community or governmentally directed needs (Doyle & Morris, 2014; Sherwood & Liu, 2005).

Resources for the consultant (office and living space, fees, and communication assistance overseas and within country through translators if necessary) should all be discussed before the onset of the consultation.

Progression

Once the consultation has begun and the traveler is in country, supports discussed in planning should be identified. Those supports may include translators, teaching and research assistants, evaluators, and collaborators. Having a cultural "touchstone" or mentor within the host country who can translate expectations and social constructs will prove to be invaluable (Kim, Woith, Otten, & McElmurry, 2006).

Progression throughout the consultation is marked by timeline, benchmarks, and deliverables. All of these should be clearly delineated in the planning stages but may need to be shifted once the consultation is under way. Keeping in mind the scope, purpose, and deliverables of the consultation will keep the project on track. Doing so while attuned to the cultural climate will make the project successful. Clearly identifying the end of the consultation before beginning will help to bound expectations.

Culmination

As the consultation draws to a close, all involved should evaluate the effectiveness of the project. Scheduling for formative and summative evaluations should be set up before beginning the consultation. Several points to consider during evaluation are the following:

- Were there any secondary responsibilities for program planning, development, or delivery that needed to be met that were not discussed initially?
- Are any return trips needed?
- What follow-up work is needed to foster the consultor's success?
- Does the team that was assembled have plans for other work?
- Are there plans to gauge how the project is doing 3, 6, and 12 months out?
- Did the consultation meet its benchmarks?
- Did the consultation meet the consultor's expectations?
- What were the strengths and weaknesses of the project?
- Can any lessons learned be generalized?

Additional Considerations

Several additional points should be considered when preparing for international educational consultation. The first is to be on guard against cultural tone deafness. The WHO has passed a resolution to set global standards for professional preparation of nurses (Nursing & Midwifery Human Resources for Health, 2009). All nurses practice in a local setting, with each setting having different boundaries for nursing and different expectations of nursing care. In addition, each setting has specific resources. Those resources determine not only care provision but also the sustainability of education and training for the care providers. Sustainability of projects that come out of the consultation process should be a key consideration in design (Mullan & Kerry, 2014).

Along the lines of sustainability, a point to consider within the consultation planning or delivery is what method or program has the sustainable potential for a "ripple effect," that is, a far-reaching capacity for change and professional development (Memmott et al., 2010).

Finally, both the consultant and consultor should enter into their relationship with a clear understanding of the ground rules governing their partnership and an appreciation of potential power sharing that may need to occur within the team (Hunter et al., 2013). As international cooperation and collaboration are critical items necessary to expand both the supply of nurses and nursing faculty, educational consultation has the potential to expand and flourish for the advancement of all involved (Haq et al., 2008).

SUMMARY

Many countries are advancing and expanding nursing practice, including efforts for APRNs/APNs who want to practice, teach, or conduct research in international settings. Pressing global healthcare needs and proven APRN/APN track records in healthcare delivery, education, and research demonstrate this is a time for APRNs/APNs to collaborate with colleagues and other medical professionals to improve health for individuals and communities everywhere. Certainly, the challenges and obstacles are great, but few professions are as flexible, dynamic, and urgently needed as that of the APRN/APN.

ACKNOWLEDGMENTS

The authors would like to thank Beverley Bird, Gene Harkless, Catherine Ling, and Patricia Maybee for their contributions to the previous edition.

REFERENCES

American Association of Nurse Practitioners. (2018). ICNNP/APN network. Retrieved from https://www.aanp.org/international/international-nursing-network

Anjana, R. M., Ali, M. K., Pradeepa, R., Deepa, M., Datta, M., Unnikrishnan, R., ... Mohan, V. (2011). The need for obtaining accurate nationwide estimates of diabetes prevalence in India: Rationale for a national study on diabetes. *Indian Journal of Medical Research*, 133(4), 369–380. Retrieved from http://www.ijmr.org.in/article.asp?issn=0971-5916;year=2011;volume=133;issue=4;spage=369;epage=380;aulast=Anjana

Appiagyei, A. A., Kiriinya, R. N., Gross, J. M., Wambua, D. N., Oywer, E. O., Kamenju, A. K., ... Rogers, M. F. (2014). Informing the scale-up of Kenya's nursing workforce: A mixed methods study of factors affecting pre-service training capacity and production. *Human Resources for Health*, 12(1), 47. doi:10.1186/1478-4491-12-47

APRN Consensus Work Group & National Council of State Boards of Nursing APRN Advisory Committee. (2008). Consensus model for APRN regulation: Licensure, accreditation, certification & education. Retrieved from https://www.ncsbn.org/aprn-consensus.htm

Batancourt, J. R., Green, A. R., Carrillo, J. E., & Owusu, A. (2003). Defining cultural competence: A practical framework for addressing racial/ethnic disparities in health and health care. *Public Health Reports, 118*, 292–302. doi:10.1016/S0033-3549(04)50253-4

Bell, S. A., Rominski, S., Bam, V., Donkor, E., & Lori, J. (2013). Analysis of nursing education in Ghana: Priorities for scaling-up the nursing workforce. *Nursing & Health Sciences, 15*(2), 244–249. doi:10.1111/nhs.12026

Bolwell, A. (2016). Using global trends to chart our course. Retrieved from http://www8.hp.com/us/en/hp-labs/innovation-journal-issue2/megatrends-shaping-the-future.html

Chase, S., & Hunter, A. (2002). Cultural and spiritual competencies: Curricular guidelines [Monograph]. *National Organization of Nurse Practitioner Faculties*, 19–28.

Digital Learning Compass. (2017). Digital learning compass: Distance education state almanac 2017. Retrieved from http://digitallearningcompass.org

Doyle, M.-J., & Morris, C. (2014). Development of mental health nursing education and practice in Somaliland. *Nurse Education in Practice, 14*(1), 1–3. doi:10.1016/j.nepr.2013.11.007

George, E. K., & Meadows-Oliver, M. (2013). Searching for collaboration in international nursing partnerships: A literature review. *International Nursing Review, 60*(1), 31–36. doi:10.1111/j.1466-7657.2012.01034.x

Haq, C., Baumann, L., Olsen, C. W., Brown, L. D., Kraus, C., Bousquet, G., . . . Easterday, B. C. (2008). Creating a center for global health at the University of Wisconsin-Madison. *Academic Medicine, 83*(2), 148–153. doi:10.1097/ACM.0b013e318160af6b

Hatzichristou, C., & Rosenfield, S. (2017). *The international handbook of consultation in educational settings.* New York, NY: Routledge.

Hay Group. (2018). The six global megatrends you must be prepared for. Retrieved from http://www.haygroup.com/en/campaigns/the-six-global-megatrends-you-must-be-prepared-for/

Hunter, A., & Crabtree, K (2010). Global health and international opportunities. In J. Stanley (Ed.), *Advanced practice nursing: Emphasizing common roles* (pp. 327–348). Philadelphia, PA: F. A. Davis.

Hunter, A., Wilson, L., Stanhope, M., Hatcher, B., Hattar, M., Hilfinger Messias, D. K., & Powell, D. (2013). Global health diplomacy: An integrative review of the literature and implications for nursing. *Nursing Outlook, 61*(2), 85–92. doi:10.1016/j.outlook.2012.07.013

International Council of Nurses. (2017). ICN 2017 international workforce forum communique. Retrieved from http://www.icn.ch/images/stories/documents/networks/IWFF%20Communique%202017.pdf

International Council of Nurses Nurse Practitioner/Advanced Practice Nursing Network. (2018). Frequently asked questions of the ICN International NP/APN network. Retrieved from http://international.aanp.org/home/faq

Kim, M. J., Woith, W., Otten, K., & McElmurry, B. J. (2006). Global nurse leaders: Lessons from the sages. *Advances in Nursing Science, 29*(1), 27–42. doi:10.1097/00012272-200601000-00004

Krogstad, D. J., Diop, S., Dialto, A., Mzayek, F., Keating, J., Koita, O. A., & Toure, Y. T. (2010). Informed consent in international research: The rationale for different approaches. *American Journal of Tropical Medicine, 83*(4), 743–747. doi:10.4269/ajtmh.2010.10-0014

Laman, M., Pomat, W., Siba, P., & Betuela, I. (2013, July 26). Ethical challenges in integrating patient-care with clinical research in a resource-limited setting: Perspectives from Papua New Guinea. *BMC Medical Ethics, 14*(29). Retrieved from http://www.biomedcentral.com/1472-6939/14/29 doi:10.1186/1472-6939-14-29

Lancefield, D., & Sviokla, J. (2018). Megatrends. Retrieved from https://www.pwc.co.uk/issues/megatrends.html

Lasater, K., Upvall, M., Nielsen, A., Prak, M., & Ptachcinski, R. (2012). Global partnerships for professional development: A Cambodian exemplar. *Journal of Professional Nursing, 28*(1), 62–68. doi:10.1016/j.profnurs.2011.10.002

Lassi, Z. S., Cometto, G., Huicho, L., & Bhutta, Z. A. (2013). Quality of care provided by mid-level health workers: Systemic review and meta-analysis. *Bulletin of the World Health Organization, 3*(91), 824–833. doi:10.2471/BLT.13.118786

Martiniuk, A. L. C., Manouchehrian, M., Negin, J. A., & Zwi, A. B. (2012). Brain gains: A literature of medical missions to low- and middle-income countries. *BMC Health Services Research, 12*, 134. doi:10.1186/1472-6963-12-134

Massachusetts Institute of Technology. (2014). Disruptive demographics. Retrieved from http://agelab.mit.edu/disruptive-demographics

McKinnon, T. H., & Fealy, G. (2011). Core principles for developing global service-learning programs in nursing. *Nursing Education Perspectives, 32*(2), 95–101.

Memmott, R. J., Coverston, C. R., Heise, B. A., Williams, M., Maughan, E. D., Kohl, J., & Palmer, S. (2010). Practical considerations in establishing sustainable international nursing experiences. *Nursing Education Perspectives, 31*(5), 298–302.

Mullan, F., & Kerry, V. B. (2014). The global health service partnership: Teaching for the world. *Academic Medicine, 89*(8), 1146–1148. doi:10.1097/ACM.0000000000000283

Nardi, D. A., & Gyurko, C. C. (2013). The global nursing faculty shortage: Status and solutions for change. *Journal of Nursing Scholarship, 45*(3), 317–326. doi:10.1111/jnu.12030

National Center for Cultural Competence. (n.d.). Welcome. Retrieved from https://nccc.georgetown.edu/

Nichols, B. L., Davis, C. R., & Richardson, D. R. (2011). International models of nursing. In the Institute of Medicine's (Eds.), *The future of nursing: Leading change, advancing health* (pp. 565–642). Washington, DC: National Academies Press.

Nursing & Midwifery Human Resources for Health. (2009). Global standards for the initial education of professional nurses and midwives (No. WHO/HRH/HPN/08.6). World Health Organization. Retrieved from http://www.who.int/hrh/nursing_midwifery/hrh_global_standards_education.pdf

O'Brien, P., & Gostin, L. O. (2011). The global health worker crisis—Executive summary. *Health worker shortages and global justice.* New York, NY: Milbank Memorial Fund.

Ordway, D., & Sokol, N. (2016). Global trends in human infectious disease: Rising number of outbreaks, fewer per-capita cases. Retrieved from https://journalistsresource.org/studies/society/public-health/global-rise-human-infectious-disease-outbreaks

Palmer, S. P., & Heaston, S. (2009). Teaching the teacher program to assist nurse managers to educate nursing staff in Ecuadorian hospitals. *Nurse Education in Practice, 9*(2), 127–133. doi:10.1016/j.nepr.2008.10.002

Pulcini, J., Jelic, M., Gul, R., & Loke, Y. (2009). An international survey on advanced practice nursing education, practice, and regulation. *Journal of Nursing Scholarship, 42*(1), 31–39. doi:10.1111/j.1547-5069.2009.01322.x

Samaritans Now. (2014). Healthcare mission trips: A manual for healthcare mission leaders. Retrieved from http://www.missiongoal.org/files/resources/Organizing_A_Med_Mission.pdf

Scanlan, J. M., & Abdul Hernandéz, C. (2014). Challenges of implementing a doctoral program in an international exchange in Cuba through the lens of Kanter's empowerment theory. *Nurse Education in Practice, 14*(4), 357–362. doi:10.1016/j.nepr.2014.01.003

Sherwood, G., & Liu, H. (2005). International collaboration for developing graduate education in China. *Nursing Outlook, 53*(1), 15–20. doi:10.1016/j.outlook.2004.08.006

Sigma Theta Tau International. (2014). Sigma Theta Tau International organizational fact sheet. Retrieved from http://www.nursingsociety.org/aboutus/mission/Pages/factsheet.aspx

United Nations. (2013, June 13). World population projected to reach 9.6 billion by 2050—UN Report. Retrieved from http://www.un.org/apps/news/story.asp?NewsID=45165#.VBMUzqOdJ8E

United Nations. (2018). From MDGs to SDGs. Retrieved from http://www.sdgfund.org/mdgs-sdgs

U.S. Department of State. (2018). The Fulbright program. Retrieved from https://eca.state.gov/fulbright/about-fulbright

Weller, C. (2018). These mega-trends could change the world by 2030. Retrieved from https://www.weforum.org/agenda/2017/08/4-mega-trends-that-could-change-the-world-by-2030

World Health Organization. (2006). The world health report 2006: Working together for health. Retrieved from http://www.who.int/whr/2006/en

World Health Organization. (2008). The world health report 2008: Primary health care, now more than ever. Retrieved from http://www.who.int/whr/2008/en

World Health Organization. (2018). *Global action plan for the prevention and control of NCDs 2013-2020.* Retrieved from http://www.who.int/nmh/events/ncd_action_plan/en

Zackowitz, M. G. (2014, March). Medical migration. Retrieved from http://ngm.nationalgeographic.com/2008/12/community-doctors/follow-up-text

Rebecca M. Patton, Margarete L. Zalon, and Ruth Ludwick

7

LEADERSHIP FOR COMPETENCIES FOR APRN: CHALLENGES AND OPPORTUNITY

Never in the history of nursing has there been a more optimal time to be an APRN. There are over a quarter million APRNs in the U.S. workforce (National Council of State Boards of Nursing, 2014). These numbers and the studies on the effectiveness of the APRN role, patient safety and cost containment, and evidence that backs full-practice authority combined with changing health demographics and reimbursement practices are providing some of the leverage needed for APRNs to lead the way in reshaping healthcare. Leadership by nurses in practice, education, research, and administration have been instrumental in finding, disseminating, and supporting the effectiveness, full practice authority, and reimbursement of APRNs. This demonstrates how APRNs can be effective in inspiring, innovating, and influencing health across the broad spectrum of care.

Two of many examples of APRN effectiveness are found in primary care and care transitions. More than 87% of nurse practitioners (NPs), are prepared in primary care (American Association of Nurse Practitioners [AANP], 2018). Currently, more than two-thirds of all Americans have seen an APRN for their primary healthcare needs, with more than 1.02 billion visits to APRNs each year (AANP, 2014; AANP, 2018). By far the largest group of APRNs in primary care is the certified nurse practitioner and this number is expected to grow in the 15-year span (2010–2025) by an amazing 84% so that, if these numbers hold, the percentage of primary care physicians will drop to 60% in 2025 (Bodenheimer & Bauer, 2016, p. 1016). The confluence of an aging and increasingly large population with chronic diseases, the growth of the APRN workforce, and the shortage of primary care physicians provide opportunities for leadership across the healthcare environment beyond one's organization.

Care transition management is another arena in which APRNs have shown distinguished leadership, especially in the management of chronic disease care. "Care transition" is defined as a "broad range of services designed to ensure health care continuity, avoid preventable poor outcomes among at risk populations, and promote the safe and timely transfer of patients from one level of care to another or from one type of setting to another" (Naylor, Aiken, Kurtzman, Olds, & Hirschman, 2011, p. 747). APRNs are not only leading care transition teams, but it is the research and policy making of APRNs that have led to the strides made in improving the health outcomes of patients with a variety of conditions and across the life span.

The early roots can be found in the work by Dorothy Brooten, PhD, RN, FAAN, who pioneered transitional care for very low-birth-weight infants. This work has expanded to include transition care by APRNs in other high-risk and high-cost populations. Mary Naylor and the research team at the University of Pennsylvania have conducted extensive work on care transition. This work has resulted in the Transitional Care Model (TCM) and the addition of at-risk populations who receive Medicare or Medicaid (Hirschman, Shaid, McCauley, Pauly, & Naylor, 2015; Naylor et al., 2017).

Thus, leadership has been a critical driver in the evolution of the APRN role and will continue to be vital not only in role development but also in success of redesigning the healthcare system. Transitional care as described previously is part of that redesign. Another example of innovation in redesigning the healthcare delivery system is the growth of retail-based clinics that provide convenient access for the management of common everyday illnesses at lower cost without compromising care.

Each APRN has a unique leadership role to cultivate regardless of title (clinical nurse specialist [CNS], certified nurse-midwife [CNM], certified registered nurse anesthetist [CRNA], or NP). All APRNs should exhibit leadership qualities that influence and empower others. Empowerment is central to the APRN role and is necessary to the work environment for APRNs and the teams that they lead. Two types of complementary empowerment are discussed in the literature: structural and psychological (Steward, McNulty, Quinn Griffin, & Fitzpatrick, 2014). Structural empowerment is a process that facilitates individuals and/or groups having sufficient resources, information, and backing to carry out expected roles. Psychological empowerment encompasses motivation. Empowering patients, other nurses, or other professionals is basic to safe, effective care. Empowerment is essential to inspiration, innovation, and influence.

Leadership is a team sport that includes not only self-development but mentoring, coaching, fostering, and facilitating leadership in others. APRNs as leaders will bring a unique lens that will help envision the reshaping of healthcare so that ease of access, safety and quality, reduced costs, and an improved work life of providers become a reality. Whether you are a CRNA, CNM, CNS, or NP, your specialty organization outlines leadership as an expected competency for the role. Equally important, graduate-level competencies delineated for APRN education at both the master's level and the doctoral level clearly emphasize the importance of leadership preparation.

In 2011, the American Association of Colleges of Nursing (AACN) published *The Essentials of Master's Education in Nursing*, which explicitly focuses on leadership competencies for all the Master's of Science in Nursing (MSN)-prepared nurses. Essential II, "Organizational and Systems Leadership," identifies that any MSN program "recognizes that organizational and systems leadership are critical to the promotion of high quality and safe patient care. Leadership skills are needed that emphasize ethical and critical decision making, effective working relationships, and a systems-perspective" (p. 4). AACN further defines leadership as an influencing process that can be either formal (e.g., based on title) or informal (e.g., influencing others without holding a formal position of power). Both are critical to the APRN role.

In the AACN, *The Essentials for Doctoral Education for Advanced Nursing Practice* (AACN, 2006) delineates the importance of leadership knowledge and skills throughout the document and specifically addresses leadership in Essentials II, VI, and VIII. Essential II is focused on organizational and systems leadership for quality improvement and systems thinking. Graduates must have advanced communication skills to lead quality improvement and patient safety initiatives. Essential VI is focused on interprofessional collaboration for improving patient and population health outcomes. To be successful, graduates must demonstrate the ability to employ effective communication and collaborative skills, lead interprofessional teams, and employ consultative and leadership skills with intraprofessional and interprofessional teams to create change in healthcare and complex healthcare delivery systems. Essential VIII is focused on advanced practice nursing. Among other requirements, doctor of nursing practice (DNP) graduates must be able to demonstrate advanced levels of systems thinking and guide, mentor, and support other nurses to achieve excellence in nursing practice (AACN, 2006). While leadership is not directly mentioned in this essential, advanced systems thinking and and guidance of nurses requires leadership.

This chapter discusses the responsibilities and competencies of APRNs related to three overlapping and complementary arenas including clinical leadership, health environment, and the nursing profession. The content highlights the opportunities APRNs have in this new world if they embrace this moment with the strong leadership competencies and skills necessary to inspire, innovate, and influence the future of healthcare. We emphasize the importance of leadership competencies for APRNs who have major responsibilities for delivery of quality care, evidence-based practice (EBP), patient safety, innovations in nursing practice, and leadership in systems. The chapter builds on the leadership content presented earlier in the book. See Chapter 3.

CLINICAL LEADERSHIP

APRNs have an essential leadership role that starts in the practice setting. This leadership role is multifaceted and is critical to the achievement of healthcare redesign and the achievement of the Quadruple AIM. The latter is an expansion of the more often recognized Triple Aim set forth by the Institute for Healthcare Improvement's (IHI), by adding the improvement of the work life of healthcare providers to the aims of quality and safety, improved health, and reduced costs (Bodenheimer & Sinsky, 2014). No one is more equipped to lead this charge in the work setting than nurses who have the education and knowledge of the policies, regulations, culture, and their own work environment.

APRNs can make the difference in accomplishing these aims where they work if and only if they develop leadership competencies needed for the current environment. The changes in healthcare restructuring, as well as revolutionary advances in technology, pharmaceutical research, and surgical innovations, coupled with the organizational complexities and fierce competition for resources, have created unprecedented challenges as well as opportunities for the APRN. In the midst of these awe-inspiring advances, it is clear that the sobering unintended consequences of a complex, highly regulated, and yet fragmented system, first identified by the Institute of Medicine (IOM, now the National Academy of Medicine [NAM]) more than 15 years ago (IOM, 1999, 2001, 2004), have not yet been solved. At a time when the cloning of a human is possible, ensuring the basics, such as hand washing for all providers and preventing falls, remains, at times, elusive. In addition, the incentive structure of the reimbursement system is finally holding providers accountable to keep communities healthy by preventing illness and supporting wellness, creating both intended and unintended consequences. Lack of leadership has been shown to be an instrumental influence in the occurrence of sentinel events (Joint Commission, 2017). APRNs have incredible opportunities but still face obstacles related to the hierarchy of the healthcare system that has plagued nurses for decades.

Pursuing your graduate education and APRN specialty is foundational to your growth as a nurse leader. Becoming a leader is process and can build on the leadership experiences you have had. Conduct a self-assessment for your current leadership in practice and school. Consider taking an inventory of leadership projects that you may have already experienced, for example: committee/council work; managing a unit; leading a team; implementing a change process; carrying out research, evidence-based or research project; and or coaching, precepting, or mentoring others such as students or new RNs. These experiences can be appointed, elected, or volunteer.

Preparation and action are required to cultivate your role as a leader in anticipation of your new work role. Self-awareness is basic to planning and taking action steps. Krejci and Malin (2001, 2006) developed a model based on more than 20 years of teaching and consulting in the area of leadership development with nurses in a variety of roles (Krejci & Malin, 1997). The model encompasses leadership development for all nurses, not just those in formal leadership positions. The foundation of the model is self-awareness, which the literature on leadership has consistently identified as being a prerequisite for successful leadership. The components in this model are congruent with the master's and DNP essentials documents (AACN, 2006, 2011; see Figure 7.1). Self-awareness, self-efficacy, and mission occupy the

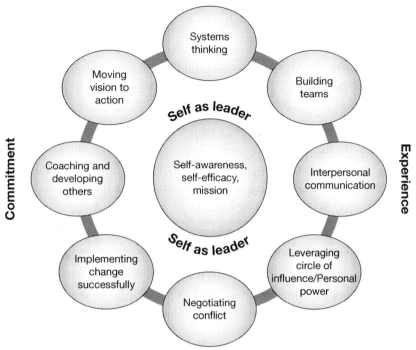

FIGURE 7.1 Krejci and Malin's leadership model of competencies.

center of the model, surrounded by supporting competencies of systems thinking, circle of influence (personal power), interpersonal communication, building teams, negotiating conflict, moving vision to action, coaching and developing others, and implementing change.

Although there seems to be much agreement that leadership competencies are a prerequisite for success as an APRN. As basic APRN education moves more fully to DNP programs, nursing education has a stunning opportunity to build a strong foundational curriculum that seeds stronger leaders.

The development of future APRN leaders is double-pronged and requires both leadership in everyday practice and a plan to take on formal leadership roles. In fact, the IOM report (2011) sets the expectation that all nurses develop as leaders "from bedside to boardroom" (IOM, 2011). However, as we look forward to the roles nurses have in leadership in healthcare today, those with advanced education, like APRNs, will be more critical than ever. The many strides that have come in the exponential growth of APRNs will not be sustained without strong leadership, given the ever-changing health, demographic, and political landscape.

The challenge for APRNs, those who educate them, and those executives to whom they report, is understanding the leadership implications of the APRN role in their day-to-day work practice. Given the primacy of leadership in the APRN role, across practice and even countries, much more work is needed to understand APRN leadership (Elliott, Begley, Sheaf, & Higgins, 2016).

Much as the barriers to APRN practice have been discussed throughout the book and your education, there are numerous barriers that exist to fully embrace and develop APRN leadership. In a scoping review, Elliott et al. (2016) identified not only 13 barriers to practice, but they categorized 11 enablers to leadership practice. The latter is a critical step to examining the ways to build on existing strengths. This study is important as leadership is discussed as a concept across types of advanced practice nursing. Both the barriers and enablers were categorized into four broad levels: healthcare system, organization, team, and advanced practitioner. Most barriers and enablers are found at the organizational level, showing how structural empowerment is essential to APRN leadership as noted by Steward et al. (2014). Interestingly at the APRN level, several barriers are noted specifically to leadership, the very focus of this chapter. Issues related to the healthcare system are discussed in Chapter 10.

Thus, within the APRN everyday work role, there are many opportunities as well as obstacles to being a leader. While you may have an APRN role that focuses on executive leadership or advancement of evidence like research or quality improvement, most entry APRN roles are in direct clinical care. Clinical leadership at the front lines is equally needed for solving everyday problems of care related to a variety of seemingly disparate topics ranging from adopting new practice guidelines to reducing readmission rates. Many thousands of articles are found in the literature that highlight specific clinical projects like EBP, quality that was carried out under the leadership of CNMs, CNPs, CRNAs, or CNSs individually, in groups, or across categories of APRNs like CNSs and NPs. The projects evolve from everyday practice like common health problems (e.g., heart failure), deficiencies identified from root cause analyses (e.g., work-arounds or hand-off failures), and high-profile national problems (e.g., hospital-acquired complications). One example can be seen in the work to decrease readmissions, costs, and adverse events by an interdisciplinary team led by CNSs in a small community hospital. The team developed the program called the At Risk Care Plan (ARCP) as a partial result of safety analyses. High-end users of care were often patients who were repeatedly readmitted and experiencing adverse events like falls while hospitalized. The ARCP is a care coordination tool that is incorporated into the patient's chart and details a tailored care plan for each patient designated at risk. Written and verbal communication both in person and electronically are essential to the ARCP (Bahle, Majercik, Ludwick, Bukosky, & Frase, 2014). Often a small project, especially when disseminated, will lead to the expansion of efforts beyond the work setting.

HEALTHCARE ENVIRONMENT

The virtues of leadership and the need for leadership are extolled within the profession and beyond through seminal documents such as the American Nurses Association's (ANA's) scope and standards of nursing practice

(2015a), the AACN Essentials documents (AACN, 2006, 2011), the IOM *Future of Nursing: Leading Change, Advancing Health Report* (2011) as well as in the competencies for each of the APRN roles. The need for APRNs to assume a leadership role in healthcare is further exemplified by the National Organization of Nurse Practitioner Faculties (NONPF) recommendation to move NP education to the DNP level by 2025 so that all NP students achieve doctoral-level core and population-focused competencies (NONPF, 2018). APRNs can exert leadership in the healthcare environment to improve outcomes in each of the domains of the Quadruple Aim through inspiration, innovation, and influence.

Operationalizing leadership for each of the APRN roles within the healthcare environment does not have clear definition nor are there specific competencies. This is in part due to the fact that the primary focus of CNMs, NPs, and CRNAs is in the direct provision of care related to their specialization. For CNSs, while they include the three spheres of patient, nurse, and system, their daily work often focuses on supporting system efforts to improve patient outcomes at the organizational level. These roles do not often translate into direct formal and visible leadership roles. Not having direct leadership responsibility limits the vision of a preferred future for nursing, and specifically, APRN roles in leading and advancing change in the healthcare system.

The need for APRNs to assume visible leadership roles within the healthcare environment is critical, given the rapidly increasing number of APRNs, the need for APRN services, and the complexity of healthcare. Formal leadership roles within one's organization may include direct management responsibility, advancement of research and quality improvement, interprofessional collaboration, and mentoring. Within the larger healthcare environment, these arenas include being a citizen leader to foster interdisciplinary collaboration and partnerships with consumers to achieve common healthcare objectives and the advancement of health for the public.

The landmark *Future of Nursing*: *Leading Change, Advancing Health* report (IOM, 2011) indicates that nurses along with physicians need to be leaders in reforming the healthcare system, which directly aligns with the Quadruple Aim of healthcare. It requires thinking more strategically about APRNs' leadership roles. The 5-year report on the *Future of Nursing* (Altman, Butler, & Shern, 2016) outcomes indicates that a major means of accomplishing this objective is for nurses to serve on boards, commissions, and advisory panels. The *Nurses on Boards Coalition (NOBC)* is one tangible initiative to increase nursing's influence at high policy levels in the healthcare environment.

The NOBC was formed by nurses from across the nation and other organizations with support from the Robert Wood Johnson Foundation and the AARP as part of the implementation of the *Future of Nursing* report under the aegis of the Future of Nursing: Campaign for Action. The goal is to increase nurse representation on corporate, health-related and other boards, panels, and coalitions by having 10,000 nurses on such boards and groups by 2020 (NOBC, 2017). As of this writing, only one APRN associa-tion, the National Association of Pediatric Nurse Practitioners (NAPNAP), is a member of this group indicating that this a potential area of growth and need for APRN organizational leadership commitment.

The NOBC philosophy is that nurses have the qualifications to serve as integral members of healthcare decision-making groups including skills in communication, finance, quality improvement, strategic planning, and management (NOBC, 2017). Nurses bring the "nursing lens," which includes their perspective on the intricacies and complexities of the human condition acquired during their nursing careers (Disch, 2019). APRNs bring their clinical focus and expertise to board service. Hospital boards that have a greater emphasis on the use of clinical quality metrics are perceived as having higher performance (Tsai et al., 2015). Dramatically increasing the number of nurses on boards has the potential to turn around the findings of a Gallup poll finding that only 14% of American opinion leaders thought that nurses were likely to exert a great deal of in-fluence on healthcare reform and eliminate some of the barriers to nurses exerting a greater influence in the healthcare system (Khoury, Blizzard, Wright Moore, & Hassmiller, 2011). Board service provides opportunities for nurses to influence healthcare, enhance care at the local or regional level, enhance the public's trust in nursing, and provide opportunities for nurses to fulfill their societal obligations (Sundean, Polifroni, Libal, & McGrath, 2017, 2018). These high-level decision-making opportunities position APRNs to fully participate in the redesign of the healthcare system.

The NOBC created a database of nurses serving on boards to track pro-gress. However, the most recently available data indicates that in 2014 only 5% of hospital boards had registered nurse (RN) members (American Hospital Association Center for Healthcare Governance, 2014). Although hospitals and large healthcare systems are one arena for board service, there are numerous other healthcare and community boards that would benefit from the expertise of APRNs. Resources for nurses serving on boards are available on the NOBC (https://www.nursesonboardscoalition.org/) and Campaign for Action websites (https://campaignforaction.org/).

APRNs can also provide leadership in achieving the Quadruple AIM through clinical processes related to their practice to improve quality. Today's healthcare environment requires the generation of new research, the evaluation of evidence, and efforts to put evidence into practice through quality improvement. APRN leadership in this arena is a two-pronged ap-proach. It has been conceptualized as a continuum between production of research and the production and implementation of EBP (Hølge-Hazleton, Kjerholt, Berthelsen, & Thomsen, 2016). APRNs, regardless of their educa-tional preparation and because of their extensive practice expertise, should be engaged in thoughtful analysis of the need for research in an area in which APRNs can partner with researchers, provide leadership in the re-search enterprise of a healthcare system, or evaluate proposed research within their organizational setting. Many practice groups have joined practice-based research networks (PBRNs) to address specific healthcare research questions and translate evidence into practice (Agency for Research and Healthcare Quality [AHRQ], n.d.). APRNs have the potential to take on a leadership role in evaluating the feasibility of joining such a network and managing the oversight in applying the information obtained through participation in a PBRN.

Leadership in quality improvement and EBP is inextricably intertwined. Although each of the APRN roles may be at different stages of development with regard to overall leadership in this arena, there is ample opportunity for APRNs to become thought leaders and experts in improving patient outcomes contributing to the achievement of the Quadruple Aim. APRNs can provide EBP and quality improvement leadership at the micro and macro levels (Finkelman, 2013). At the micro level, these activities may include identification of problems, proposing quality improvement and EBP projects working with members of interdisciplinary teams to achieve specific goals; at the macro level, it may include participation in these initiatives at the state and national levels (Finkelman, 2013).

Improving quality on a broader basis requires a focus on population health; the health of a population is intertwined with health inequities. One cannot achieve population health goals when large segments of the population do not have access to healthcare. Achieving population health goals will involve efforts to address the underlying health inequities with local engagement and commitment (Williams & Phillips, 2019). Access to healthcare means addressing the needs of vulnerable populations.

APRNs have traditionally served vulnerable populations (Xue & Intrator, 2016). APRNs may often be the only healthcare providers in their communities, in nursing homes, and other settings serving low-income patients; federally qualified community health centers are twice as likely to employ NPs, CNMs, and physicians' assistants as other settings (National Association of Community Health Centers, 2014). The Comprehensive Addiction and Recovery Act (CARA) of 2016, which expands substance use treatment services, also provides additional prescribing privileges to NPs (Substance Abuse and Mental Health Services Administration, 2018), thus facilitating access to care.

Although many APRNs are in settings that serve vulnerable populations, every day they may face challenges in subtle biases hindering access to care and impacting the experience of care which in turn impacts quality and safety. Fitzgerald, Myers, and Clark (2017) propose using Bardaracco's model of quiet leadership (2002) to address the needs of vulnerable populations such as immigrants by taking action to stop injustice, being persistent in solving a problem, and using an incremental approach to work a problem through the organizational hierarchy. APRNs can address the needs of vulnerable populations not only by the type of work settings and their location (e.g., rural), but also by exerting leadership and taking action to ensure that their patients receive the care that is intended.

With care shifting to outpatient and community settings, organizations at the state and national levels are setting policy, and creating standards and guidelines. Advancement of this leadership role includes engaging staff in these processes and providing guidance to enhance the development of collective EBP and quality improvement expertise within healthcare systems, thus directly impacting overall quality of care. Including cost analyses for the implementation of new practices and/or new ways of utilizing healthcare personnel has the potential to reduce the cost of healthcare.

Nursing has a long history of demonstrating the overall benefit of APRNs for the quality of care, as well as real and potential cost savings (Newhouse et al., 2011; Rantz, Birtlely, Flesner, Crecelius, & Murray, 2017). For example, the Family Health and Birth Center in Washington, DC, addresses the needs of a vulnerable population by using a midwifery/NP model to provide low-income women with access to care. This has resulted in a reduction of preterm births and cesarean section rates with more than $1.6 million in savings annually for the Washington, DC healthcare system (American Academy of Nursing, 2015). These types of efforts need to be expanded to all areas of practice with the inclusion of financial analyses. There are considerable challenges in conducting economic analyses for NPs and CNSs: the use of standard guidelines has the potential to enhance the comprehensiveness of such economic evaluations (Lopatine et al., 2017).

As the utilization of APRNs becomes more widespread, it is also important for APRNs to take on leadership roles in fostering positive work environments and responsibilities commensurate with their education to contribute to the fourth aim of healthcare. This can involve a variety of formal leadership roles as well as participation in shared governance at the direct care level. An extensive body of research indicates that a positive work environment, job satisfaction, and autonomy for nurses are critical to improve outcomes for hospitalized patients. When NPs serve as primary care providers with their own patient panels, they have more positive perceptions of their work environment, and NP job satisfaction is linked with being less likely to report intention to leave and organizational support of NP practice (Poghosyan, Liu, & Norful, 2017; Poghosyan, Liu, Shang, & D'Aunno, 2017). This research is being expanded to the nurse anesthetist arena as well (Boyd & Poghosyan, 2017).

APRNs can also provide expertise in the credentialing process as well as in the regulatory and legislative environment to enhance more effective utilization of APRNs (Anen & McElroy, 2017). APRNs should examine their work responsibilities to ensure that they are practicing at the top of the license and not engaging in work that is more appropriately carried out by other healthcare professionals. Nurses transitioning to their APRN role may have traditionally carried out non-nursing activities as staff nurses, and thus, may not realize the implications of continuing that practice in their new realm by engaging in traditional nursing responsibilities when functioning as an APRN. This will allow for greater efficiencies, thereby enhancing access to care while allowing APRNs to focus on improving outcomes directly related to their care.

LEADERSHIP AND ADVOCACY FOR THE PROFESSION

Within nursing, there is no argument that APRNs possess expert knowledge, skill, and have unique roles in healthcare. Regardless of their roles and practice specialties, all APRNs are RNs first; one cannot become an APRN without being licensed as an RN. Recognizing that, APRN roles and responsibilities extend to some basic aspect that applies to all RNs regardless of their positions. ANA's core documents, *Code of Ethics for Nurses with Interpretative Statements* (ANA, 2015a), and *Nursing: Scope and Standards of Practice* (2015b) describe the responsibility for all nurses to be advocates (Patton, Zalon, & Ludwick, 2019). These levels include nurse-to-patient, nurse-to-nurse, nurse-to-self, nurse-to-others, nurse-to-profession, nurse-to-society, and nursing-to society (Badzek & Turner, 2015). A first step in the advocacy role is membership in and involvement with professional associations. A professional association like the International Council of Nurses (ICN), the ANA, or state or territorial nurses associations are designed to represent all nurses in the profession no matter the level of education. Equally important, APRNs should also be members of and be involved with their specialty associations that address their specific needs. This is not an either/or responsibility to meet the APRNs ethical obligations to the profession and society. APRNs may belong to other nursing organizations (e.g., Sigma Theta Tau, American Academy of Nursing), interdisciplinary professional groups, and consumer organizations.

As addressed in Chapter 9, APRNs need to see their advocacy responsibilities beyond their patients. Although each APRN association has a proud history where its leaders made a difference, needed APRN leadership is not just for role-specific issues but for the profession as a whole. Each APRN role is unique and can be complementary in addressing issues that impact the profession as a whole. Addressing just one APRN role or a single-issue focus creates unintended consequences for the profession. This siloed approach limits the larger nursing profession's visibility, influence, and ultimate ability to further a broader agenda to advance the role of nurses in providing quality, safe, cost-effective healthcare for all. Whether at the bedside or the boardroom, when nurses work collaboratively with each other and speak with a shared voice, individual APRNs and the profession benefit.

This siloed focus has been a concern among nursing leaders for years. A strategy for organizing established in 2009 is the Nursing Community Coalition that includes 58 national nursing associations. Through an organizational consensus decision-making model, the Nursing Community Coalition advocates for and provides leadership on a wide spectrum of policy issues. Established during healthcare reform discussions, the Nursing Community Coalition recently worked together and identified key provisions that they together could support in the Patient Protection and Affordable Care Act. Today, the Nursing Community Coalition is committed to collaborating on issues that support the education, practice, and research of RNs and APRNs.

Although APRN membership and leadership in coalitions in the United States have produced limited success, Canadian nurses have undertaken an unusual action to exercise their leadership and strengthen their unity and advocacy. Four nurses associations representing NPs, RNs, licensed practical nurses, and registered psychiatric nurses will become a new organization, the Nurses and Nurse Practitioners of British Columbia (NNPBC; *Canadian NURSE*, 2018). This recent action has the potential to reduce the ongoing issues with too many nursing associations speaking without clear consensus and agreement, therefore minimizing intended influence and success. A lesson may be learned here about a united front as Congressional legislators have been known to tell nurses "to come back when you can agree on what you need."

Leadership competencies learned during formal APRN education establish foundational skills to lead the profession on issues of importance to all RNs. Indeed, the *Future of Nursing* landmark report called for strong and qualified leadership in key positions in policy, politics, organizations, and practice (IOM, 2011). See Exhibit 7.1 for APRNs who have assumed leadership roles in national nurses associations that are beyond their APRN focus.

APRNs associations' websites describe numerous activities where the association was providing leadership addressing issues of concerns not just within their scope of practice but beyond in society and the larger nursing profession. The following sections focus on just three high-profile areas that impact society and where APRNs are uniquely positioned to provide leadership: the opioid crisis, gun violence and gun safety, and Healthy Nurse, Healthy Nation (HNHN).

Opioid Crisis

As one of today's most pressing healthcare issues, the opioid addiction crisis requires effective strategies to reverse the growing addiction epidemic and preventable deaths. The statistics are alarming and are a serious global crisis that affects health, social, and economic interests. Both prescribed and nonprescribed usages have contributed to the severity of the brutal consequence of the opioid abuse problem. Pain management choices and consequences are increasingly of importance to providers and consumers. The fundamental goal of pain management is striking the right balance between providing maximum relief while minimizing associated risks and adverse effects of prescription drug abuse. Although NPs are positioned to lead successful strategies mitigating the effects of the opioid epidemic in direct care settings, and CNSs are positioned to lead in developing system solutions, we highlight the unique role of CRNAs and CNMs in addressing opioid management.

CRNAs are well-educated and highly-qualified anesthesia providers working with patients to offer holistic, patient-centered, multimodal pain management during the perioperative period both in and out of hospital settings. The American Association of Nurse Anesthetists (AANA) acknowledges that the overprescription of pain medications has fueled patients'

Exhibit 7.1   APRNS' LEADERSHIP IN NATIONAL NURSING ASSOCIATIONS (MAY, 2018)

Association	APRN and Board Role
ANA	Director Mary Lee Pakieser, MSN, RN, BC-FNP
ANF	Chairperson Timothy Porter-O'Grady, DM, EdD, APRN, FAAN, FACCWS
AACN	President Christine S. Schulman, MS, RN, CNS, CCRN-K
AORN	Secretary Lizz Pincus, MSN, MBA, RN, ACNS-BC, CNS-CP, CNOR
	Director Lisa A Miller, JD, CNM
ENA	Director Gordon Gillespie, PhD, DNP, RN, CEN, CNE, CPEN, PHCNS-BC, FAEN, FAAN
National Council of State Boards of Nursing	Director Valerie Fuller, PhD, DNP, AGACNP-BC, FNP-BC, FAANP
ONS	Director Heather Mackey, MSN, RN, ANP-BC, AOCN
Sigma Theta Tau International Honor Society of Nursing	President Beth Baldwin Tigges, PhD, RN, PNP, BC

ANA, American Nurses Association; ANF, American Nurses Foundation; AACN, American Association of Critical-Care Nurses; AORN, Association of periOperative Registered Nurses; AWHONN, Association of Women's Health, Obstetric and Neonatal Nurses; ENA, Emergency Nurses Association; ONS, Oncology Nursing Society.

medication dependence when alternative solutions are available (Rechtoris, 2017). To address the opioid crisis, anesthesia providers are making a concerted effort to address prevention of opioid addiction with the judicious use of multimodal pain management strategies. These strategies, which are often part of an Enhance Recovery After Surgery (ERAS) protocol, include the use of regional anesthesia, peripheral nerve blocks, nonpharmacological approaches, and nonopioid medications for pain reduction and management (AANA, 2018). Additional strategies directed to CRNAs include (a) careful preoperative evaluation; (b) formulation of institutional policies related to responsible prescribing practices; (c) continuing education; (d) support of local, state, and federal efforts directed toward the availability of naloxone; (e) adherence to opioid prescription practice standards; and (f) use of AANA resources (Griffis, Grion, & Darna, 2017).

Opioid addiction and pregnancy create additional concerns for healthcare providers. Pregnant women with an opioid use disorder need a safe environment that protects their health and the health of their fetuses.

Additionally, criminal retribution with criminal charges, incarceration, and temporary or permanent loss of parental rights is a real fear for these women when seeking care. Protecting the rights of these women to healthcare provides another leadership opportunity. Understanding the law, knowing the availability of resources, and supporting these women may reduce their fears so they will be more likely to access healthcare services. CNMs can exhibit leadership by advocacy at the individual level as well as broader policy advocacy for access to services. One arena is the collaborative work of the American College of Nurse-Midwives and the American College of Obstetricians and Gynecologists to amend the CARA Act to expand prescriptive authority that was granted to NPs and physicians' assistants for buprenorphine to include CNMs and certified midwives and also allow them to prescribe medication-assisted treatment for pregnant women with opioid use disorders (Murphy, Goodman, Johnson, & Terplan, 2018). This also illustrates the importance of all APRNs and nurses working together to achieve professional and societal goals for access to quality care.

Moving From Gun Violence to Gun Safety

Similar to opioid addiction, gun violence has reached national attention impacting thousands in all economic and social classes with approximately 30,000 deaths annually; there is a death from gun violence every 15 minutes (Gelinas, 2017). Gun violence is a complex social and psychological issue that requires multiple strategies to address this public health threat. Medscape Medical News found that 71% of APRNs and RNs polled indicated that gun violence is a public health problem, but only 39% of nurses reported ever having a conversation with patients about gun violence, and 29% indicated that they were not prepared to have those conversations (Frellick, 2017).

Nurses associations are beginning to make more forceful efforts to address gun violence. The American Academy of Nursing took the lead in delivering a letter to Congress with 96 nursing organization signatories calling for the creation of a national bipartisan commission on mass shootings. This effort has been echoed with policy statements and press releases from nurses associations, including APRN professional groups. The AANP called policy makers to address gun violence by focusing on common sense reforms, investing in research, and expanding access to mental health services both nationally and in each state to address this national crisis (AANP, 2018). The NAPNAP has begun to partner with the American Academy of Pediatrics to address child health and safety, including gun violence (Zielinski, 2017). APRNs can take the lead in joining these initiatives on a state and national level to lend strength and voice to these efforts.

Grassroots efforts are underway across the country such as EVERYTOWN For Gun Safety (n.d.) which works in local communities, and the Sandy Hook Promise (n.d.), which works to prevent gun-related deaths due to crime, suicide, and accidental discharge. Partnering with consumer advocacy groups strengthens these efforts also. APRNs gain expertise in working with people from diverse backgrounds and perspectives. Just as noted by the NOBC, APRNs bring their nursing lens and have the trust of the public, which facilitates opportunities for leadership.

Organized nursing has addressed some of these issues over the years with position statements, press releases, and lobbying efforts. However, these efforts have not been as much as one would expect as pointed out by Odom-Forren, then president of the American Society of Perianesthesia Nurses (2016) "Nursing as a whole has been rather silent on the issue of gun violence." This void provides opportunities for APRNs to take on leadership in practice, education, research, and also in policy at the grassroots level and beyond at the state and national levels.

Healthy Nurse, Healthy Nation

It is well known that nurses are committed to caring for their patients, families, and their communities. It is less known and understood that unfortunately, many nurses struggle to take care of themselves. The 4 million nurses are known to have health measures less healthy than the average American (see Exhibit 7.2). More likely to be overweight, nurses have higher levels of stress and fewer hours of recommended sleep. For years, nurses have sustained more occupational injuries than many other industries. Annually nurses and some other healthcare workers experience the highest rate of nonfatal occupational injuries and illnesses of any sectors (ANA, 2017). Nurses exceed injury rates for construction workers. In addition, hazards

The health of nurses is suffering

In most indicators, the health of a registered nurse is worse than that of average Americans.

	BMI	Sleep	Nutrition	Stress
NURSES	28	7.0 hours	16%	81%
Average American	26.6	7.8 hours	23%	29%

Body mass index: BMI in the 25–29.9 range are classified as "overweight"
Sleep: Number of hours of sleep in a 24-hour period
Nutrition: % eating recommended servings of five fruits and vegetables daily
Quality of Life: % reporting high levels of stress

EXHIBIT 7.2 The Health of Nurses Is Suffering.
Source: Judge, K. (2018). *Healthy nurse, healthy nation*. Presented at the meeting of Frances Payne Bolton School of Nursing Case Western Reserve University, Cleveland, Ohio.

such as workplace violence and musculoskeletal injuries are contributing factors to poorer health.

In 2017, the ANA launched a new initiative designed to transform the health of the nation by improving the health of America's registered nurses. HNHN is designed to engage individual and groups of nurses to address factors that impact their health (ANA, 2017). Often in the past, workplace and professional initiatives like HNHN required champions and leadership to benefit stakeholders. Today, APRNs are ideal to lead HNHN programs. One example that stands out is the president of the West Virginia Nurses Association, Toni DiChiacchio, DNP, APRN, FNP-BC, CEN. Using the slogan "Balance Your Life for a Healthier You" in her presidential report, she addresses strategies nurses can undertake to improve their personal health (DiChiacchio, 2017). Not alone in this effort, other APRNs have been noted online advocating for healthy behavior and calling for nurses to address health and find strategies to address their personal needs. While not as well known, the HNHN staff have recognized individuals for their leadership in their communities (personal communication, K. Judge, 2018). APRNs across the country have utilized and promoted the HNHN resources. These are all issues that require leadership in multiple arenas, boots on the ground, research, and policy.

SUMMARY

Although the ability to operationalize leadership in a measurable way remains elusive, there is now a growing body of literature that has correlated outcomes with leadership, even when measured or articulated in different ways (Burgess & Curry, 2014; Kelly, Kutney-Lee, Lake, & Aiken, 2013; Wong, Cummings, & Ducharme, 2013). AACN has identified a need for stronger leadership presence in the healthcare system in order to enhance quality care by mandating preparation at the DNP level for advanced practice after 2015 (AACN, 2006).

APRNs may gain skills in a variety of ways: by reading, attending workshops and training, taking courses, and/or working with a mentor. Porter-O'Grady (2011), a leadership expert, interprets the 2011 IOM *The Future of Nursing: Leading Change, Advancing Health* report to mean that each of us as nurses has a fundamental responsibility "for personal and professional growth through efforts that continue individual education and opportunities that develop and advance the exercise of leadership skills."

Second, APRNs need to understand the system and the system politics. APRNs need to be socialized in their graduate education as well as in their professional organizations to study the systems where they are or will be employed. All APRNs should understand the organizational formal and informal aspects of their organizations and reporting relationships. APRNs should carefully review their job descriptions and ascertain how words such as "supervision" and "collaboration" are defined. In essence, how APRNs are described, where they sit in the organization, and what decisions they make and influence are just as important as their clinical expertise in terms of affecting outcomes of care and access to it.

Finally, and quite simply, APRNs need to *show up* at the table. APRNs are often so immersed in practice that they may make the mistake of being unintentionally absent at, or even intentionally avoiding, important system decision-making bodies (formal and informal) because they do not want to engage in "politics." APRNs need to network with their colleagues to ensure adequate representation through themselves or other strong nursing leaders, when discussions or decisions are being carried out that affect their role and the patients for whom they provide care. APRNs must take every opportunity to be present, particularly when invited to the table. Missing these opportunities unfortunately signals disinterest, and lack of professional involvement and allows others to make decisions for them and their patients. Taking these lessons to heart will allow APRNs to inspire, innovate, and influence.

REFERENCES

Agency for Research and Healthcare Quality. (n.d.). Practice-based research networks: Research in everyday practice. Retrieved from https://pbrn.ahrq.gov

Altman, S. H., Butler, A. S., & Shern, L. (Eds.). (2016). *Assessing progress on the Institute of Medicine report: The future of nursing.* Washington, DC: National Academies Press.

American Academy of Family Physicians. (2018). 2018 Match® results for family medicine. Retrieved from https://www.aafp.org/medical-school-residency/program-directors/nrmp.html

American Academy of Nursing. (2015). Raise the voice Edge Runner: Family health and birth center in the developing families center. Retrieved from http://www.aannet.org/initiatives/edge-runners/profiles/edge-runners--family-health-and-birth-center-in-the-developing-families-center

American Association of Colleges of Nursing. (2006). *The essentials of doctoral education for advanced nursing practice.* Washington, DC: Author. Retrieved from http://www.aacnnursing.org/Education-Resources/AACN-Essentials

American Association of Colleges of Nursing. (2011). *The essentials of master's education in nursing.* Washington, DC: Author. Retrieved from http://www.aacnnursing.org/Education-Resources/AACN-Essentials

American Association of Nurse Anesthetists. (2018). AANA calls on healthcare community to use opioid-sparing pain management to prevent addiction and abuse. Retrieved from https://www.aana.com/news/press-releases/2018/05/09/aana-calls-on-healthcare-community-to-use-opioid-sparing-pain-management-to-prevent-addiction-and-abuse

American Association of Nurse Practitioners. (2014). NP infographic. Retrieved from http://www.aanp.org/images/about-nps/npgraphic.pdf

American Association of Nurse Practitioners. (2017). More than 234,000 license nurse practitioners in the United States. Retrieved from https://www.aanp.org/press-room/press-releases/173-press-room/2017-press-releases/2098-more-than-234-000-licensed-nurse-practitioners-in-the-united-states

American Association of Nurse Practitioners. (2018, February 23). Statement by the American Association of Nurse Practitioners on gun violence. Retrieved from

https://www.aanp.org/press-room/press-releases/173-press-room/2018
-press-releases/2181-statement-by-the-american-association-of-nurse
-practitioners-on-gun-violence

American Hospital Association Center for Healthcare Governance. (2014). *2014 National Health Care Governance Survey report.* Retrieved from http://trustees .aha.org/envtrends/Governance-Survey-Report-update.pdf

American Nurses Association. (2015a). *Code of ethics for nurses with interpretive statements.* Silver Spring, MD: Nursebooks.org.

American Nurses Association. (2015b). *Nursing: Scope and standards of practice* (3rd ed.). Silver Spring, MD: Nursebooks.org.

Anen, T., & McElroy, D. (2017). The evolution of the new provider team: Driving cultural change through data. *Nursing Administration Quarterly, 41*(1), 4–10.

Badzek, L., & Turner, M. (2015). 2015 Code of ethics for nurses with interpretive statements: Summary boards: An integrative review. *Nursing Outlook, 65*(4), 361–371. doi:10.1016/j.outlook.2017.01.009

Bahle, J., Majercik, C., Ludwick, R., Bukosky, H., & Frase, D. (2014). At risk care plans: A way to reduce readmissions and adverse events. *Journal of Nursing Care Quality, 30*(3), 200–204. doi:10.1097/NCQ.0000000000000106

Bodenheimer, T., & Bauer, L. (2016). Rethinking the primary care workforce: An expanded role for nurses. *New England Journal of Medicine, 375*(11), 1015–1017. doi:10.1056/NEJMp1606869

Bodenheimer, T., & Sinsky, C. (2014). From triple to quadruple aim: Care of the patient requires care of the provider. *Annals of Family Medicine, 12*(6), 573–576. doi:10.1370/afm.1713

Boyd, D., & Poghosyan, L. (2017). Measuring certified registered nurse anesthetist organizational climate: Instrument adaptation. *Journal of Nursing Measurement, 25*(2), 224–237. doi:10.1891/1061-3749.25.2.224

Burgess, C., & Curry, M. (2014). Transforming the health care environment collaborative. *AORN Journal, 99*(4), 529–539. doi:10.1016/j.aorn.2014.01.012

Canadian NURSE. (2018, January). Amalgamation the next step for B.C.'s professional associations. Retrieved from https://www.canadian-nurse .com/articles/issues/2018/january-february-2018/amalgamation-the-next -step-for-bcs-professional-associations

DiChiacchio, T. (2017). President's message: Reflections on "Healthy Nurse, Healthy Nation". *West Virginia Nurse, 20*(4), 1. Retrieved from https:// www.nursingald.com/uploads/publication/pdf/1579/West_Virginia_ Nurse_11_17.pdf

Disch, J. (2019). Applying a nursing lens to shape policy. In R. M. Patton, M. L. Zalon, & R. Ludwick (Eds.), *Nurses making policy from bedside to boardroom* (2nd ed, pp. 329–356). New York: Springer/Silver Spring, MD: American Nurses Association.

Elliott, N., Begley, C., Sheaf, G., & Higgins, A. (2016). Barriers and enablest to advanced practitioners' ability to enact their leadership role: A scoping review. *International Journal of Nursing Studies, 60,* 24–45. doi:10.1016/j .ijnurstu.2016.03.001

EVERYTOWN For Gun Safety. (n.d.). We are Everytown for Gun Safety. Retrieved from https://everytown.org/who-we-are

Finkelman, A. (2013). The clinical nurse specialist: Leadership in quality improvement. *Clinical Nurse Specialist, 27*(1), 31–35. doi:10.1097/ NUR.0b013e3182776d8f

Fitzgerald, E. M., Myers, J. G., & Clark, P. (2017). Nurses need not be guilty bystanders: Caring for vulnerable immigrant populations. *The Online Journal of Issues in Nursing, 22*(1), 8. doi:10.3912/OJIN.Vol22No01PPT43

Frellick, M. (2017, December 28), Most healthcare providers see gun violence as a public threat. *Medscape Medical News-Clinician Insights.* Retrieved from https://www.medscape.com/viewarticle/890677

Gelinas, L. (2017). Guns and nurses. *American Nurse Today, 12*(1), 4.

Griffis, C., Giron, S., & Darna, J. (2017). The opioid crisis and the certified registered nurse anesthetist: How can we help? *AANA Journal Online,* August, 2017. Retrieved from https://www.aana.com/docs/default-source/aana-journal-web-documents-1/guest-editorial---the-opioid-crisis-and-the-certified-registered-nurse-anesthetist---how-can-we-help.pdf?sfvrsn=76ad4ab1_4

Hirschman, K. B., Shaid, E., McCauley, K., Pauly, M. V., & Naylor, M. D. (2015). Continuity of care: The transitional care model. *Online Journal of Issues in Nursing, 20*(3), 1. doi:10.3912/OJIN.Vol20No03Man01

Hølge-Hazleton, B., Kjerholt, M., Berthelsen, C. B., & Thomsen, T. G. (2016) Integrating researchers in clinical practice: A challenging, but necessary task for nurse leaders. *Journal of Nursing Management, 24*, 464–474. doi:10.1111/jonm.12345

Institute of Medicine. (2001). *Crossing the quality chasm: A new health system for the 21st century.* Washington, DC: National Academies Press.

Institute of Medicine. (2004). *Insuring American's health: Principles and recommendations.* Washington, DC: National Academies Press.

Institute of Medicine. (2011). *The future of nursing: Leading change, advancing health.* Washington, DC: The National Academies Press.

The Joint Commission. (2017). Sentinel event alert 57: The essential role of leadership in developing a safety culture. Retrieved from https://www.jointcommission.org/sea_issue_57/

Judge, K. (2018). *Healthy nurse, healthy nation.* Presented at the meeting of Frances Payne Bolton School of Nursing Case Western Reserve University, Cleveland, Ohio.

Kelly, D., Kutney-Lee, A., Lake, E., & Aiken, L. H. (2013). The critical care work environment and nurse reported health care associated infections. *American Journal of Critical Care, 22*(6), 482–489. doi:10.4037/ajcc2013298

Khoury, C. M., Blizzard, R., Wright-Moore, L., & Hassmiller, S. (2011). Nursing leadership from bedside to boardroom: A Gallup national survey of opinion leaders. *Journal of Nursing Administration, 41*(7–8), 299–305. doi:10.1097/NNA.0b013e3182250a0d

Kohn, L. T., Corrigan, J. M., & Donaldson, M. S. (Eds.). (2000). *To err is human: Building a safer health system.* Washington, DC: National Academies Press.

Krejci, J. W., & Malin, S. (1997). Impact of leadership development on leadership competencies. *Nursing Economic$, 15*(5), 235–241.

Krejci, J. W., & Malin, S. (2001, October). *Leadership critical incidents, before and after leadership development.* Presented at the National Nursing Administration Research Conference, Cincinnati, OH.

Krejci, J. W., & Malin, S. (2006). Leadership skills and expertise: Keys to APN success in health care systems. In M. P. Mirr Jansen & M. Zwygart-Stauffacher (Eds.), *Advanced practice nursing: Core concepts for professional role development* (3rd ed., pp. 61–78). New York, NY: Springer Publishing.

Lopatine, E., Donald, F., DiCenso, A., Martin-Misener, R., Kirkpatrick, K., Bryant-Lukosius, D., . . . Marshall, D. A. (2017). Economic evaluation of nurse practitioner and clinical nurse specialist roles: A methodological review. *International Journal of Nursing Studies, 72,* 71–82. doi:10.1016/j .ijnurstu.2017.04.01

Murphy, J., Goodman, D., Johnson, M. C., Terplan, M. (2018). The comprehensive addiction and recovery act: Opioid use disorder and midwifery practice. *American Journal of Obstetrics & Gynecology, 131*(3), 542–544. doi:10.1097/ AOG.0000000000002493

National Association of Community Health Centers. (2013). Expanding access to primary care: The role of nurse practitioners, physician assistants, and certified nurse midwives in health center workforce. Fact Sheet. Retrieved from http://www.nachc.org/wp-content/uploads/2016/02/Workforce_FS_0913.pdf

National Council of State Boards of Nursing. (2014). APRN consensus model. Retrieved from https://ncsbn.org/aprn-consensus.htm

National Organization of Nurse Practitioner Faculties. (2018, May). The doctor of nursing practice degree: Entry to nurse practitioner practice by 2025. Retrieved from https://cdn.ymaws.com/www.nonpf.org/resource/resmgr/ dnp/v3_05.2018_NONPF_DNP_Stateme.pdf

Naylor, M. D., Shaid, E. C., Carpenter, D., Gass, B., Levine, C., Li, J., . . . Williams, M. D. (2017). Components of comprehensive and effective transitional care. *Journal of the American Geriatrics Society, 65*(6), 1119–1125. doi:10.1111/jgs.14782

Newhouse, R. P., Stanik-Hutt, J., White, K. M., Johantgen, M., Bass, E. B., Zangaro, G., . . . Weiner, J. P. (2011). Advanced practice nurse outcomes 1990–2008: A systematic review. *Nursing Economic$, 29*(5), 230–250.

Nurses on Boards Coalition. (2017). About. Our story. Retrieved from https:// www.nursesonboardscoalition.org/about

Odom-Forren, J. (2016). Gun violence: A public health concern. *Journal of Perianesthesia Nursing, 31*(4), 463–464. doi:10.1016/j.jopan.2016.06.003

Patton, R., Zalon, M., & Ludwick, R. (2019). Implementing the plan. In R. Patton, M. Zalon, & R. Ludwick (Eds.), *Nurses making policy: From bedside to boardroom.* (pp. 261–290) New York, NY: Springer Publishing; Silver Spring, MD: American Nurses Association.

Poghosyan, L., Liu, J., & Norful, A. A. (2017). Nurse practitioners as primary care providers with their patient panels and organizational structures: A cross-sectional study. *International Journal of Nursing Studies, 74,* 1–7. doi:10.1016/j .ijnurstu.2017.05.004

Poghosyan, L., Liu, J., Shang, J., & D'Aunno, T. (2017). Practice environments and job satisfaction and turnover intentions of nurse practitioners: Implications for primary care workforce capacity. *Healthcare Management Review, 42*(2), 162–171. doi:10.1097/HMR.0000000000000094

Porter-O'Grady, T. (2011). Leadership at all levels. *Nursing Management, 42*(5), 32–27. doi:10.1097/01.NUMA.0000396347.49552.86

Rantz, M. J., Birtley, N. M., Flesner, M., Crecelius, C., & Murray, C. (2017). Call to action: APRNs in U.S. nursing homes to improve care and reduce costs. *Nursing Outlook, 65*(6), 689–696. doi:10.1016/j.outlook.2017.08.011

Rechtoris, M. (2017). 3 Key thoughts from American Association of Nurse Anesthetists incoming president Bruce Weiner. *Becker's ASC Review.* June 22, 2017. Retrieved from https://www.beckersasc.com/anesthesia/3-key -thoughts-from-american-association-of-nurse-anesthetists-incoming -president-bruce-weiner.html

Steward, J. G., McNulty, R., Quinn Griffin, M. T., & Fitzpatrick, J. J. (2014). Psychological empowerment and structural empowerment among nurse practitioners. *Journal of the American Academy of Nurse Practitioners, 22*(1), 27–34. doi:10.1111/j.1745-7599.2009.00467.x

Substance Abuse and Mental Health Services Administration. (2018). Qualify for nurse practitioners (NP) and Physician Assistants (PAs) waiver. Retrieved from https://www.samhsa.gov/programs-campaigns/medication-assisted-treatment/training-materials- resources/qualify-np-pa-waivers

Sundean, L. J., Polifroni, E. C., Libal, K., & McGrath, J. M. (2017). Nurses on health care governing boards: An integrative review. *Nursing Outlook, 65*(4), 361–371. doi:10.1016/j.outlook.2017.01.009

Sundean, L. J., Polifroni, E. C., Libal, K., & McGrath, J. M. (2018). The rationale for nurses on boards in the voices of nurses who serve. *Nursing Outlook, 66*(3), 222–232. doi:10.1016/j.outlook.2017.11.005

Tsai, T. C., Jha, A. K., Gawande, A. A., Huckman, R. S., Bloom, N., & Sadun, R. (2015). Hospital board and management practices are strongly related to hospital performance on clinical quality metrics. *Health Affairs, 34*(8), 1304–1311. doi:10.1377/hlthaff.2014.1282

Williams, S. D., & Phillips, J.M. (2019). Eliminating health inequities through national and global policy. In R. M. Patton, M. L. Zalon, & R. Ludwick (Eds.), *Nurses making policy from bedside to boardroom* (2nd ed, pp. 391–423). New York: Springer; Silver Spring, MD: American Nurses Association.

Wong, C. A., Cumming, G. G., & Ducharme, L. (2013). The relationship between nursing leadership and patient outcomes: A systematic review update. *Journal of Nursing Management, 21*(5), 709–724. doi:10.1111/jonm.12116

Xue, Y. & Intrator, O. (2016). Cultivating the role of nurse practitioners in providing primary care to vulnerable populations in an era of health-care reform. *Policy, Politics and Nursing Practice, 17*, 24–31. doi: 10.1177/1527154416645539

Zielinski, T. E. (2017, October 10). Gun violence and working together. President's message. *National Association of Pediatric Nurse Practitioners.* Retrieved from https://www.napnap.org/gun-violence-and-working-together

IMPLEMENTATION OF THE APRN ROLE

Kathryn A. Blair

8

ADVANCED CLINICAL DECISION MAKING

Medical errors are the third leading cause of death in the United States (Makary & Daniel, 2016). Every day, nurses, including APRNs, are required to make clinical decisions that impact patient care. Clinical decisions are based on clinical or diagnostic reasoning and clinical decision-making skills. Clinical decision making in advanced practice nursing occurs as a continuous, purposeful, theory- and knowledge-based process of assessment, analysis, strategic planning, and intentional follow-up. It is both a cognitive and affective problem-solving activity for defining patient problems and selecting appropriate management approaches (Buckingham & Adams, 2000; Tiffen, Corbridge, & Slimmer, 2014).

The role of the APRN is multifaceted, and the scope of decision making is similarly complex. It incorporates health promotion, disease prevention, risk reduction, management of functional health needs, subjective concerns, program planning, biomedical diagnostics, and disease management. Large amounts of data are elicited, sorted, and organized into meaningful patterns. Conducted within the context of nurse–patient relationships, APRN clinical decision making is frequently characterized by changing health circumstances and complex social variables. The nursing and biomedical decision making involved may be straightforward or of low, moderate, or high complexity.

DECISION-MAKING PROCESSES: RESEARCH IN CLINICAL REASONING

Research in clinical judgment and decision making has been an important area of study for more than 50 years. Much of the decision-making and problem-solving research began in the cognitive sciences (Newell & Simon, 1972; Tversky & Kahneman, 1974), with early application to diagnostic reasoning and clinical problem solving in nursing and medicine (Elstein, 1976; Elstein, Shulman, & Sprafka, 1978; Hammond, 1964;

Hammond, Kelly, & Castellan, 1966). Strong interest in this field of study has continued with distinctions between clinical reasoning in nursing and in medicine. Clinical reasoning is the cognitive processes used to make a diagnosis and treatment plan (Pinnock, Young, Spence, Henning, & Hazell, 2015). Nursing clinical reasoning is based on the interrelatedness of intuition, analytical processes, context, and experience (Cappelletti, Engel, & Prentice, 2014). Medical reasoning is based on knowledge, experience, and pattern recognition with validation through confirmatory evidence and intuition (Pinnock et al., 2015). As can be seen, there is considerable overlap in clinical reasoning processes used by medicine and nursing. Advanced practice nursing involves a complex blending of both nursing and medical clinical reasoning and decision making.

COMMONALITIES IN CLINICAL REASONING ACROSS HEALTH DISCIPLINES

Clinical reasoning is fundamental to clinical decision making in that it is the antecedent to a decision and action (Simmons, 2010). Several common or core features of clinical reasoning across health disciplines have been identified in the research (Higgs & Jones, 2008). One core element is clinical knowledge that is interdependent and fundamental to clinical reasoning. As clinical knowledge expands, the complexity of knowledge structures increases (Higgs & Jones, 2008) resulting in refinement of clinical reasoning skills.

A second core feature of clinical reasoning is an array of higher-order cognitive skills and processes. Various theorists identify these higher order cognitive skills differently, but some that are emphasized include *clinical appraisal* (Brookfield, 2008), *categorization* (Loftus & Higgs, 2008), and *propositional knowledge* (Titchen & Higgs, 2000). "Clinical appraisal" consists of critically evaluating the totality of presenting information for the most relevant clinical features and accurately defining what those features represent. An example of critical appraisal is assessing a patient to determine the pertinent positives or negatives. "Categorization" is a way of both learning complex content and using relevant features and pattern recognition to relate novel instances to known categories. For instance, categorization would be used to judge the level of severity or acuity of patient presentation. Risk stratification is an important application of categorization, selecting management approaches based on the level of severity or risk and statistically predicted patient care outcomes. "Propositional knowledge" incorporates hypothesis generation and the development of plausible and probabilistic relationships between events. For example, the APRN uses propositional knowledge to hypothesize the most probable diagnosis, given a certain patient presentation. When clinicians make prospective predictions about the likely course of a condition based on clinical signs and symptoms, they are engaging in a combination of categorization and probabilistic reasoning.

The third feature associated with clinical reasoning is that it is highly context dependent. The context within which clinical reasoning occurs is determined by the patient's health concern(s), the specific health setting, the care provider's disciplinary background and level of experience, the patient's unique personal context, the stage of case management (e.g., initial diagnosis vs. long-term stabilization vs. exacerbation management), and elements of the wider healthcare environment (Higgs & Jones, 2008). Research attending to context-specific factors demonstrates that expert clinical reasoning is complex, interpretive, and personalized. Other clinicians have likened this to good clinical jazz (Hamm Flynn & Becker, 2004). Good jazz needs structure and improvisation. Structure in healthcare is the clinical evidence, and improvisation is the patient's personal situation. A good clinician blends these two components uniquely for each patient as a part of clinical reasoning and decision making.

Finally, information storage and retrieval or script theory (Lubarsky, Dory, Audétat, Custers, & Charlin, 2015) can be applied to clinical reasoning. Script theory offers a means to explain how information is saved and recovered to be used in the interpretation of events. Healthcare providers use "illness scripts" to identify symptom patterns, recognize similarities and differences in disease states, and make predictions (Lubarsky et al., 2015). As with all elements of clinical reasoning, knowledge organization or networks are expanded through experience and education.

Clinical Decision Making

Multiple approaches have been used to study clinical decision making. Repeated themes in the literature include information processing model, intuitive-humanistic model, and cognitive continuum model (Tanner, 2006).

Information processing model uses hypothetico-deductive approach (Banning, 2008), which uses rational logic. This process includes cue recognition and interpretation, hypothesis generation, and evaluation (Chen, Hsu, Chang, & Lin, 2016; Thompson, Moorley, & Barratt, 2017). This model requires using propositional representation (i.e., if A then X; Abuzour, Lewis, & Tully, 2018). The process begins with identifying facts (history), generating a hypothesis based on observations combined with knowledge and experience, then assessment (physical examination) resulting in the final hypothesis. Information processing provides a better theoretical match for the dynamic environments and ambiguity of decisions in clinical practice, because it logically moves from identification of cues, step-by-step analysis, evaluation, and reevaluation until the problem is solved (Chen et al., 2016; Thompson et al., 2017).

The intuitive-humanistic model uses intuition and experience. Intuition refers to the capacity of the expert clinician to process quickly large amounts of complex data, simultaneously discern patterns, and act on hypotheses without consciously naming all the factors involved in his or her decision making. An intuitive decision is made on the basis of sudden awareness of knowledge, which is based on cues and pattern recognition (Banning, 2008; Hedberg & Larsson, 2003). It is the highly expert application of rational processes and cue analysis, occurring at a pace too rapid for each step to be discretely named or recognized.

How different professionals use intuition varies. For example, nurse-midwives use intuition as a way of knowing, while physicians use intuition when analytical thinking is inadequate (Rosciano, Lindell, Bryer, & DiMarco, 2016; Woolley & Kostopoulou, 2013).

Cognitive continuum model suggests a range of analytical thinking approaches with varying combinations of intuitive and analytical thinking (Rycroft-Malone, Fontenla, Seers, & Bick, 2009). In this theory, the task structure (weighing and combining information to make judgments) and cognitive processes determine the degree of intuition and/or analysis used by the decision maker (Cader, Campbell, & Watson, 2005). Particularly salient here are these three features of task properties: (a) the complexity of task structure (number and redundancy of cues, form of an accurate organizing principle), (b) the ambiguity of task content (availability of organizing principles, familiarity with the task, and possibility of high accuracy), and (c) the form of task presentation (task decomposition, cue definition, and response time). The task structure (well structured vs. ill structured) governs the mode cognition. If a person weighs certain cues incorrectly (ill-structured task structure) then the judgment is flawed (Cader et al., 2005). For example, a patient presents with normal vital signs, no acute distress but is having indigestion. Here if the clinician weighs the vital signs and presentation greater than the history or risk factors then the clinician could miss the acute myocardial infarction (MI) because of the atypical presentation. In this model, greater analytical thinking is assumed to be related to fewer cues, less redundancy of cues, and more complex procedures for combining evidence to result in correct answers. The availability of organizing principles, greater task familiarity, and the possibility for high accuracy also contribute to greater use of formal reasoning.

Analytical decision making as related to clinical decision making relies on a more structured process of identifying options and possible outcomes, assigning values to the outcomes, and determining probability relationships between the options and anticipated outcomes. Formal (mathematically based) or informal (conceptually based) models are used to systematize decision making using decision trees, grids, or decision flow diagrams (Narayan, Corcoran-Perry, Drew, Hoyman, & Lewis, 2003). Decision analysis is useful for evaluation of medical treatment options, cost analysis, sensitivity analysis, quality improvement decisions, and policy decisions (Narayan et al., 2003).

Moving from data collection to diagnosis is difficult for novice APRNs. As with all nurses, APRNs move from using domain-general knowledge to domain-specific knowledge in clinical decision making (Pretz & Folse, 2011). Novices will rely more on analytic process with common situations and rely more on intuition with novel problems (Price, Zulkosky, White, & Pretz, 2016). For the inexperienced APRN, every judgment or decision has some degree of uncertainty, which is the probability that specific signs and symptoms are associated with particular conditions (Thompson,

Aitken, Brown, & Dowding, 2013). Ways to foster and support clinical decision making in the novice APRNs can be found in using clinical practice guidelines to reduce the uncertainty and mentoring.

Experience in the role of an RN is an important variable in examining factors that influence level of decision making. In a study of 70 entry-level nurse practitioners, Sands (2001) found that entry-level nurse practitioners with at least 5 years of RN experience demonstrated stronger scores on the test of diagnostic reasoning. Participants with less than 2 years of RN experience were at increased risk for inadequate reasoning through the clinical problem.

APRN Practice Focus

One factor that can be used to distinguish clinical decision making in advanced practice nursing from other autonomous healthcare providers is the focus of APRN practice. Smith (1995) identified the core of advanced practice nursing as lying within nursing's disciplinary perspectives on health, healing, person–environment interactions, and nurse–patient relationships. Huch (1995) echoes this in identifying the need to use nursing theory as the basis for advanced nursing practice.

APRNs focus their clinical decision making on health promotion, health protection, disease prevention, and management of health concerns (National Association of Clinical Nurse Specialists [NACNS], 2017; National Organization of Nurse Practitioner Faculties [NONPF], 2017). As outlined by nurse practitioner and clinical nurse specialist organizations, health promotion activities include lifestyle concerns, principles of lifestyle change, and behavioral change. Health protection includes knowledge of health risks, use of epidemiologic principles, and community/population-level measures to protect health. Disease prevention includes primary and secondary prevention measures addressing major chronic illness, disability, and communicable disease. Management of health concerns focuses on assessing, diagnosing, monitoring, and coordinating the care of individuals and populations (NACNS, 2017; NONPF, 2017). Depending on the APRN's role and specialty preparation, the practice focuses include both disease- and non-disease–based etiologies that affect health, wellness, and quality of life. For nurse practitioners, the focus is generally on providing direct patient care. For clinical nurse specialists, the focus tends to be on influencing the outcomes of care more widely within an area of population focus, at individual patient, population, and health system levels. With the advent of the doctorate of nursing practice (DNP), practice doctorate APRNs are educated to practice with increased emphasis on the healthcare system and population healthcare outcomes (American Association of Colleges of Nursing [AACN], 2004; NONPF, 2017).

APRN Practice Frameworks

Advanced practice nursing is holistic, patient-centered, theory-driven, population- and evidence-based practice that incorporates professional autonomy, application of knowledge, critical analysis, and synthesis of data in decision making. Some of these characteristics are built into nationally recommended educational guidelines for advanced practice educational programs (AACN, 2006; NACNS, 2017; NONPF, 2017). For example, the core competencies for nurse practitioner and clinical nurse specialist clinical decision making incorporate the following expectations for practice: critical analysis of data (NONPF, 2017) and synthesis of data, knowledge, and expertise (NACNS, 2017). Like NONPF and NACNS, the American College of Nurse-Midwives (ACNM) core competencies include evaluation and application of clinical knowledge in management of patients (ACNM, 2014). AACN's (2006) *The Essentials of Doctoral Education for Advanced Practice Nursing* outlines advanced clinical decision making as part of the core of APRN work: "Demonstrate sound critical thinking and clinical decision making" (p. 23).

An important feature of clinical decision making in advanced practice nursing is that the nursing focus continues to be evident in daily practice. This can be done, for example, by making an effort to understand the meanings that patients attribute to their health situation; by learning about the patients' lived social world, support systems, and role responsibilities; and by working with patients to identify personal and social health obstacles or facilitators. Several additional approaches for incorporating basic nursing perspectives into APRN care are listed in Exhibit 8.1.

In addition to the specialty knowledge required for health and illness management, these patient-centered, holistic dimensions of clinical decision making are necessary to maintain the quality of APRN care and the ability to distinguish advanced practice nursing from other forms of autonomous health practice.

Exhibit 8.1 APPROACHES FOR INCORPORATING CORE NURSING PERSPECTIVES INTO APRN CARE

- Make an effort to understand meanings that patients attribute to their health situation.
- Learn about patients' lived social world, support systems, and role responsibilities.
- Work with patients to identify their personal and social health obstacles or facilitators.
- Determine patients' preferences for and abilities to participate in healthcare decision making and self-health management.
- Jointly determine appropriate healthcare goals and priorities.
- Work with patients as they struggle through personal crises, losses, or transitions.
- Learn about patients' spiritual points of view and how they view the relationship between their health status and spirituality.

CLINICAL DECISION MAKING AS UNDERSTOOD FROM PRACTICE

In addition to influences from nursing research, theory, and professional organizations, much has been learned about APRN clinical decision making directly from clinical practice as well as research and practice experiences from other disciplines.

Skilled communication and interaction are essential components of clinical decision making at all levels, whether the APRN is posing wide-field or focused inquiries, clarifying diverse perspectives, providing guidance for lifestyle health behaviors, or evaluating a patient's responses to treatment. As Chase (2011) points out, clinical decision making is not a process that occurs with the APRN in isolation. It occurs as dialogue and interaction between the patient and provider, with experiences of satisfaction significantly influenced by the quality of communication and engagement with the clinical situation (Benner, Stannard, & Hooper, 1996).

Most descriptions of APRN clinical decision making begin with an expanded nursing process model that integrates elements of hypothetico-deductive reasoning. Carnevali and Thomas (1993) describe the diagnostic reasoning process in nursing as reviewing pre-encounter data, entering into the assessment situation, collecting the database, coalescing cues into working clusters, selecting pivotal cues or cue clusters, determining possible diagnostic explanations, further comparing the clinical situation with diagnostic categories, and assigning the diagnosis.

White, Nativio, Kobert, and Engberg (1992) and Noon (2014) outline a clinical decision-making framework for APRNs that adds elements from hypothetico-deductive reasoning. Hypotheses formed are used to guide the process of inquiry (i.e., decisions about how to focus the history, examination, and diagnostic testing). The process outlined by White et al. adds many of these elements to nursing clinical decision making: reviewing pre-encounter data, generating early hypotheses, engaging in clinical inquiry, determining working hypotheses, conducting diagnostic testing, testing the final hypothesis, specifying the diagnosis, determining patient management, and evaluating the total clinical situation.

Chase (2004) configures this process specifically for nurse practitioner practice. She lists the phases of clinical judgment as follows: conducting an early wide-field search for the primary concerns, generating an early hypothesis on probable causes of the concerns, engaging in focused data acquisition related to supporting the active hypotheses and ruling out other serious conditions, evaluating various hypotheses by clustering and analyzing the data for the appropriate fit with diagnostic categories, naming the priority problems, determining appropriate therapeutic goals, determining an appropriate management plan, evaluating the effectiveness of the clinical process, and confirming or revising the diagnoses and plans.

In advanced practice nursing, each of these approaches might be appropriate for differing clinical scenarios or problems and stages. The decision-making processes can be used with both disease- and non-disease–based concerns, as well as with medical or nursing diagnoses. Hypothetico-deductive models are perceived generally to be more useful during data collection and implementation. Intuitive–interpretive models are reported in use more during data processing, whereas during planning both models are perceived to be equally in use (Bjork & Hamilton, 2011). Clinical nurse specialists might place less relative emphasis on the biomedical diagnostic content, tending more often to work collaboratively with medical care providers for these decision-making components. Nurse practitioners emphasize greater autonomy in medical diagnostic and treatment elements, but place less overall emphasis on specialty nursing care and system-level thinking. With either role, however, keys to the process are clinician characteristics of perception and engagement, discipline-specific knowledge, commitment to quality practice, and know-how related to "think clinically" under differing clinical role expectations. Skilled clinical decision making occurs as an intentional process of problem solving, critical thinking, and reflection in action (Benner et al., 1996). It is guided by content expertise and deliberate decisions about how to proceed through the current clinical encounter as well as reasoning through the anticipated trajectory of the health concern.

Relationship Between Critical Thinking and Clinical Decision Making

Critical thinking skills can assist with sorting out the aforementioned complexities. In a 1990 consensus statement on critical thinking, Facione (1990) defines "critical thinking" as a tool of inquiry characterized by "purposeful, self-regulatory judgment" resulting in "interpretation, analysis, evaluation, and inference" (p. 3). It is not "rote, mechanical, unreflective" (p. 8) or disconnected from other thought activities. Critical thinkers are able to examine and evaluate their own reasoning processes and apply critical thinking skills in a variety of contexts. The consensus components of critical thinking are provided in Table 8.1.

Scheffer and Rubenfeld (2000) used a Delphi method to develop a consensus statement on critical thinking in nursing, describing both its affective and cognitive components. In addition to the components described by Facione (1990), the nursing study identified creativity and intuition as two additional affective components.

Although "critical thinking" is defined by educators as a broad set of cognitive skills and habits of mind, applying these skills in clinical practice requires large amounts of discipline-specific knowledge. Research-based understandings of relationships between critical thinking and clinical decision making are not yet well developed. Clearly, however, the skills of interpretation, analysis, evaluation, and inference are highly necessary in advanced clinical practice, where both nursing and medical knowledge must be distinguished and applied. Well-developed critical thinking skills and habits of mind are an important foundation for the

TABLE 8.1 Consensus Components of Critical Thinking

Critical Thinking Skill	Identified Components of the Skill
Interpretation evaluation	Categorizing Clarifying meanings Assessing claims and arguments
Inference	Examining evidence Drawing conclusions Proposing alternatives
Explanation	Stating results Presenting arguments Justifying procedures
Self-regulation	Self-examination Self-correction
Dispositional skills	Inquisitiveness Eagerness for reliable information

discipline-specific processes of clinical thinking required in advanced practice nursing.

Organizing Clinical Knowledge for Practice

Ultimately, cognitively organizing diagnostic and treatment concepts for clinical practice is hard work that individual practitioners must do for themselves (Carnevali & Thomas, 1993). A systematic approach is recommended, based on building a repertoire of specific diagnostic/prognostic/treatment concepts and exemplars from practice. For knowledge from nursing, such cognitive categories could be built around human response categories, broad nursing diagnostic categories, functional health patterns, or population health needs. As the depth of knowledge increases with various phenomena, increasing expertise is developed relating to manifestations, underlying mechanisms, risk factors and complications, prognostic variables and anticipated trajectories, and efficacy of treatment options. Increasing depth of medical knowledge, on the other hand, relates to the complexity of pathophysiologic explanations and relationships, variations in disease attributes and manifestations, use and interpretation of diagnostic tests, increasingly precise probabilistic and prognostic thinking, and increasingly sophisticated risk–benefit analyses.

Building interprofessional and nursing knowledge for advanced clinical practice is an ongoing process of study and practice. The complexity of the healthcare system and patients requires interprofessional collaboration and communication to ensure sound clinical decision making resulting in patient-centered care (ten Ham, Ricks, Rooyen, & Jordan, 2017).

Clinical Decision Making in Health–Illness Management

In the realm of biomedical knowledge, diagnosis and management of health–illness place greater emphasis on probabilistic thinking and inferential or inductive reasoning, with greater attention to the specificity of the data and the precision of decisions. Rational justification, confirmation and elimination strategies, and judgment of value are critical reasoning skills within this domain. The first step in the diagnostic process is hypothesis activation or the identification of diagnostic possibilities. Hypothesis activation is based on preliminary information such as the patient's age, medical history, clinical appearance, and presenting concerns. The next step is information gathering and interpretation. This step is strongly influenced by probabilistic thinking and inductive reasoning. The likelihood of various diagnostic hypotheses is carefully considered, with new data used to assist with confirming, eliminating, or discriminating between diagnoses. The working diagnosis is then selected based on causal attribution (i.e., whether all physiologic features are consistent with the favored diagnosis and underlying cause).

This hypotheses generation and revision occur in both novices and experienced clinicians, although the experienced clinicians' hypotheses are of higher quality. It is also noted that some of diagnostic reasoning variation between novices and experts does not appear to be problem-solving variations but instead dependent on the experts' increasing use of pattern recognition based on their knowledge organization and experiences. Retrieval of those patterns can be based on previously experienced exemplars or more abstract prototypes. Thus, expert–novice differences can be somewhat explained in terms of the volume of experts' experienced exemplars available for pattern recognition (Schwartz & Elstein, 2008).

The working diagnosis becomes the basis for therapeutic action, prognostic assessment, or further diagnostic testing. Final verification of the diagnostic hypothesis is determined through tests of adequacy and coherence. "Adequacy" ascertains whether the suspected disease process encompasses all of the patient's findings. "Coherence" determines whether all the patient's illness manifestations are appropriate for the suspected health concern. The final diagnostic hypothesis then becomes the basis for treatment decisions, in combination with evidence-based analysis of treatment options and patient-specific cost–benefit analyses for each of the treatment options.

Probability decision making is used to narrow the hypotheses. As new data are obtained, each diagnostic probability is recalculated. The posttest probability is then used to guide additional data collection and to generate the pretest probability of the usefulness of that data. The formal mathematical rule for this process is Bayes's theorem. Inaccurate application of Bayes' theorem explains some of the errors that occur in the diagnostic reasoning process, such as overestimation of pretest probability. The clinician tends to overemphasize rare conditions with inflation of pretest probabilities because those are the cases most memorable. In general, small probabilities are overestimated and large probabilities are underestimated by clinicians. Experience and mentoring are clearly necessary to learn biomedical decision making.

Errors in Clinical Reasoning

Several types of clinical practice errors are described in the literature, broadly grouped as skill-based errors, knowledge-based errors, and errors caused by psychoemotional factors. Skill- and knowledge-based errors in this context are not the same as not possessing the necessary skills or knowledge. Rather, the assumption is made that the necessary skills and knowledge are present, but errors are made in their application. Skill-based failures include lack of attention at crucial moments, distraction or preoccupation resulting in missed crucial events, failure to carry out specific activities or intentions, and errors resulting from mixing up behaviors or activities.

Knowledge-based failures include errors resulting from the use of heuristics. Despite the value of heuristics, overuse has the potential to increase errors in clinical judgment. Care must be taken to maintain a reflective balance between formal reasoning and the use of knowledge from practice. Being overconfident about the correctness of one's knowledge (overconfidence bias), using personal case experience alone as the basis for a decision (hindsight bias), and neglecting the underlying base rate of a health condition when diagnosing or treating (base rate neglect) are three common types of errors in the application of practice knowledge (Thompson, 2002). Conservatism is the failure to revise diagnostic probabilities as new data are presented. Confirmation bias is the tendency to seek information that confirms a diagnosis but failing to efficiently test competing hypotheses (Schwartz & Elstein, 2008). Psychological commitment takes place early in the hypothesis generation process, and clinicians find it difficult to restructure the problem. A psychoemotional error occurs (value-induced bias) when the clinician exaggerates the probability of a diagnosis when one possible outcome is perceived as exceedingly unfavorable compared with others (Buckingham, 2002).

Errors in the information-processing components of practice are also categorized using terminology from hypothesis testing. Type I errors, claiming a significant difference when there is none (analogous to rejecting a true null hypothesis), occur in clinical decision making through naming a clinical problem when there is none. In this situation, the disease model used by the clinician may be too broad, perhaps causing the clinician to overestimate the allowable range of variation for findings in a given diagnosis and not recognizing that the actual findings are at odds with the favored diagnosis.

Type II errors, claiming no significant difference when there is one (analogous to accepting a false null hypothesis), occur with failing to name a clinical problem when there is one. This may occur through missing significant clinical indicators of a health problem or failing to realize the significance of specific signs or symptoms. A correct diagnosis may have been eliminated even though the findings are consistent with the diagnosis.

Type III errors occur in solving the wrong problem, phrasing the problem incorrectly, setting the boundaries or scope of the problem too narrowly, or failing to think systematically (Kassirer & Kopelman, 1991). Based on this information, habits of practice that promote sound clinical reasoning can be cultivated by the APRN. These are summarized in Table 8.2.

Evidence Practice

A final aspect of APRN decision making is the increasingly important role of a variety of tools that can be used to support and enhance clinical decision making. A listing of these tools is provided in Exhibit 8.2.

Multiple nursing standards of practice have been developed by the American Nurses Association and by specialty nursing organizations. These are organized both by specialty practice areas and by practice-related frameworks, such as the nursing code of ethics and the nursing social policy statement. They continue to serve as basic frameworks for nursing practice and are especially important documents for clinical nurse specialists. The North American Nursing Diagnosis Association (NANDA)/Nursing Intervention Classification (NIC)/Nursing Outcomes Classification (NOC) taxonomies, although not necessarily complete and not universally used, help organize ways of naming nursing diagnoses and begin the process of building common expectancies for nursing interventions and outcomes. Midlevel theories help guide practice by addressing the needs or experiences of specific populations, typically relative to one or more human responses or areas of concern. Incorporating information or concepts from midlevel theories is an excellent way to begin addressing the holistic care considerations of healthcare populations and build depth at an advanced practice level.

Evidence-based practice has been described as basing clinical decisions and practice on the best available evidence (Melnyk & Fineout-Overholt, 2011). Not all elements of practice are based on empirical evidence, however. Many areas of practice do not have adequate bodies of evidence. In addition, context-specific problems sometimes warrant decisions not addressed by the research literature. Thus, it is imperative that critical thinking, research appraisal, and clinical decision-making skills be used in combination with one another. Typically, evidence-based practice is assumed to refer to external, population-based evidence derived through systematic research. There is the expectation that APRNs will seek the available evidence and use this evidence to inform their decision making in the context of a patient's unique situation.

Evidence-based practice guidelines can be formalized by specific managed care organizations with the expectation that the guidelines are used to direct practice, or they may simply refer to concise informational outlines and algorithms intended to assist clinicians with the massive

TABLE 8.2 Habits That Promote Sound Clinical Reasoning in Advanced Practice Nursing

Phase of Clinical Reasoning	Habits That Promote Sound Reasoning
Data acquisition	Use a systematic and comprehensive approach. Use nursing and medical hypotheses in combination with a systems approach to focus the data collection. Integrate new findings into the emerging model. Search for and attend to both confirming and disconfirming data. Critically evaluate the significance and reliability of findings. Attend to variations in clinical attributes and manifestations.
Hypothesis generation	Formulate preliminary hypotheses early in the encounter. Develop reasonable competing hypotheses. Remain vigilant for serious or life-threatening conditions. Use the hypotheses as models against which to seek and compare findings. Adjust the hypotheses as new data emerge. Carefully compare the hypotheses to reliable information on manifestations, prevalence, and probability. Eliminate hypotheses that fail to remain tenable.
Diagnostic testing	Consider test results as further probability information. Decide whether a test result could alter the probability of disease enough to alter management. Use highly sensitive tests (low rate of false-negative results) to exclude serious disease. Use highly specific tests (low rate of false-positive results) to confirm a diagnosis.
Hypothesis evaluation	Determine the "working hypothesis." If competing hypotheses remain, determine a strategy for discriminating between them. Test the hypothesis for coherence, adequacy, and parsimony. Avoid premature closure. Continue testing the working hypothesis against test results, clinical course, and response to therapy.
Comprehensive care	Identify the most fundamental problems and concerns. Incorporate risk stratification. Include disease- and non-disease–based perspectives. Incorporate nursing theory, human responses, and personhood. Include health promotion, disease prevention, and risk reduction. Engage the patient as a partner in care.
Goal setting	Include the patient in establishing goals. Determine management priorities and plan care accordingly. Identify specific and realistic goals for treatment. Incorporate clinical standards in goal setting.

(continued)

TABLE 8.2   Habits That Promote Sound Clinical Reasoning in Advanced Practice Nursing
(continued)

Phase of Clinical Reasoning	Habits That Promote Sound Reasoning
Determination of management plans	Employ intervention modalities from both nursing and medical perspectives. Initiate effective care for emergency or life-threatening conditions. Consult with appropriate colleagues in complex care situations. Consider patient's social context, preferences, abilities, lifestyle, and individual needs. Anticipate and discuss possible conflicts in values, priorities, and beliefs. Use evidence-based therapies appropriately. Consider treatment efficacy as compared to risks, costs, and desired outcomes. Think ahead to probabilistic disease progression needs. Incorporate evidence-based approaches, accepted treatment guidelines, and current standards of care. Provide effective and appropriate management for comorbidities.

Source: Adapted from Chase, S. K. (2004). *Clinical judgment and communication in nurse practitioner practice*. Philadelphia, PA: F. A. Davis.

Exhibit 8.2 TOOLS TO SUPPORT AND ENHANCE CLINICAL DECISION MAKING IN ADVANCED CLINICAL PRACTICE

Nursing Standards of Practice

NANDA/NIC/NOC

Midlevel theories

Evidence-based practice guidelines

Web-based information systems

Smartphone applications (apps)

Electronic health record systems

NANDA, North American Nursing Diagnosis Association; NIC, Nursing Intervention Classification; NOC, Nursing Outcomes Classification.

---

amounts of diagnostic and management information available. Utilization of practice guidelines does assist in minimizing cognitive and systemic sources of clinician error such as the bias that occurs from overemphasizing risk for rare conditions and the potential for the clinician to overreact to that perceived risk. They can also constrain and oversimplify practice by focusing on more common problems (Tracy, 2009). If they are overly relied on, practice guidelines can result in failing to attend to the individual needs and nuanced presentations of a patient's condition. Many web-based information systems have been developed that are now viewed as part of the standard support tools for practice. These include intranet and Internet systems, as well as online journals and texts, databases, and governmental and organizational websites. The advent of smartphone and associated apps has provided the opportunity to have support tools in all clinical settings at the point of care. One entry-level advanced practice competency is the ability to access, search, and critically evaluate the appropriateness of practice guidelines and electronic resources for practice (AACN, 2006).

SUMMARY

Expertise in clinical decision making is vital for clinical competency. At the advanced practice level, this is a complex undertaking for both the individual provider and the profession. Keeping the core of nursing theory and perspectives central and visible while gaining competency in the knowledge base and probabilistic thinking of advanced practice requires continual attention to practice-based cognitive skills and processes. It is recommended that advanced practice clinical decision making be approached as a continual and deliberate process of knowledge expansion and reflective practice, maintaining the personhood and holistic needs of the patient and the importance of the nurse–patient relationship central to practice. The complexity of the healthcare system and patients requires interprofessional collaboration and communication to ensure sound clinical decision making resulting in patient-centered care (ten Ham, Ricks, Rooyen, & Jordan, 2017).

ACKNOWLEDGMENT

The author acknowledges the contributions of Rhonda Squires to this chapter in the previous edition.

REFERENCES

Abuzour, A. S., Lewis, P. J., & Tully, M. P. (2018). A qualitative study exploring how pharmacists and nurse independent prescribers make clinical decisions. *Journal of Advanced Nursing, 74*, 65–74. doi:10.1111/jan.13375

American Association of Colleges of Nursing. (2004). *AACN position statement on the practice doctorate in nursing.* Washington, DC: Author.

American Association of Colleges of Nursing. (2006). *The essentials of doctoral education for advanced practice nursing.* Washington, DC: Author.

American College of Nurse-Midwives. (2014). *Competencies for master's level midwifery education.* Silver Spring, MD: Author. Retrieved from http://www.midwife.org/acnm/files/ccLibraryFiles/Filename/000000004993/Competencies-for-Master's-Level-Midwifery-Education-Dec-2014.pdf

Banning, M. (2008). A review of clinical decision making: Models and current research. *Journal of Clinical Nursing, 17*, 187–195. doi:10.1111/j.1365-2702.2006.01791.x

Benner, P., Stannard, D., & Hooper, P. L. (1996). A "thinking-in-action" approach to teaching clinical judgment: A classroom innovation for acute care advanced practice nurses. *Advanced Practice Nursing Quarterly, 1*(4), 70–77.

Bjork, I. T., & Hamilton, G. A. (2011). Clinical decision making of nurses working in hospital settings. *Nursing Research and Practice, 2011*(524918), 1–8. doi:10.1155/2011/524918

Brookfield, S. (2008). Clinical reasoning and generic thinking skills. In J. Higgs, M. A. Jones, S. Loftus, & N. Christensen (Eds.), *Clinical reasoning in the health professions* (pp. 65–75). Philadelphia, PA: Butterworth-Heinemann Elsevier.

Buckingham, C. D. (2002). Psychological cue use and implications for a clinical decision support system. *Medical Informatics and the Internet in Medicine, 27*(4), 237–251. doi:10.1080/1463923031000063342

Buckingham, C. D., & Adams, A. (2000). Classifying clinical decision making: A unifying approach. *Journal of Advanced Nursing, 32*, 981–989. doi:10.1046/j.1365-2648.2000.t01-1-01565.x

Cader, R., Campbell, S., & Watson, D. (2005). Cognitive continuum theory in nursing decision making. *Journal of Advanced Nursing, 49*(4), 397–405. doi:10.1111/j.1365-2648.2004.03303.x

Cappelletti, A., Engel, J. K., & Prentice, D. (2014). Systematic review of clinical judgement and reasoning in nursing. *Journal of Nursing Education, 53*(8), 453–458. doi:10.3928/01484834-20140724-01

Carnevali, D. L., & Thomas, M. D. (1993). *Diagnostic reasoning and treatment decision making in nursing*. Philadelphia, PA: J. B. Lippincott.

Chase, S. K. (2004). *Clinical judgment and communication in nurse practitioner practice*. Philadelphia, PA: F. A. Davis.

Chase, S. K. (2011). The art of diagnosis and treatment. In L. M. Dunphy, J. E. Winland-Brown, & D. Thomas (Eds.), *Primary care: The art and science of advanced practice nursing* (pp. 43–61). Philadelphia, PA: F. A. Davis.

Chen, S. L., Hsu, H. Y., Chang, C. F., & Lin, E. C. (2016). An exploration of the correlates of nurse practitioners' clinical decision-making abilities. *Journal of Clinical Nursing, 25*, 1016–1024. doi:10.1111/jocn.13136

Elstein, A. S. (1976). Clinical judgment: Psychological research and medical practice. *Science, 194*, 696–700. doi:10.1126/science.982034

Elstein, A. S., Shulman, L. S., & Sprafka, S. A. (1978). *Medical problem solving: An analysis of clinical reasoning*. Cambridge, MA: Harvard University Press.

Facione, P. (1990). *Critical thinking: A statement of consensus for purposes of educational assessment and instruction*. Fullerton: American Philosophical Association, California State University.

Hamm Flynn, C. A., & Becker, L. (2004). Clinical jazz: Harmonizing clinical experience with evidence-based medicine. In W. Rosser, D. Slawson, & A. Shaughnessy (Eds.), *Information mastery: Evidence based family medicine* (pp. 61–65). Hamilton, ON, Canada: BC Decker.

Hammond, K. R. (1964). An approach to the study of clinical inference in nursing: Part II. *Nursing Research, 13*(4), 315–319. doi:10.1097/00006199-196413040-00007

Hammond, K., Kelly, K., & Castellan, E. A. (1966). Clinical inference in nursing: Use of information seeking strategies by nurses. *Nursing Research, 15*(4), 330–336. doi:10.1097/00006199-196615040-00008

Hedberg, B., & Larsson, U. S. (2003). Observations, confirmations and strategies: Useful tools in decision-making process for nurses in practice? *Journal of Clinical Nursing, 12,* 215–222. doi:10.1046/j.1365-2702.2003.00703.x

Higgs, J., & Jones, M. (2008). Clinical reasoning in the health professions. In J. Higgs, M. A. Jones, S. Loftus, & N. Christensen (Eds.), *Clinical reasoning in the health professions* (pp. 3–17). Philadelphia, PA: Butterworth-Heinemann Elsevier.

Huch, M. H. (1995). Nursing science as a basis for advanced practice. *Nursing Science Quarterly, 8*(1), 6–7. doi:10.1177/089431849500800104

Kassirer, J. P., & Kopelman, R. I. (1991). *Learning clinical reasoning.* Baltimore, MD: William & Wilkins.

Loftus, S., & Higgs, J. (2008). Learning the language of clinical reasoning. In J. Higgs, M. A. Jones, S. Loftus, & N. Christensen (Eds.), *Clinical reasoning in the health professions* (pp. 339–348). Philadelphia, PA: Butterworth-Heinemann Elsevier.

Lubarsky, S., Dory, L., Audétat, M., Custers, E., & Charlin, B. (2015). Using script theory to cultivate illness script formation and clinical reasoning in health profession education. *Canadian Medical Education Journal, 6*(2), e61–e70.

Makary, M. M., & Daniel, M. (2016). Medical error: The third leading cause of death in the US. *British Journal of Medicine, 353,* i2139. doi:10.1136/bmj.i2139

Melnyk, B. M., & Fineout-Overholt, E. F. (2011). Making the case for evidence-based practice and cultivating a spirit of inquiry. In B. M. Melnyk & E. F. Fineout-Overholt (Eds.), *Evidence-based practice in nursing and healthcare: A guide to best practice* (pp. 3–24). Philadelphia, PA: Lippincott, Williams & Wilkins.

Narayan, S. M., Corcoran-Perry, S., Drew, D., Hoyman, K., & Lewis, M. (2003). Decision analysis as a tool to support an analytical pattern-of-reasoning. *Nursing and Health Sciences, 5,* 229–243. doi:10.1046/j.1442-2018.2003.00157.x

National Association of Clinical Nurse Specialists. (2017). *Draft: Clinical nurse specialist core competencies.* Philadelphia, PA: Author. Retrieved from http://nacns.org/wp-content/uploads/2017/10/2017-Draft-CNS-Core-Competencies-FINAL.pdf

National Organization of Nurse Practitioner Faculties. (2017). *Nurse practitioner core competencies contents.* Washington, DC: Author. Retrieved from http://c.ymcdn.com/sites/www.nonpf.org/resource/resmgr/competencies/2017_NPCoreComps_with_Curric.pdf

Newell, A., & Simon, H. A. (1972). *Human problem solving.* Englewood Cliffs, NJ: Prentice Hall.

Noon, A. J. (2014). The cognitive process underpinning clinical decision in triage assessment: A theoretical conundrum. *International Emergency Nursing, 22,* 40–46. doi:10.1016/j.ienj.2013.01.003

Pinnock, R., Young, L., Spence, F., Henning, M., & Hazell, W. (2015). Can *Think Aloud* be used to teach and assess clinical reasoning in graduate medical education? *Journal of Graduate Medical Education, 7*(3), 334–337. doi:10.4300/JGME-D-14-00601.1

Pretz, J. E., & Folse, V. N. (2011). Nursing experience and preference for intuition in decision making. *Journal of Clinical Nursing, 20,* 2878–2889. doi:10.1111/j.1365-2702.2011.03705.x

Price, A., Zulkosky, K., White, K., & Pretz, J. (2017). Accuracy of intuition in clinical decision-making among novice clinicians. *Journal of Advanced Nursing, 73*(5), 1147–1157. doi:10.1111/jan.13202

Rosciano, A., Lindell, D., Bryer, J., & DiMarco, M. (2016). Nurse practitioner's use of intuition. *The Journal for Nurse Practitioners, 12*(8), 560–565. doi:10.1016/j.nurpra.2016.06.007

Rycroft-Malone, J., Fontenla, M., Seers, K., & Bick, D. (2009). Protocol-based care: The standardization of decision-making? *Journal of Clinical Nursing, 18*(10), 1490–1500. doi:10.1111/j.1365-2702.2008.02605.x

Sands, H. M. (2001). *Making the diagnosis: Factors shaping diagnostic reasoning among entry level nurse practitioners* (Unpublished doctoral dissertation). University of California, Los Angeles.

Scheffer, B. K., & Rubenfeld, M. G. (2000). A consensus statement on critical thinking in nursing. *Journal of Nursing Education, 39*(8), 352–359.

Schwartz, A., & Elstein, A. S. (2008). Clinical reasoning in medicine. In J. Higgs, M. A. Jones, S. Loftus, & N. Christensen (Eds.), *Clinical reasoning in the health professions* (pp. 223–234). Philadelphia, PA: Butterworth-Heinemann Elsevier.

Simmons, B. (2010), Clinical reasoning: Concept analysis. *Journal of Advanced Nursing, 66*(5), 1151–1158. doi:10.1111/j.1365-2648.2010.05262.x

Smith, M. C. (1995). The core of advanced practice nursing. *Nursing Science Quarterly, 8*, 2–3. doi:10.1177/089431849500800102

Tanner, C. A. (2006). Thinking like a nurse: A research-based model of clinical judgment in nursing. *Journal of Nursing Education, 45*, 204–211.

ten Ham, W., Ricks, E. J., van Rooyen, D., & Jordan, P. J. (2017). An integrative literature review of the factors that contribute to professional nurses and midwives making sound clinical decisions. *International Journal of Nursing Knowledge, 28*, 19–29. doi:10.1111/2047-3095.12096

Thompson, C. (2002). Human error, bias, decision making and judgment in nursing: The need for a systematic approach. In C. Thompson & D. Dowding (Eds.), *Clinical decision making and judgment in nursing* (pp. 21–45). Edinburgh, Scotland: Churchill Livingstone.

Thompson, C., Aiken, A., Brown, D., & Dowding, D. (2013). An agenda for clinical decision making and judgment in nursing research and education. *International Journal of Nursing Studies, 50*, 1720–1726. doi:10.1016/j.ijnurstu.2013.05.003

Thompson, S., Moorley, C., & Barratt, J. (2017). A comparative study on clinical decision-making processes of nurse practitioners vs. medical doctors using scenarios in secondary care environment. *Journal of Advanced Nursing, 73*(5), 1097–1110. doi:10.1111/jan.13206

Tiffen, J., Corbridge, S. J., & Slimmer, L. (2014). Enhancing clinical decision making: Development of continguous definition and conceptual framework. *Journal of Professional Nursing, 30*(5), 399–405. doi:10.1016/j.profnurs.2014.01.00

Titchen, A., & Higgs, J. (2000). Facilitating the acquisition of knowledge and reasoning. In J. Higgs & M. Jones (Eds.), *Clinical reasoning in the health professions* (pp. 222–229). Oxford, UK: Butterworth-Heinemann.

Tracy, M. F. (2009). Direct clinical practice. In A. B. Hamric, J. A. Spross, & C. M. Hanson (Eds.), *Advanced practice nursing: An integrative approach* (pp. 123–158). St. Louis, MO: Saunders Elsevier.

Tversky, A., & Kahneman, D. (1974). Judgment under uncertainty: Heuristics and biases. *Science, 185,* 1124–1131. doi:10.1017/CBO9780511809477.002

White, J. E., Nativio, D. G., Kobert, S. N., & Engberg, S. J. (1992). Content and process in clinical decision making by nurse practitioners. *Image: The Journal of Nursing Scholarship, 24,* 153–158. doi:10.1111/j.1547-5069.1992.tb00241.x

Woolley, A., & Kostopoulou, O. (2013). Clinical intuition in family medicine: More than first impressions. *Annals of Family Medicine, 11*(1), 60–66. doi:10.1370/afm.1433

Evelyn G. Duffy

9

HEALTHCARE POLICY: IMPLICATIONS FOR ADVANCED NURSING PRACTICE

The Patient Protection and Affordable Care Act (ACA) was passed in 2010, and with that the opportunities for APRNs increased. In a subsequent tax reform bill, which was passed in December 2017, the ACA requirement that all Americans purchase health insurance was repealed. APRNs need to stay vigilant and engaged in the process to prevent losing legislative ground that was gained.

In addition to the passage of the ACA in 2010, the Institute of Medicine (IOM) 2011 report, *The Future of Nursing: Leading Change, Advancing Health*, was released and has been another factor in increasing opportunities for APRNs. These events were preceded by the publication in 2008 of the *Consensus Model for APRN Regulation: Licensure, Accreditation, Certification & Education*, completed through the work of the APRN Consensus Work Group and the National Council of State Boards of Nursing (NCSBN) APRN Advisory Committee. Initially to comply with the recommendations of the *Consensus Model*, educational programs, certification examinations, and the accreditation processes were modified. Although changes in state laws are still in process, significant advances have occurred. The NCSBN keeps a record of the implementation status of the *Consensus Model* as states update their laws to fully implement all the changes proposed. The NCSBN map, which is an overview of each state's status, is accessible at www. ncsbn.org/5397.htm. The scoring grid for this map provides points for incorporation of *Consensus Document* recommendations including use of the APRN title, recognition of all roles, use of the term "license" in recognizing APRN practice, requirement of a graduate or postgraduate degree, national certification required for practice, and APRNs practicing and prescribing independently. For practice and prescribing, each role is scored individually. The passage of the ACA, the IOM Report, and the *Consensus Model* combined to advance the opportunities for APRNs and helped unify their voices and purpose.

As the public has become better informed of the full capacity of APRNs to provide healthcare, groups outside of healthcare have advocated for the removal of boundaries that prevent APRNs from practicing to the full extent of their education and training. Improving access to care is a major objective of the Center to Champion Nursing in America, a joint initiative of the Robert Wood Johnson Foundation (RWJF) and the American Association of Retired Persons (AARP). Their Campaign for Action (accessible at www.campaignforaction.org) works nationally to implement the recommendations of the IOM report on the *Future of Nursing: Leading Change, Advancing Health* (2011). They help to form coalitions of professionals, the public, and businesses to remove barriers to practice and care.

The variation in state's scope of practice (SOP) laws for APRNs are cited as a barrier to access to care. In 2012, the National Governors Association released a well-researched document addressing the role of nurse practitioners (NPs) in meeting the demand for primary healthcare. A review of the existing evidence of NP quality outcomes and issues of access resulted in the conclusion that restrictions on the practice of NPs be eased and reimbursement policies be modified to increase the access to NPs to meet the increasing demand for primary care in the states. A study of the growth of care provided by NPs found that in states with the least restrictive regulations, Medicare patients were 2½ times more likely to be receiving care from an NP than in more restrictive states (Kuo, Loresta, Rounds, & Goodwin, 2013). Another study of the impact of restrictive regulations noted that states with full practice authority had lower hospitalization rates and improved health outcomes (Oliver, Pennington, Revelle, & Rantz, 2014). Another key contribution supporting the removal of barriers to full SOP came from the 2014 Federal Trade Commission (FTC) report, *Policy Perspectives: Competition and the Regulation of Advanced Practice Nurses,* which addressed the threat to competition in the marketplace that results from the requirement for physician supervision of APRNs.

The consolidation in 2012 of the two largest NP organizations, the American College of Nurse Practitioners and the American Academy of Nurse Practitioners, into one organization: the American Association of Nurse Practitioners (AANP) has matured over the past 5 years and it has worked to leverage its voice addressing issues that affect practice. In 2017, AANP celebrated reaching the 75,000-member milestone. This is a 25,000-member increase since the 50,000 milestone of 2014. Like the map accessible on the NCSBN website, the AANP has a map of the State Practice Environments accessible at www.aanp.org/legislation-regulation/state-legislation/state-practice-environment. The AANP definition of "full practice authority" is: "State practice and licensure laws provide for all NPs to evaluate patients, diagnose, order and interpret diagnostic tests, initiate and manage treatments—including prescribing medications and controlled substances—under the exclusive licensure authority of the state board of nursing." This is the model recommended by the National Academy of

Medicine, formerly called the IOM, and NCSBN. Because of the slight variation in definition of "independent authority," the NCSBN and AANP maps do classify practice environment in some states differently. APRNs today more than ever before need to be informed health professionals who are aware of the current health policy issues, the process necessary to make change happen, and the advocacy groups for nursing and advanced practice nursing that are working to remove barriers and support policy that will allow them to provide the best care to their patients. Patient-centered care is the hallmark of nursing and has become the focus of healthcare nationally and the motivation for the formulation of coalitions to support the advancement of APRN practice.

No matter the scale of the health policy issue or the size of the community it affects, the process of creating health policy is basically the same on the local, state, and national levels. Knowing how that process works and ways to influence it empowers the APRN to stand up for health policies on any level. The purpose of this chapter is to help the APRN understand and engage in that process.

APRNs provide excellent patient care with quality comparable to or better than that of physicians; this is supported by multiple studies with the earliest work commissioned by the U.S. Congress in the 1980s (Lenz, Mundinger, Kane, Hopkins, & Lin, 2004; Mundinger et al., 2000; Newhouse et al., 2011; Stanik-Hutt et al., 2013; U.S. Congress, Office of Technology Assessment [OTA], 1980; U.S. Congress, OTA, 1986). The physician community has often cited the small sample sizes and the lack of more recent work as a reason to refute the conclusion regarding quality and safety of APRN practice. An Evidence Brief was commissioned by the Veteran's Administration (VA) in preparation for the proposed changes to the VA Nursing Policy Manual, which allowed for full practice authority for NPs, clinical nurse specialists (CNSs), and certified nurse-midwives (CNMs). A thorough review of evidence available to answer the question of quality and safety of NP care concluded that:

> The generally low strength of evidence outlined in this brief does not necessarily mean that additional randomized trials are necessary to prove comparable health outcomes among patients cared for by APRNs and physicians. Data on performance measures and provider errors, which is routinely collected by the VA, may be a better source of information on the actual quality of care provided by independent VA APRNs. (McCleery, Christensen, Peterson, Humphrey, & Helfand, 2014, p. 13)

LEADERSHIP AND HEALTH POLICY

Although APRNs are comfortable advocating for their patients, they may not see the connection between advocating for health policy and providing quality care. Without the development of leadership competencies and influence at decision-making tables, clinical competence will not be enough to affect care. Leadership skills that are especially important in advocacy for health policy include vision, timing, risk-taking, communication, and relationship building. Nursing education emphasizes the importance of communication and collaboration skills as crucial in influencing policy makers. The example of Florence Nightingale and her use of evidence to change the healthcare systems of her day serves as a model for leadership in health policy development today. Her vision for change was informed by her practice on the battlefields in Crimea. Her use of statistics to support her theories allowed her to realize her vision. APRNs today also bring their nursing skills of communication, use of evidence, and their practice experience to the policy tables. Their stories from practice personalize for decision makers the impact of the policies they are working to create.

The National Organization of Nurse Practitioner Faculties (NONPF) in 2017 published updated *Nurse Practitioner Core Competencies Content* that include suggested curriculum content. At least four leadership competencies directly relate to leadership in health policy:

1. Assumes complex and advanced leadership roles to initiate and guide change
2. Provides leadership to foster collaboration with multiple stakeholders (e.g., patients, community, integrated healthcare teams, and policy makers) to improve healthcare
4. Advocates for improved access, quality, and cost-effective healthcare
7. Participates in professional organizations and activities that influence advanced practice nursing and/or health outcomes of a population focus (p. 4).

These competencies reflect NONPF's endorsement of the doctorate of nursing practice (DNP) as entry level for NP practice. In *The Essentials of Doctoral Education for Advanced Nursing Practice* (American Association of Colleges of Nursing [AACN], 2006), the ability to influence policy is a central theme throughout the document. Essentials II (Organization and systems leadership for quality improvement and systems thinking), V (Healthcare policy for advocacy in healthcare), VI (Interprofessional collaboration for improving patient and population health outcomes), and VIII (Advanced nursing practice), all address various aspects of leadership in policy development and implementation to improve healthcare quality and access. Specifically, Essential V outlines in more detail the expectation that APRNs prepared at the DNP level will be involved in policy development at the governmental, institutional, and organizational level. Essential V emphasizes the role of the APRN as political activist on behalf of their patients as well as the profession.

Why should APRNs care about becoming leaders in health policy? For many APRNs, moving from leadership in clinical practice to leadership in health policy is not an obvious choice. However, APRNs need to understand how the skills used in motivating patients to improve their health are the same skills that can move legislatures to pass laws and develop rules that will allow APRNs to practice to their full scope and remove the barriers to providing quality care to their patients. Policy makers at the federal, state, and local levels as well as in institutions influence what nursing professionals can do, how they do it, and what they are paid. Public policies dictate who has insurance and what insurance will pay. Public policies and how they are implemented shape the direction of healthcare delivery. They affect the experience of providers as they practice and the experience of consumers as they attempt to receive care in an increasingly complex and expensive system. APRNs need to have the resources to stay informed and respond to proposed changes to federal, state, local, and institutional policies that will affect their practice and the care their patients receive.

PUBLIC POLICY: THE PROCESS

The U.S. Constitution was written by men of vision. Their ability to frame a document that not only addressed current issues but provided for adaptation to challenges faced in the future has been cited as the reason the Constitution has remained relevant. The document utilized broad principles that allowed for the future development of laws, rules, and actions based on the context at that time (Stone & Marshal, 2011). When laws contain specific language, adaptation to changes in the future environment may be stymied. Medicare Law P.L. 89–97, passed in 1965, specified that authority for many actions was limited to physicians. Lawmakers did not envision future changes to a physician-dominated healthcare system because most of the advanced practice roles did not exist at that time. This limitation resulted in a number of barriers to APRN practice and helped to support the argument for the inclusion of provider-neutral language in more recent laws and rulemaking. Inclusion of provider-neutral language is one of the key priorities of the APRN *Health Affairs* agenda today.

The Constitution describes three branches of government and delineates the responsibilities of each. The *legislative branch,* which includes the Senate and the House of Representatives, creates the laws, confirms presidential appointments, and has the power to declare war. The *executive branch* includes the president, the vice president, and the cabinet and is charged with carrying out and enforcing the laws, including the responsibility for rulemaking. The *judicial branch* includes the Supreme Court and other federal courts; it is responsible for settling conflicts that occur over the law, interpreting the law, and deciding whether a law is constitutional (Govetrack.us, 2018).

Process Models

Work by Kingdon (2011), Wakefield (2006), and Longest (2016) identify key factors in moving legislation forward and understanding the process. Kingdon identified agenda setting as the initiation of the policy process. His policy stream included the identification of a problem, development of a proposal, and evaluation of the political factors. The work of Kingdon

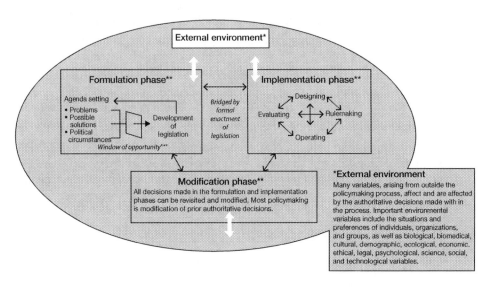

FIGURE 9.1 Three phases of the policy-making process.
Source: Longest, B. B. (2016). *Health policy making in the United States* (6th ed.). Chicago, IL: Health Administration Press.

influenced Longest's (2016) "Three Phases of the Policymaking Process" (p. 86; Figure 9.1), which provides a map of the process of decision making. Although the model was designed around the federal system, it is also applicable to state, county, and local governments and the concepts could be applied at the institutional level as well. The three interrelated phases include formulation, policy making, and modification. The process is cyclical, which underscores the fact that laws are subject to change. Laws introduced each year generally are modifications of some existing law.

Influential Factors: Lessons for APRNs

The Longest (2016) model also emphasizes the influence that individuals, organizations, and special interest groups have on every aspect of the process. Wakefield (2006) and Kingdon (2011) also describe the environment that informs the policy-making process. Mary Wakefield became the first nurse appointed as the director of the Health Resources and Services Administration (HRSA) in 2009. Her leadership in health policy helped to guide others in advocacy. Wakefield defined nine factors that influence legislation including constituents (the public), research findings (the experts), special interest groups, the media, crisis, market forces, fiscal pressures, personal experience, and political ideology (Figure 9.2). Kingdon (2011) describes the "actors" that influence the agenda, including elected officials,

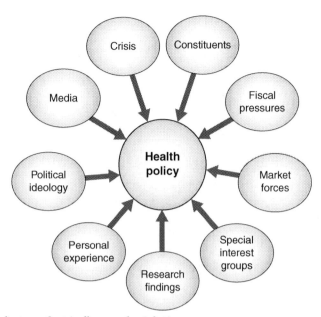

FIGURE 9.2 Nine factors that influence legislation.
Source: Wakefield, M. (2006, February 19). So you want to be an advocate? Strategies for advocacy, knowledge, resources, colleagues and actions (PPT slides). In: *Presented at the American College of Nurse Practitioners health policy conference,* Washington, DC.

the public, the media, experts, and interest groups. There is overlap between Longest's external environment, Kingdon's actors, and Wakefield's nine factors that influence legislation, but understanding the influence of each can help APRNs as they scan the environment to assess for opportunities for change.

For Kingdon (2011), the foremost actors in the policy-making process are the *elected officials.* At the federal level, the president and members of Congress set the national agenda. The governor and legislature serve the same role on a state level. Members of Congress decide what proposals or bills will be introduced, which will have public hearings, and which will be debated.

The role of the public (constituents) is not insignificant. Constituents have the ability to influence what policies are discussed and ultimately what policy changes occur, when they support candidates who represent their perspectives and values. The fear of displeasing constituents and risking reelection often exceeds their responsibility to govern the country. APRNs become engaged citizens when they use their voices to communicate with legislators, attend and testify in hearings, and are involved in events that legislators hold.

Elected officials may gain awareness about certain issues through their own personal experiences. They may become acutely aware of a problem or develop a unique insight because of personal events. Rob Portman, a Republican senator from Ohio, went against his party in March 2013 and supported same-sex marriage after his son told his parents that he was gay. Senator Portman wanted to think that his son could experience the same supportive relationship that he shared with his wife (Portman, 2013). Portman did not cite any other compelling argument for this shift in his support of this initiative. Without the context of his personal experience, it is not clear whether he would have made that policy shift.

Media are in a powerful position to shape the national discussion of issues and get these onto the policy-making agenda. When Dr. Sam Foote resigned from the Phoenix VA hospital in December 2013 after 24 years, he used the media to inform the public of the corruption he had observed. Before he resigned, he sent two letters to the VA inspector general requesting an investigation into the secret waiting lists, but his requests fell on deaf ears. After he resigned, he contacted the House Veteran Affairs Committee and a reporter with the *Arizona Republic* to discuss the problems at the Phoenix VA (Foote, 2014). The news stories about the corruption enraged the public, and the investigation that occurred in the wake of this public outcry uncovered a widespread problem involving a number of VA hospitals across the country. In response, multiple actors worked together to create and pass legislation—that is, the Veterans' Access to Care through Choice, Accountability and Transparency Act of 2014, P.L. 113–146, which was signed into law by President Obama on August 7, 2014. The bipartisan support in both the House and the Senate was a highly unusual occurrence for this 113th session of Congress, "the least productive Congress ever" (Cillizza, 2014). APRNs need to learn to use the media to advance their agendas. Education of the public regarding APRN practice and the barriers APRNs face to providing optimal care to their patients may be as effective in accomplishing policy change as contacting their representatives. Social media can also be a useful tool for APRNs. For example, by acquiring Twitter followers, APRNs are able to get their messages out, and if they become recognized by their tweets, APRNs may be sought out by the media for their expertise and commentary.

Experts from governmental agencies, universities, think tanks, congressional committees, and associations provide advice and counsel to the elected officials, and much of this is based on research findings. Experts often disagree, and ultimately, the elected officials who make the laws will choose the expert advice that most closely aligns with their personal agenda. Special interest groups look after their constituents and advocate for preferred policy choices based on the preferences of their members. An important distinction should be made between advocacy, lobbying, and working as a lobbyist. Anyone can lobby for their position, but lobbyists must be registered with the government. There were nearly 11,143 lobbyists registered with the government in 2016, and they received $3.15 billion in fees (Statista, 2018).

Nursing has created several special interest groups; the Nurse Practitioner Roundtable (NPRt), the Extended Roundtable, the APRN Workgroup, and the Nursing Community Coalition are of particular interest to APRNs. When O'Grady (2011) noted the importance of a coordinated front by nursing, she did not recognize the many nursing health advocacy groups that work together to present a unified message to policy makers. The NPRt advocacy groups include the AANP, Gerontological Advanced Practice Nurses Association, National Association of Pediatric Nurse Practitioners, NONPF, and Nurse Practitioners in Women's Health. Representatives from each of the organizations, as well as their lobbyists, meet twice a month by conference call to review current issues and develop a coordinated message to present to policy makers. They advocate not only to legislatures but also to federal agencies such as the Centers for Medicare & Medicaid Services (CMS) and the HRSA.

The extended NPRt expands the NPRt membership to include the American Nurses Association, the AACN, and the American Academy of Nursing. This group also meets twice a month by conference call, which provides an opportunity for the agenda agreed on by the NPRt to be shared and discussed with these other influential professional organizations. These conversations help coordinate the messages that are presented and resolve differences when they exist.

The APRN Workgroup originated in 2009 to develop a document that would describe the barriers to APRN full practice authority and includes the organizations in the NPRt and the extended NPRt, as well as the American Association of Nurse Anesthetists; Association of Women's Health, Obstetric and Neonatal Nurses; American College of Nurse-Midwives; and the National Association of Clinical Nurse Specialists. The "barriers" document identified federal regulatory, statutory, and policy barriers to the use of APRNs. This document has been used by the member groups for organizing advocacy efforts on Capitol Hill and in agencies. The group meets face to face in various locations in Washington, DC, and by conference call on a monthly basis. Issues may arise with a very short turn-around time, and the APRN Workgroup drafts letters and documents to send to policy makers expressing the unified voice of the members of the group. This rapid response cycle would be difficult for one organization to track, and again the unified message is important in communicating concerns to policy makers.

The Nursing Community Coalition (www.thenursingcommunity.org) expands the reach of the APRN organizations by including a total of 58 national professional nursing organizations. A typical letter from the Nursing Community Coalition begins with the words:

> On behalf of the undersigned organizations representing the Nursing Community, we write in support of…Collectively, our organizations represent over one million registered nurses, advanced practice registered nurses, nurse faculty, researchers, and students, and we are committed to promoting efforts that advance the health of our nation through nursing care.

An individual professional organization, even one with 75,000 members, does not have the impact of a coalition of professional organizations representing more than 1 million members. Each of these advocacy groups needs the stories from APRNs in practice to help to put a context around the list of barriers to providing quality patient care. The link to this critical resource is membership and involvement in professional nursing organizations.

Kingdon's (2011) actors and Wakefield's (2006) factors do not work in isolation. It is the combination of these influences that ultimately result in setting the agenda. When APRNs understand the multiple forces involved in the development of health policy, they are better equipped to find ways to become involved and to work to accomplish their professional agenda.

Policy Formulation Phase: Agenda Setting

Setting the political agenda prioritizes concerns and guides the policy-making process. Many problems require solutions, and there is a limited amount of time to address those problems. In developing his model of public policy-making process, Longest (2016) drew on the prior work of Kingdon, which was first published in 1984. Kingdon noted that public policy starts with agenda setting. His work addressed the questions of how issues come to the attention of lawmakers, how the agenda is set, and why an issue is chosen when its "time has come." With so many voices and influences, how does a single idea move to the top of the agenda? Kingdon's second edition was published in 2011 and expanded on the earlier work. Kingdon described three Ps—problems, possible solutions, and political circumstances—that are involved in setting the agenda. For policy change to occur, policy makers must be convinced that a problem is serious. Reaching agreement on what constitutes a serious problem can be a challenging task among policy makers. Crisis, one of Wakefield's (2006) factors, is clearly influential. The rapid bipartisan response from an otherwise underperforming legislature to a crisis in the Middle East in 2014 is an excellent example of the impact of crisis on legislative priority. When Americans were being beheaded by a radical Islam faction in September 2014, within a span of 3 days, an amendment went from the House of Representatives to the Senate to the president and became part of the continuing budget resolution, P.L. 113–164, and signed into law. A crisis can create a sense of urgency or the desire to get something done. As Rahm Emanuel, President Barack Obama's thenchief of staff, said shortly before the president's inauguration, "You never want a serious crisis to go to waste" (Seib, 2008).

Policy Formulation Phase: Development of Legislation

The possible solutions are the policy proposals that are created, debated by committees, and presented to the legislative body. The less conflict there is regarding a possible solution to a serious problem, the more likely it will actually be heard in Congress. There is a strong relationship between the problems and the solutions that are proposed. How a problem is defined influences and limits the solutions that are proposed to address it. Two policy makers can look at the same problem and describe it differently because they are defining the problem based on what *they* think the solution ought to be.

A well-defined problem and reasonable solution are not enough to guarantee that a policy proposal will move forward. A third factor, the political circumstances, is also involved in opening the window of opportunity. When there is a recognized problem, a solution available in the policy community to solve that problem, and a favorable political environment, a policy window is open. Kingdon (2011) writes, "Policy windows open infrequently, and do not stay open long. Despite their rarity, the major changes in public policy result from the appearance of these opportunities" (p. 166). When the ACA was passed in 2010, it was the result of a unique combination of problem, proposal, and political circumstances. Democrats had a majority in the both the House of Representatives and the Senate, and President Obama had identified healthcare as his top priority. After the midterm elections, the control of the House shifted to the Republican Party, and the window was closed, not only for legislation about healthcare, but for almost any legislation at all. APRNs need to use the open window when it exists to help remove barriers to their practice and allow them the opportunity to care for their patients as they were prepared to do.

Creation of a Bill

When a problem has been identified as important and a reasonable solution is proposed, a congressperson introduces a bill. Only a congressperson may introduce a bill, but he or she may receive the language of the bill from interested parties who ask the congressperson to sponsor the legislation. The bill is evaluated by the Office of Legislative Counsel to put it into proper legislative language. There is a separate legislative counsel for the House and the Senate. The counsel consists of groups of lawyers with specific expertise who will aid in the development of the bill and identify what current laws the bill will affect. The law or laws the bill affects will determine to which committee the bill will be assigned. There are 20 standing committees in the House and 16 in the Senate; in addition there are special committees and numerous subcommittees. Healthcare policies usually involve either Medicare or Medicaid law. In the Senate, bills affecting either of these laws would be sent to the Senate Finance Committee. In the House, bills that affect Medicare law would go to the House Ways and Means Committee, and those that affect Medicaid law go to the House Energy and Commerce Committee. Depending on the issue, other committees may get involved as well.

A committee chair calls the committee together, sets the committee agenda, and prioritizes the bills that will be addressed by the committee. The majority party appoints the committee chairs, so party politics has a strong influence on which bills will be addressed by the committee and the amount of time given to the hearings. Each year thousands of bills are introduced to committee, but less than 10% of them find that "policy window" that allows them to go to the floor for debate (www.govtrack.us).

Committees hold hearings to address bills, and during the interaction between committee members and interested parties, it may be obvious that there are issues in common with other bills. When a bill is important but does not have the urgency to bring it to the top of the political agenda, it may be included in a bill that does reach the level of introduction; the new bill is a vehicle for the less important bill; looking for a vehicle is a way to get your agenda addressed. Bills can also be "packaged" so that less popular bills are combined with bills that are more likely to be passed. They may be included in other legislation as amendments or written into "clean bills."

Bills must pass both the House and the Senate to become law. In the 114th Congress from January 6, 2015, to January 3, 2017, only 3% of bills that were introduced became law. Bills that are passed go from the Congress to the president for his signature. When the president signs a bill, it becomes law. If the president does not sign the bill, it may still become law after 10 days as long as Congress is still in session. If Congress adjourns before the 10 days pass, the bill is "pocket vetoed" and does not become law. The president may also actively veto the bill, but the bill may still become law if a two-thirds majority in both the House and the Senate override the presidential veto.

Incrementalism

Laws are imperfect, and the cyclical process allows for modifications over time. The small changes that are made in laws define the concept of incrementalism. Kingdon (2011) describes "incrementalism" as a strategy used to enact policy change a little piece at a time. As legislation is debated and competing proposals are presented, compromise is necessary to make change happen. If one group refuses to accept the compromise, the important problem may not get any solution at all. Through incremental changes, some aspect of the problem may be solved now, which will open the policy window for more complete change in the future. Even though it can succeed, the strategy of incrementalism is controversial. It can achieve results in the long run, but it may seem as if not enough is being done in the short term to solve the big problems of the day. Advocates of all or nothing should understand that compromise is the best method of achieving change and that they should not allow the perfect to become the enemy of the good.

Incrementalism is the way that APRNs have achieved increasing independence in practice. In 1997, APRNs in the state of Ohio first received license recognition, the Certificate of Authority (COA) for Advanced Practice, but this did not include prescriptive authority. APRNs were allowed to order laboratory tests and could prescribe medications that were available over the counter. In January 2000, Ohio granted prescriptive authority to APRNs who held a COA. This included the ability to prescribe Schedules III through V drugs with limited authority for prescribing Schedule II drugs. In 2011, the Ohio legislature expanded the authority of APRNs to prescribe Schedule II drugs. The latest legislation, House Bill 216, which was passed in 2016, provides for licensure with the title APRN, the creation of an APRN advisory board to the Board of Nursing and the elimination of a 1,500 hour supervision requirement for prescribing. Now APRNs have prescriptive authority when they are first licensed. The goal of independent authority is still not a reality in Ohio, but with each of the incremental steps that have spanned over two decades, soon that may become a reality.

Policy Implementation Phase: Rulemaking

After a bill becomes law, it is assigned to the appropriate federal agency for rulemaking. Rulemaking authority was defined by the Administrative Procedure Act of 1946, which governs the way an agency may propose regulations. An agency may not exceed statutory authority in writing the rules and may not violate the Constitution. All proposed and final rules must be published in the *Federal Register* (available online at www.federalregister. gov). The *Federal Register* is published every business day by the Government Printing Office and includes the Federal Agency Regulations, Proposed Rules and Public Notices, Executive Orders, Proclamations, and other presidential documents. Important resources for information about rulemaking include the review of federal regulations available on the Office of Information and Regulatory Affairs website (www.Reginfo.gov) and the website that provides a venue for the public to submit comments regarding the proposed rules and regulations (www.regulations.gov). APRNs engaged in health policy should be aware of these resources. Typically, there is a 30- to 60-day window of opportunity for the public to provide feedback regarding the proposed rule. Advocacy groups inform organizations, which in turn can inform members of important actions that would benefit from their comments. Sending letters to legislatures is one avenue, but posting comments is another way to influence policy.

There is an important distinction between law and regulation. APRNs need to be mindful of this difference when advocating for change locally or nationally. When an issue is specifically addressed in the law or statute, it requires a new law to make a change in the existing statute, as illustrated in Longest's (2016) cyclical model. However, if the issue is specified in regulation, it can be changed by a revision of the regulation using the rulemaking process. The less detail that is included in the statute, the more opportunity there will be for response to changes in the future environment by the use of rulemaking. One example that directly affects APRNs is the stipulation in the Medicare Law of 1965 that only physicians can certify a patient for home healthcare. Because it is in the law, it cannot be changed by rulemaking; it requires a new law. Each year, the CMS develops *The Physician Fee Schedule*, which specifies what services under Medicare Part B will be covered and reimbursed. It is a regulation that is published in the *Federal Register* and provides an opportunity to change rules that have been created in the past. In contrast to the law regarding certification for home healthcare, a regulation that prohibited APRNs from ordering portable x-rays, which resulted from the 1969 *Conditions for Coverage* (CMS, 2012) was removed in July 2012, with the *Proposed Rule for Revisions to Payment Policies Under the Physician*

Fee Schedule. The new regulation stated, "we propose revisions to the Conditions for Coverage at § 486.106(a) and § 486.106(b) to permit portable x-ray services to be ordered by a physician or nonphysician practitioner in accordance with the ordering policies for other diagnostic services under § 410.32(a)." Once a rule is finalized, it is reviewed by the House and the Senate. The House and Senate can pass a resolution of disapproval, which then can be approved or vetoed by the president. This review process began in 1996, and since then, only one rule has been disapproved by Congress (Office of the Federal Register, 2011).

THE APRN AS ENGAGED CITIZEN

Scanning the Environment

For APRNs to make an impact in health policy requires the engagement of each individual (see Table 9.1). Developing leadership skills and increasing the understanding of the political process will support the effectiveness of APRNs as they seek to increase their engagement. Business theory has described the concept of "scanning the environment," the monitoring of the organization's internal and external environment. APRNs can use this concept in the monitoring of the local and national health policy environment. The individual APRN can extend his or her reach at the federal and state levels by participating in professional organizations whose staff scan the environment daily. Scanning the local environment is just as important and provides an opportunity for direct involvement, especially for the fledgling political activist. Political process occurs in institutions as well, and engaging locally in small ways can be an avenue to increase confidence in advocacy that will extend to a larger stage.

Locally, APRNs can scan for opportunities to educate others about their role and respond to barriers when identified. It may be as simple as having the language on the school health form changed from physician to provider. When institutional policies set up barriers to full practice authority, the well-informed APRN is positioned to respond. Institutional policies that are more restrictive than necessary may be a result of a knowledge gap. The administrators who created the policy may lack an understanding of changes in federal and state laws that govern APRN practice. When an informed APRN presents data with a request for a change in policy and emphasizes the effect on improved patient care and the benefit to the organization, that APRN will be presenting a strong argument in support of his or her agenda. The uninformed APRN is at the mercy of policies from others that may not represent the current regulations. For example, a portable x-ray company, unaware of the change that occurred in the regulation in the physician fee schedule, may refuse to accept an order from an APRN. This may negatively affect the patient of an uninformed APRN who acquiesces to the policy. However, an informed APRN could use the strategy of providing data, emphasizing the effect on the patient and the benefit to the organization, and may successfully accomplish the objective and benefit colleagues as well.

TABLE 9.1 Policy Resources

	Websites	Description
LEGISLATIVE BRANCH		
Federal Legislative Information	www.congress.gov	Is the official website for up-to-date information on legislation presented by the Library of Congress
Library of Congress	www.loc.gov	Serves as an archival resource
House of Representatives	www.house.gov	Provides a directory of Representatives, leadership, committees, and legislation
U.S. Senate	www.senate.gov	Provides a directory of Senators, committees, and legislation
GovTrack.us	www.govtrack.us	Is not a government site but independently tracks the bills that are considered by Congress
Countable	www.countable.us	Provides updates on the bills being addressed daily in the U.S. Congress. Provides an avenue for contacting your representatives and informs you of how they voted. Includes an APP for your phone or tablet.
EXECUTIVE BRANCH		
White House	www.whitehouse.gov	Provides a directory of the executive branch, the executive offices, the White House schedule, and issues
HHS Administration	www.hhs.gov	Cabinet department
Centers for Disease Control and Prevention	www.cdc.gov	A department under HHS resource for many health statistics; publishes the *Morbidity and Mortality Weekly Report*
Centers for Medicare & Medicaid Services	www.cms.gov	Provides comprehensive information on Medicare, Medicaid, CHIP, and resource for statistics
Food and Drug Administration	www.fda.gov	Provides safety information, regulatory information
Substance Abuse and Mental Health Services Administration	www.samhsa.gov	Is a resource for mental health services and data
Health Resources and Services Administration	www.hrsa.gov	Provides information on National Health Service Corps, loans and scholarships, federally qualified health centers

(continued)

TABLE 9.1   Policy Resources *(continued)*

National Institute of Nursing Research	www.ninr.nih.gov	Provides funding for nursing scientists

RULEMAKING AND REGULATION

Federal Register	www.federalregister.gov	Includes all proposed and final rules; is published daily
Office of Information and Regulatory Affairs	www.Reginfo.gov	Publishes the *Unified Agenda and Regulatory Plan*
Regulations.gov	www.regulations.gov	Provides access to federal regulatory content; submits comments on documents published in the *Federal Register*

STATE RESOURCES

National Conference of State Legislatures	www.ncsl.org	Provides information and resources to state legislatures
National Governors Association	www.nga.org	Bipartisan coalition of governors to create a unified response to national issues

RESEARCH AND POLICY INSTITUTES

Cato Institute	www.cato.org	A public policy research organization focused on a wide variety of topics, including healthcare and welfare
Center on Budget and Policy Priorities	www.cbpp.org	Works on federal and state fiscal policies and programs that affect low- and moderate-income people
The Commonwealth Fund	www.commonwealthfund.org	Private foundation that supports healthcare systems
The Heritage Foundation	www.heritage.org	Mission is to formulate and support conservative public policies
Kaiser Family Foundation	www.kff.org	Provides policy analysis on national health issues

COALITIONS

Future of Nursing Campaign for Action	http://campaignforaction.org	An initiative of AARP, AARP Foundation, and the Robert Wood Johnson Foundation to implement the recommendations in the Institute of Medicine report on nursing

(continued)

TABLE 9.1	Policy Resources *(continued)*	
Robert Wood Johnson Foundation	www.rwjf.org	Shares evidence and promotes change in healthcare through partnerships and collaboration
The Nursing Community	www.thenursingcommunity.org	A coalition of 61 national nursing organizations that strive to "Speak With One Voice"

CHIP, Children's Health Insurance Program; HHS, Health and Human Services.

Working Collaboratively

Collaboration with other APRNs through professional engagement in nursing organizations (see Table 9.2) and with other healthcare providers and stakeholders will be a growing requirement in new regulatory models. New delivery models include accountable care organizations, medical/health homes, and retail clinics. These models are intended to be patient centered and to help contain costs. The Center for Medicare and Medicaid Innovation at the CMS was an agency created as a result of ACA. The center is charged with testing new healthcare delivery models. APRNs need to be aware of these initiatives and become active participants in the development of the models. Remember the warning: If you're not at the table you're on the menu.

As the public became more aware of the value of the patient-centered care provided by APRNs, coalitions formed outside of healthcare to support expansion of advanced practice nursing. It is equally important for APRNs to articulate their expertise and the contribution that advanced practice nursing can make to the success of the new delivery models, working together with other professionals to meet the objectives of improved quality at cost savings. With increased emphasis on interprofessional collaboration and new graduates who are prepared with interprofessional educational experiences, obstacles that have separated professionals in the past will hopefully be removed. Interprofessional models emphasize collaboration and increase the understanding of the expertise that each profession brings to the care of the patient.

The Policy Process and the Nursing Process

The cyclical nature of Longest's (2016) Health Policy Making Model has similarities with the nursing process: assessment, planning, intervention, and evaluation. The policy-making process, moving from a problem to the implementation of a program that aims to fix it, requires the separation of one problem from another. It requires us to understand that many solutions exist, to prioritize our needs, to interact and compromise with many other interests, and to be ready to respond to change, which is certain to come in a highly dynamic environment. With a more in-depth understanding of the legislative process, the rulemaking, and the development of regulation that follows, APRNs are prepared to apply that understanding to address their own concerns. Developing their leadership ability and connecting to their colleagues at the local, state, and national levels are essential to accomplishing policy change.

A Story of Successful Advocacy

On May 24, 2016, a rule to amend the VA's Medical Regulations to permit full practice authority for all four roles of advanced practice nurses was published in the *Federal Register* (APRN, 2016). This policy window was opened as a result of the problem of corruption that was revealed in 2014 with secret waiting lists created to disguise the lack of access available to veterans needing care. The VA treats 9 million veterans and is the largest healthcare system in the United States. In introducing the rule change, the VA cited the long wait times that had led to some deaths. They reported that more than a half million veterans were waiting at least 30 days for care, and another 300,000 were waiting 31 to 60 days. As nursing groups activated their membership to comment on the rule in Regulations.gov, the response was incredible. The document received 225,000 comments and the AANP reported that 88% of Americans surveyed agreed veterans should have direct access to APRNs.

The rationale for the move to allow APRNs full practice authority was all about access and not an ideological statement regarding APRN quality. The greatest resistance to the rule came from the anesthesiologists, and a key argument from them was the lack of a problem with access to anesthesia services. Their opposition was successful and certified registered nurse anesthetists (CRNAs) were removed from the final rule. This final rule was published on December 14, 2016, and included three APRN roles, NPs, CNSs, and CNMs. Of interest is the fact that currently the VA does not have CNMs on their staff, but they are exploring including them in the future.

The final rule became effective on January 13, 2017. In an article by GraduateNursingEDU (2017), the question was raised if this change, which allows for APRNs in all 1,500 VA medical facilities to practice to the full extent of their education and training regardless of the law of the state where the facility is located, would be a tipping point for APRN practice in the private sector as well. As each individual VA facility implements this new regulation, it will become one of the best demonstration models available to support future efforts in states still striving for APRNs' ability to practice to their full scope. This is an important time for APRNs to be vigilant and watch for open policy windows in their community.

TABLE 9.2 National APRN Professional Organizations

Organization	Website
American Academy of Emergency Nurse Practitioners	www.aaenp-natl.org
American Academy of Nursing	www.aannet.org
American Association of Colleges of Nursing	www.aacnnursing.org
American Association of Critical Care Nurses	www.aacn.org
American Association of Nurse Anesthetists	www.aana.com
American Association of Nurse Practitioners	www.aanp.org
American College of Nurse-Midwives	www.acnm.org
American Nurses Association	www.nursingworld.org
Association of Women's Health, Obstetric, and Neonatal Nurses	www.awhonn.org
Gerontological Advanced Practice Nurses Association	www.gapna.org
Hospice & Palliative Care Nurses Association	www.hpna.org
National Association of Clinical Nurse Specialists	www.nacns.org
National Association of Pediatric Nurse Practitioners	www.napnap.org
National Organization of Nurse Practitioner Faculties	www.nonpf.org
National Organization of NPs in Women's Health	www.npwh.org
Oncology Nurses Society	www.ons.org

SUMMARY

Healthcare policy is a moving target for each new administration. Although there was progress made with the Affordable Care Act, much is needed to fix the healthcare system. APRNs should and must be at the table when the reforms are suggested, made, and implemented. This can be accomplished only by becoming engaged in the political process at the local, state, and national levels. Involvement will require knowledge of legislation that impacts healthcare and APRN practice, how to engage politicians, participation in professional organizations, and becoming immersed in the politics of healthcare.

REFERENCES

Advanced Practice Registered Nurses, Vol #81 Fed Reg2016-12227. (May 24, 2016). (to be codified at 38 C. F. R pt. 17).

American Association of Colleges of Nursing. (2006). The essentials of doctoral education for advanced nursing practice. Retrieved from http://www.aacn.nche.edu/publications/position/dnpessentials.pdf

APRN Consensus Workgroup and APRN Joint Dialogue Group. (2008). Consensus model for APRN regulation: Licensure, accreditation, certification & education. Retrieved from http://www.aacn.nche.edu/Education/pdf/APRNReport.pdf

Centers for Medicare & Medicaid Services. (2012). Medicare program; revisions to payment policies under the physician fee schedule, proposed rules. *Federal Register*. Retrieved from https://www.federalregister.gov/articles/2012/07/30/2012-16814/medicare-program-revisions-to-payment-policies-under-the-physician-fee-schedule-dme-face-to-face#h-138

Cillizza, C. (2014, April 10). Yes, President Obama is right. The 113th Congress will be the least productive in history. *The Washington Post*. Retrieved from http://www.washingtonpost.com/blogs/the-fix/wp/2014/04/10/president-obama-said-the-113th-congress-is-the-least-productive-ever-is-he-right

Federal Trade Commission. (2014). Policy perspectives: Competition and the regulation of advanced practice nurses. Retrieved from http://www.ftc.gov/system/files/documents/reports/policy-perspectives-competition-regulation-advanced-practice-nurses/140307aprnpolicypaper.pdf

Foote, S. (2014, May 23). Why I blew the whistle on the VA. *The New York Times*, p. A 21.

Govtrack.us. (2018). Statistics and historical comparisons. Retrieved from https://www.govtrack.us/congress/bills/statistics

GraduateNursingEDU. (2017). The VA is now granting full practice authority to APRNs despite state laws—does this signal a tipping point? Retrieved from http://www.graduatenursingedu.org/2017/02

Institute of Medicine. (2010). *The future of nursing: Leading change, advancing health*. Retrieved from http://books.nap.edu/openbook.php?record_id=12956&page=R1

Kingdon, J. W. (2011). *Agendas, alternatives, and public policies* (2nd ed.). New York, NY: Longman.

Kuo, Y. F., Loresta, F. L., Rounds, L. R., & Goodwin, J. S. (2013). States with the least restrictive regulations experienced the largest increase in patients seen by nurse practitioners. *Health Affairs* 32(7), 1236–1243. doi:10.1377/hlthaff.2013.0072

Lenz, E. R., Mundinger, M. O., Kane, R. L., Hopkins, S. C., & Lin, S. X. (2004). Primary care outcomes in patients treated by nurse practitioners or physicians: Two-year follow-up. *Medical Care Research and Review, 61*, 332–351. doi:10.1177/1077558704266821

Longest, B. B. (2016). *Health policy making in the United States* (6th ed.). Chicago, IL: Health Administration Press.

McCleery, E., Christensen, V., Peterson, K., Humphrey, L., & Helfand, M. (2014). Evidence brief: The quality of care provided by advanced practice nurses. In: VA evidence-based synthesis program evidence briefs [Internet]. Washington DC: Department of Veterans Affairs.

Mundinger, M. O., Kane, R. L., Lenz, E. R., Totten, A. M., Tsai, W. Y., Cleary, P. D., ...Shelanski, M. L. (2000). Primary care outcomes in patients treated by nurse practitioners or physicians. *Journal of the American Medical Association, 283*, 59–68. doi:10.1001/jama.283.1.59

National Organization of Nurse Practitioner Faculties. (2017). Nurse practitioner core competencies content. Retrieved from http://www.nonpf.org/resource/resmgr/competencies/2017_NPCoreComps_with_Curric.pdf

Newhouse, R. P., Stanik-Hunt, J., White, K. M., Johantgen, M., Bass, E. B., Zangaro, G., . . . Weiner, J. P. (2011). Advanced practice nurse outcomes 1990-2008: A systematic review. *Nursing Economic$, 29,* 230–250.

Office of the Federal Register. (2011). A guide to the rulemaking process. Retrieved from https://www.federalregister.gov/uploads/2011/01/the_rulemaking_process.pdf

O'Grady, E. T. (2011). Advanced practice nursing and health policy. In J. M. Stanley (Ed.), *Advanced practice nursing: Emphasizing common roles* (pp. 351–377). Philadelphia, PA: F. A. Davis.

Oliver, G. M., Pennington, L., Revelle, S., & Rantz, M. (2014). Impact of nurse practitioner on health outcomes of Medicare and Medicaid patients. *Nursing Outlook, 62*(6), 440–447. doi:10.1016/j.outlook.2014.07.004

Portman, R. (2013, March 15). Gay couples also deserve a chance to get married. *The Plain Dealer.* Retrieved from http://www.dispatch.com/content/stories/editorials/2013/03/15/gay-couples-also-deserve-chance-to-get-married.html

Seib, G. (2008). In crisis, opportunity for Obama. *The Wall Street Journal.* Retrieved from http://online.wsj.com/article/SB122721278056345271.html

Stanik-Hutt, J., Newhouse, R. P., White, K. M., Johantgen, M., Bass, E. B., Zangaro, G., Wilson, R., . . . Weiner, J. P. (2013). The quality and effectiveness of care provided by nurse practitioners. *Journal for Nurse Practitioners, 9*(8), 492–500. doi:10.1016/j.nurpra.2013.07.004

Statista—The portal for statistics. Retrieved from https://www.statista.com/statistics/257337/total-lobbying-spending-in-the-us/

Stone, G. R., & Marshall, W. P. (2011). The framers constitution. *Democracy Journal. org,* pp. 61–66. Retrieved from http://www.democracyjournal.org/pdf/21/the_framers_constitution.pdf

USA.gov. (2018). U.S. federal government. Retrieved from http://www.usa.gov/Agencies/federal.shtml

U.S. Congress, Office of Technology Assessment. (1980). *The implications of cost-effectiveness analysis of medical technology.* GPO stock No. 052-003-00765-7. Washington, DC: U.S. Government Printing Office.

U.S. Congress, Office of Technology Assessment. (1986). *Nurse practitioners, physician assistants, and certified nurse-midwives: A policy analysis* (Health Technology Case Study37), OTA-HCS-37. Washington, DC: U.S. Government Printing Office.

Wakefield, M. (2006, February 19). So you want to be an advocate? Strategies for advocacy, knowledge, resources, colleagues and actions (PPT slides). In: *Presented at the American College of Nurse Practitioners health policy conference,* Washington, DC.

10

Kathryn A. Blair

PRACTICE ISSUES: REGULATION INCLUDING PRESCRIPTIVE AUTHORITY AND TITLE PROTECTION, CERTIFICATION, CLINICAL PRIVILEGES/CREDENTIALING, AND LIABILITY

APRNs encounter or will encounter a variety of professional issues during their careers. Most questions focus on what APRNs are permitted to do within the scope of nursing practice. Although APRNs have made progress in removing barriers to practice, many continue to exist. As healthcare reform evolves in individual states and on a national level, APRNs need to be fully cognizant of legislative or regulatory activity that may impede their ability to perform within their full scope of practice. In an ideal world, APRNs would have the same privileges and legal and prescriptive authority across all states.

As APRNs seek employment, they must consider what regulations will allow or limit their practice in their specific states. In doing so, they can choose positions that are congruent with their educational scope of practice. They should also know what credentials might be needed to practice in a certain state, institution, or organization. For example, if they choose to practice in a selected state, would they be able to prescribe medications, sign death certificates, admit patients to hospitals, sign worker's compensation claims or disabled parking permits? Would they be required to be supervised by a physician, develop a collaborative agreement, or have restrictions placed on their billing? These are all practice issues that surround regulation, certification, scope of practice, and liability.

The terms "regulation," "certification," and "credentialing," as they apply to all APRNs, can be misunderstood by the public as well as healthcare providers. There are distinct differences in the meaning of each term and understanding these terms will help APRNs carry out their roles while avoiding any barriers that may exist.

REGULATION

The development of regulation begins with the legislative process. Once legislation is passed, most laws go to an administrative rules committee comprising legislators who develop rules for interpreting the law. Administrative rules committees often seek input from professionals, consumers, and parties affected by the law. It is extremely important for APRNs to be "at the table" during these discussions. The absence of APRN input during the rulemaking can result in special interest groups influencing whether rules are broadly or literally interpreted.

Regulation is a mechanism to define scope of practice, level of educational requirements, the degree of prescriptive authority, and level of physician involvement. "Scope of practice" encompasses who can practice as an APRN (legal authority), who can prescribe (prescriptive authority), and who can receive reimbursement (Sonenberg & Knepper, 2016). "Title protection" is a necessary component of regulatory function to protect the public from those who are not authorized to use the APRN title.

Nursing practice is regulated by each state in accordance with state statutes and interpreted through administrative rules. In most states, APRNs are regulated under the authority of a board of nursing. The major functions of the boards of nursing are to provide scope and standards of nursing practice and education, licensure requirements, title, and rules for disciplinary action and remedies.

Annual legislative updates published in the *Nurse Practitioner* highlight the state regulations for APRNs. As of 2018, 14 states (AK, AZ, DC, HI, IA, ID, MT, ND, NH, NM, OR, RI, WA, and WY) have independent practice without physician supervision, delegation or collaboration, and full prescriptive authority; 11 states (CO, CT, DE, MD, ME, MN, NE, NV, SD, VT, and WV) have independent practice with full prescriptive authority after post-licensure/certification period of supervision; and 26 states (AL, AR, CA, FL, GA, IL, IN, KS, KY, LA, MA, MI, MO, MS, NC, NJ, NY, OH, OK, PA, SC, TN, TX, UT, VA, and WI) have limited practice and prescriptive authority under a physician supervision (Phillips, 2018). Additional resources are available that elaborate further whether APRNs are eligible for medical staff membership (Barton Associates, 2017).

This variability of state regulation of APRNs inhibits APRNs from moving from state to state with the same authority and scope of practice. As of 2015, 25 states have enacted a Nurse Licensure Compact for registered nurses to increase employment between states (National Council of State Boards of Nursing, 2015). More recently the enhanced nurse licensure compact (eNLC) implementation date of January 2018 will replace the original nurse licensure compact and enable registered nurses and APRNs greater mobility (National Council of State Boards of Nursing, 2017).

The road to removing regulatory barriers for APRNs has been a daunting journey. However, due to the perseverance and endless efforts of individual and professional advanced practice advocates, APRNs can practice in every state. However, much more work needs to be done to educate legislators, interprofessional groups, and the public to provide access to safe, competent care for all consumers.

A hallmark publication by the committee on the Robert Wood Johnson Foundation Initiative on the *Future of Nursing* at the Institute of Medicine (IOM) has provided support and foundation for state legislatures to update nurse practice acts to allow APRNs to practice to the full extent of their licenses. The publication, *The Future of Nursing. Leading Change, Advancing Health* (IOM, 2011), makes four recommendations:

1. Nurses should practice to the full extent of their education and training.
2. Nurses should achieve higher levels of education and training through an improved education system that promotes seamless academic progression.
3. Nurses should be full partners, with physicians and other health professionals, in redesigning healthcare in the United States.
4. Effective workforce planning and policy making require better data collection and an improved information infrastructure (p. S-3).

The implications of this publication continue to unfold and provide a positive forum for APRNs to remove barriers from practice. The timing of this publication, along with the Patient Protection and Affordable Care Act of 2010 (ACA), has been helpful for nursing and APRNs to promote legislation in their states and encourage provider-neutral terminology.

Prescriptive Authority

Historically, the issue of prescriptive authority has been a barrier to autonomy in advanced nursing practice. The ability to prescribe medications allows the APRN more flexibility in implementing holistic care for patients. Although great strides have been made legislatively to allow full prescriptive authority in each state, there continues to be inconsistency among states.

Prescriptive authority can be granted in several ways. The greatest independence is in those states where APRNs have full practice authority and can prescribe medications, including controlled substances, independent of any required physician involvement. The first states to provide legislation granting prescriptive authority were Washington, Oregon, and Alaska during the 1970s. All states allow APRNs to prescribe medications, including controlled substances, but some states require some degree of physician collaboration or delegation or limit controlled substances (Phillips, 2018).

Another issue surrounding prescriptive authority is the language used in regulations and legislation. Some rules and regulations specify "nurse practitioner," excluding clinical nurse specialists (CNSs), certified nurse-midwives (CNMs), and certified registered nurse anesthetists (CRNAs). Increasingly, legislation is written to reflect the expanded advanced nursing practice title. Terms that have been used include "midlevel practitioner," "midlevel provider," "advanced practice nurse," and "APRN." Terms such as "/ often refer to nurse practitioners (NPs), CNSs, CNMs, physician assistants (PAs), or anyone who is not a physician, suggesting that these providers are less than a physician rather than being identified within the context of their own profession. For example, the term "APRN" clearly identifies the nurse with advanced practice training and education within his or her profession of nursing and does not suggest a provider who is less than a physician but different from a physician. Active participation in the political process by professional nursing lobbyists and individuals has resulted in provider-neutral terminology for all APRNs.

Other trends serve to restrict or limit prescriptive practice. These include a movement toward joint regulation (a joint board with representatives from pharmacy, medicine, and nursing); reluctance to "grandfather in" nurses with existing prescriptive authority; ignoring state boards of nursing actions by other governmental agencies; restricting drug utilization review boards to pharmacists and physicians; and unwillingness by insurance companies to fill prescriptions written by APRNs.

In 1991, the U.S. Drug Enforcement Administration (DEA) proposed rules for affiliated practitioners (e.g., NPs, PAs) that would have imposed restrictive regulations for APRNs that superseded state laws. The DEA rules did not acknowledge the existing prescriptive regulations in states. Nurses in independent practice would have been affected by the ruling. However, the DEA withdrew these proposed rules after a huge protest from the nursing community. A second ruling entitled Definition and Registration of Mid-Level Practitioners was proposed in 1992 (*Federal Register*, 1992). The 1992 ruling is less restrictive regarding prescriptive authority for APRNs. DEA registration is required to prescribe controlled substances; APRNs can apply for DEA registration online at www.deadiversion.usdoj.gov. A practitioner-prescribing manual is also available through the DEA website www.deadiversion.usdoj.gov/pubs/manuals/pract/index.html.

An additional requirement governing prescriptive authority is the national provider identification number (NPI), which is a 10-digit unique identification number issued by the Centers for Medicare & Medicaid Services (CMS) to U.S. healthcare providers for submission of claims or other transactions specified by the Health Insurance Portability and Accountability Act (HIPAA). All noncontrolled substance prescriptions require the utilization of the NPI. (NPI numbers can be obtained or accessed online at nppes.cms.hhs.gov.)

Drug utilization review programs mandated by the Omnibus Budget Reconciliation Act of 1990, effective from January 1, 1993, were designed to reduce fraud, abuse, overuse, or unnecessary care among physicians, pharmacists, and patients. Currently, no state specifically provides for the inclusion of nurses or other healthcare members on the review program board. The exclusion of APRNs from these boards is a concern because prescriptive practice by APRNs will be evaluated by individuals lacking a nursing perspective.

Prescriptive authority of medications, including controlled substances, is not only a privilege; it is a responsibility that APRNs cannot take lightly. The provider is fully responsible for understanding the regulatory parameters for prescribing these drugs. Ongoing pharmacotherapeutics education is essential in safe prescribing practices. All prescribers should avoid any prescribing practices that would put their prescriptive privileges at risk.

Title Protection

One of the functions of regulation is title protection, which limits the use of a title unless the user meets the requirements mandated by state regulation. Currently, 39 states have legislation that protects the title "nurse" (American Nurses Association [ANA], 2013) through explicit or implicit language in their nurse practice act. Restriction of the term "nurse" affords reassurance to the public that the individual using that title has met all the requirements mandated for licensure in that state. Eleven states do not provide title protection; however, these states do regulate professional nursing. Of the 39 states that offer title protection for the title "nurse," only seven states specifically delineate the various APRN categories such as NP, CNM, CNS, or CRNA in the statute. Without title protection, persons can call themselves nurses without meeting the requirements in those states.

There is variability as to the title for APRN in each state. Currently, there are 13 titles associated with the recognition of APRNs by state regulatory boards. Table 10.1 provides a list of these titles. The APRN Consensus Workgroup and APRN Joint Dialogue Group (2008) identify NPs as certified nurse practitioners (CNPs), one of the four APRN roles.

Title protection is not synonymous with autonomous or uniform regulation. APRNs must continue to promote legislation to remove statutory restrictions that limit advanced practice nursing. The APRN Consensus Workgroup and APRN Joint Dialogue Group (2008) proposed the title APRN as the licensing title for the four advanced practice roles. Since the publication of this model, several states have incorporated the model and titling in their state statutes to follow the APRN regulatory model, which is one of the driving forces for revising state regulatory statutes.

Even as advanced practice education moves toward requiring the clinical doctorate for practice at the entry level, several states have statutory restrictions against doctorally prepared NPs being addressed as "doctor" (Pearson, 2009). Several advanced practice nursing organizations developed

TABLE 10.1	APRN Titles Recognized by State Regulatory Bodies
APN	Advanced practice nurse
APNP	Advanced practice nurse prescriber
APPN	Advanced practice professional nurse
APRN	Advanced practice registered nurse
ARNP	Advanced registered nurse practitioner
CNM	Certified nurse-midwife
CNP	Certified nurse practitioner
CNS	Clinical nurse specialist
CRNA	Certified registered nurse anesthetist
CRNM	Certified registered nurse-midwife
CRNP	Certified registered nurse practitioner
NA	Nurse anesthetist
RNP	Registered nurse practitioner

a unified statement outlining Doctor of Nursing Practice (DNP) certification, education, and use of the title "doctor" (Nurse Practitioner Roundtable, 2008). The unified statement acknowledges that a medical doctor or doctor of osteopathy may be title protected, but explains that "doctor" represents an academic credential and no discipline owns the title "doctor." Furthermore, the recognition of the title "doctor" for APRNs who are doctorally prepared facilitates parity within healthcare (Nurse Practitioner Roundtable, 2008).

Consensus Model for APRN Regulation, Licensure, Accreditation, Certification, and Education

The variability in scope of practice, recognized advanced practice roles, criteria for entry into advanced practice, and accepted certification examinations have created confusion for legislators and the public. A model has been developed that includes four essential elements—licensure, accreditation, certification, and education (LACE)—to protect the public and decrease barriers for APRNs who practice in multiple states. "Licensure" is the granting of authority to practice; "accreditation" is the formal review and approval by a recognized agency of educational degree; "certification" is the formal recognition of the knowledge, skills, and experience demonstrated by the achievement of standards identified by the profession; and "education" is the formal preparation of APRNs in graduate

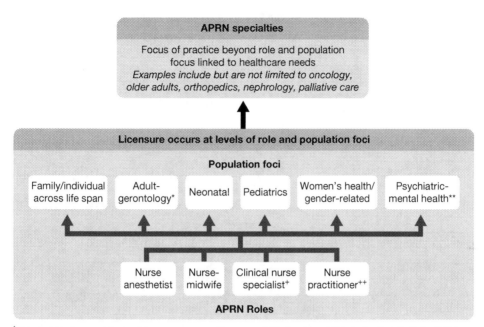

*The population focus, adult-gerontology, encompasses the young adult to the older adult, including the frail elderly. APRNs educated and certified in the adult-gerontology population are educated and certified across both areas of practice and will be titled adult-gerontology certified nurse practitioner (CNP) or clinical nurse specialist (CNS). In addition, all APRNs in any of the four roles providing care to the adult population (e.g., family or gender specific) must be prepared to meet the growing needs of the older adult population. Therefore, the education program should include didactic and clinical education experiences necessary to prepare APRNs with these enhanced skills and knowledge.

**The population focus, psychiatric/mental health, encompasses education and practice across the life span.

⁺CNS is educated and assessed through national certification process across the continuum from wellness through acute care

⁺⁺Acute or primary care CNP

FIGURE 10.1 APRN regulatory model.
Source: APRN Consensus Workgroup and APRN Joint Dialogue Group. (2008). *Consensus model for APRN regulation: Licensure, accreditation, certification and education*, p. 9. Retrieved from http://www.aacn.nche.edu/Education/pdl/APRNReport.pdf

degree-granting or postgraduate certificate programs (APRN Consensus Workgroup and APRN Joint Dialogue Group, 2008, p. 7).

The Consensus model or APRN regulatory model defines and offers title clarity. APRN is a legal title and through the Consensus model, CRNAs, CNMs, CNSs, and CNPs are acknowledged as APRNs (Stanley, 2012). The consensus group recognized that there are many nurses with graduate preparation, such as nurse educators, informatics specialists, or administrators; however, their focus is not direct care to individuals. The model provides for APRNs to "be licensed as independent practitioners for practice at the level of one of the four APRN roles within at least one of the six identified population foci. Education, certification, and licensure of an individual must be congruent in terms of role and population foci. APRNs may be specialized but they cannot be licensed solely within a specialty area" (APRN Consensus Workgroup and APRN Joint Dialogue Group, 2008, p. 5).

The APRN regulatory model (Figure 10.1) illustrates the four advanced practice roles educated by an accredited academic program in at least one

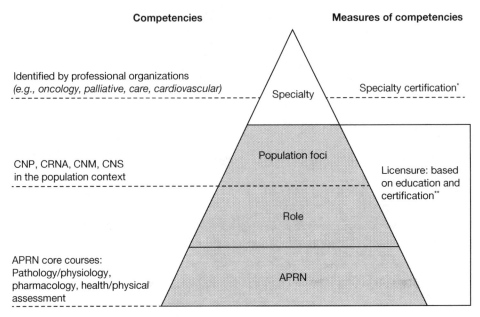

Competencies   **Measures of competencies**

Identified by professional organizations
(e.g., oncology, palliative, care, cardiovascular)   Specialty   Specialty certification*

CNP, CRNA, CNM, CNS
in the population context   Population foci   Licensure: based
on education and
certification**

APRN core courses: Role
Pathology/physiology,
pharmacology, health/physical   APRN
assessment

*Certification for specialty may include exam, portfolio, peer review, and so on.

**Certification for licensure will be a psychometrically sound and legally defensible
examination by an accredited certifying program.

FIGURE 10.2 Relationship among educational competencies, licensure, and certification in
the role/population foci, and education and credentialing in a specialty.
Source: APRN Consensus Workgroup and APRN Joint Dialogue Group. (2008). *Consensus
model for APRN regulation: Licensure, accreditation, certification and education*, p. 14. Retrieved
from http://www.aacn.nche.edu/Education/pdl/APRNReport.pdf

of six population foci: family/individual across the life span, adult/geron-
tology, neonatal, pediatrics, women's health/gender related, and psychi-
atric/mental health. Licensing will occur at the level of role and population
focus, and certification will reflect the population focus. APRN specialties are areas of focus beyond the role and population. Implementation of
the model will occur incrementally by state boards of nursing. Figure 10.2
illustrates the relationship among educational competencies, licensure, and
certification in the role/population foci and education and credentialing in
a specialty.

CERTIFICATION

The introduction of the APRN regulatory model has put a greater emphasis
on certification. Certification by a national board has been a requirement
for regulatory processes and prescriptive authority. Certification differs
from licensure in that certification is a process by which a nongovernmental agency or association certifies that an individual licensed to practice a profession has met certain predetermined standards specified by that
profession for population or specialty practice. The purpose of certification

is to assure that an individual has mastered a body of knowledge and acquired skills for a particular population or specialty.

Historically, certification in nursing has been murky with no uniform standards. Many specialty organizations certified nurses with varying educational backgrounds at one general level. Most certification agencies now require a master's or higher degree to be eligible for certification at an advanced practice level. As the APRN regulatory model is implemented, certification for licensing at an advanced practice level will reflect the six populations identified and entry level will be at the practice doctorate level. Specialty certification will occur by the same or additional certifying bodies. Specialty certification will not suffice alone for licensing as an APRN.

Certifying Bodies

American Association of Critical-Care Nurses Certification Corporation

The certification arm of the American Association of Critical-Care Nurses (AACN), the American Association of Critical-Care Nurses Certification Corporation (AACNCC), began offering certification for CNSs in 1999.

The AACN Certification Corporation now has population and specialty certifications for APRNs (AACNCC, n.d.). Their advanced practice consensus model–based certifications include acute care nurse practitioner (adult-gerontology; ACNPC-AG) and clinical nurse. AACNCC offers a certification (CCRN-K) for critical care nurses and APRNs who influence patients, nurses, and/or organizations to have a positive impact on acutely and/or critically ill adult, pediatric, or neonatal patients but do not work at the bedside.

American Association of Nurse Practitioners (AANP)—Certification Board

The AANP has an affiliated organization, the AANP Certification Board (AANPCP), that provides entry-level, competency-based examinations in three areas: adult, family, and adult-gerontology primary care. The purpose of this certification is "to provide a valid and reliable program for entry-level NPs to recognize their education, knowledge and professional expertise" (AANPCB, 2017). Medicare, Medicaid, the Veterans Administration, and private insurance companies recognize NPs in all 50 states, as well as certification by the AANPCB. NPs receiving certification by the AANPCB use NP-certified as their credential.

American Nurses Credentialing Center (ANCC)

The ANCC provides certification for the nursing profession, guaranteeing to the public that nurses have a certain level of knowledge or skill. The ANCC is an outgrowth of the ANA certification program, which was established in 1973 to function as an independent center through which the ANA would serve as its own credentialing program. ANCC certifies RNs and APRNs in specialty nursing practice ensuring competence and nursing excellence (Strickland, 2018). ANCC also recognizes healthcare organizations, which foster nursing excellence through Magnet® Recognition Program.

Historically, ANCC certified CNSs in the following areas: adult health gerontology, public/community health, child/adolescent psychiatric mental health, and adult psychiatric mental health. These certifications have been retired, however, and those currently certified in these areas need to recertify. In collaboration with the National Association of Clinical Nurse Specialist (NACNS), the ANCC formerly offered a core CNS examination that addressed competencies across the lifespan, regardless of the specialty focus; however, this exam has been retired to move certification to a population-based focus. Today ANCC offers certification for CNSs in two areas: Adult-Gerontology CNS and Pediatric CNS.

The ANCC also certifies NPs in five clinical areas: (a) adult/gerontology primary care, (b) adult/gerontology acute care, (c) family, (d) pediatric primary care, and (e) psychiatric and mental health. Certification examinations for adult, gerontology, adult psychiatric and mental health, school, and advanced diabetes management will no longer be offered, but individuals can continue to recertify.

Over the years, the ANCC has granted multiple credentials to designate certification at an advanced practice level. Over the past 15 years, APRNs have seen multiple changes in their credentials. For example, before 1993, NPs certifying with the ANCC were given in their titles "C" to indicate certification. CNSs were given the credential "CS." From 1993 to 2000, both CNSs and NPs were given "CS" as the certifying credential. After 2000, NPs and CNSs were first given the credential APRN-BC; then APRN, BC, to indicate APRN, board certified. Currently, NPs and CNSs have their own certification credential that reflects the clinical focus. For example, a family nurse practitioner (FNP) would have the following credentials: "FNP-BC" representing FNP–board certified. An adult/gerontology CNS would use the credentials "AGCNS-BC" to signify board certification for this population.

American Midwifery Certification Board (AMCB)

The AMCB is the certifying body for CNMs and certified midwives (AMCB, n.d.). Students who have completed graduate programs accredited by the Accreditation Commission for Midwifery Education (ACME) are eligible to take the examination. Certification by the AMCB is the gold standard for CNMs and is recognized in all 50 states. Certified midwives require a graduate degree, but not nursing degree, for certification and are recognized in four states. Certified professional midwives (CPMs) are certified by the North American Registry of Midwives. No educational degree is required for the CPM designation, which is regulated in 27 states.

National Board of Certification and Recertification of Nurse Anesthetists (NBCRNA)

Since 1956, CRNAs have been certified by the NBCRNA. There are more than 120 accredited CRNA programs and, of those programs, 16 award the DNP (Council on Accreditation, n.d.). CRNAs take the National Certification Exam (NCE) and are required to take a minimum of 40 hours of approved continuing education every 2 years, maintain state licensure, and document substantial anesthesia practice for a minimum of 850 hours. The NBCRNA recently increased passing standards (NBCRNA, 2017).

Other Certification Opportunities

Although most specialty organizations provide certification for professional nursing practice, few offer certifications at an advanced practice level. The organizations that offer advanced practice examinations are often at the specialty level of the APRN regulatory model. The American Psychiatric Nurses Association (APNA) considered offering certification for advanced practice psychiatric mental health nurses, but currently, the certification as a psychiatric/mental health CNS or NP comes through the ANCC.

Women's Health

The National Certification Corporation (NCC) offers certification for women's healthcare NPs and neonatal NPs. The NCC also offers a subspecialty certification in gynecologic reproductive health along with the two core certifications (NCC, 2015). The NCC was formerly known as the Nurses' Association of the American College of Obstetricians and Gynecologists (NAACOG) Certification Corporation. The NAACOG was renamed the Association for Women's Health, Obstetrics, and Neonatal Nursing and became an independent certification organization in 1991.

Pediatrics

Pediatric NPs can also be certified by the Pediatric Nursing Certification Board (PNCB). The PNCB offers certification for primary care pediatric NPs and acute care pediatric NPs. Certified pediatric NPs, pediatric CNSs, and family NPs are also eligible to take the pediatric primary mental health specialists certification examination offered by PNCB if they meet the eligibility criteria (PNCB, 2018).

Oncology

The Oncology Nursing Society through the Oncology Nursing Certification Corporation (ONCC) offers certification for NPs (Advanced Oncology Certified Nurse Practitioner [AOCNP]) and CNSs (Advanced Oncology Certified Clinical Nurse Specialist [AOCNS]). The ONCC also offers an Advanced Oncology Certification Nurse (AOCN) designation for nurses with master's degrees or higher working in administration, clinical practice, education, or research (ONCC, 2014). Other examples of specialty certification include orthopedic nurse practitioners (ONP-C) and clinical nurse specialists (OCNS-C) certified by the Orthopaedic Nurses Certification Board (ONCB, 2014).

The Council for the Advancement of Comprehensive Care (CACC), established in 2000, is a consortium of academic and health policy leaders who are committed to ensuring high standards of doctoral nursing practice. In 2007, the CACC collaborated with the Board of Medical Examiners to develop and administer a certification examination for DNPs. The comprehensive care certification examination is comparable to the performance standards in Step 3 (the final step) in the U.S. medical licensing exam (USMLE) for medical students. Although the examinations are similar, the comprehensive care certification examination is only for graduates of DNP programs, and the candidate must be certified as an APRN. APRNs who pass this examination are designated diplomats in comprehensive care by the American Board of Comprehensive Care. The AACN released a statement in March 2009 to clarify that this examination is considered a specialty exam defined by Columbia University and is not a population-based examination (AACN, 2009). The CACC examination is an examination for DNP graduates from comprehensive care programs.

Criteria for Certification

Each certifying body has its own set of eligibility criteria. Certification corporations that certify NPs, CNSs, and CRNAs require a master's degree. Some of the early NPs and CRNAs graduated from nonmaster's certificate programs and have been "grandfathered in." In the future, eligibility criteria may require a practice doctorate to apply for certification.

Each certification area (e.g., family, adult, acute care, women's health) may have different practice or recertification requirements. Given the dynamic nature of certification and professional standards, the reader is referred to the specific certification website for the desired advanced practice role. Exhibit 10.1 provides a list of some websites offering information on eligibility and the application process.

Accreditation of Educational Programs

Accreditation of educational programs for APRNs will become integrated with the APRN Regulation Model. The American Association of Colleges of Nursing (AACN) has developed *Essentials* documents that provide guidance for baccalaureate (AACN, 2008), master's (AACN, 2011), and DNP programs (AACN, 2006). The DNP *Essentials* was followed by a white paper clarifying recommendations (AACN, 2015). These *Essentials* provide the roadmap for nursing programs and accreditation organizations.

The Commission on Collegiate Nursing Education (CCNE) and National League for Nursing Commission for Nursing Education Accreditation (NLNCNEA) are the major accrediting organizations for all nursing education. In addition, each APRN role has developed standards

---

Exhibit 10.1 CERTIFICATION WEBSITES

- American Association of Critical-Care Nurses Certification: www.aacn.org/certification
- American Board of Comprehensive Care: http://abcc.dnpcert.org/
- American Midwifery Certification Board: www.amcbmidwife.org
- American Nurses Credentialing Center: www.nursecredentialing.org
- American Academy of Nurse Practitioners Certification Program: www.aanpcert.org
- Oncology Nursing Certification Corporation: www.oncc.org
- Orthopaedic Nurses Certification Board: www.oncb.org
- National Board of Certification and Recertification for Nurse Anesthetists: https://thecrna.com/recertification
- National Certification Corporation: www.nccwebsite.org
- Pediatric Nursing Certification Board: www.pncb.org

---

or competencies that are used in the evaluation of specific programs. The American College of Nurse-Midwives developed competencies for basic midwifery (ACNM, 2012) and the American Association of Nurse Anesthetists (AANA) developed guidelines for core clinical privileges (AANA, 2013). Competencies for NPs and CNSs have been developed by the NACNS and the National Organization of Nurse Practitioner Faculties (NONPF), respectively (NACNS, 2009; NONPF, 2017). The NONPF has also developed criteria for evaluation of NP programs (NONPF, 2016). CNM and CRNA programs are also accredited by the ACME and the Council on Accreditation of Nurse Anesthesia Educational Programs (COA), respectively.

Credentials

One of the concerns related to certification is the multiplicity of acronyms that are used to indicate certification and that each certifying body uses its own credentials. The frequent change in credentials, as well as the variety of terms used to indicate advanced practice nursing, is confusing for the consumer as well as other healthcare professionals. As regulatory bodies become more uniform and as certification corporations align their examinations with the APRN regulatory model, there may be more consistency and understanding of the titles that reflect advanced practice.

In the interim, APRNs can facilitate common terminology within their organizations. For example, having a common format for name badges that is consistent with documentation signatures would be a first step. The American Nurses Credentialing Center (2013) provides guidance for listing credentials in the following order: degree, licensure, state designation or requirement, national certification, honors or awards, then other certifications. An illustration of this titling is as follows: Jane Doe, DNP, APRN, FNP-BC, FAAN.

Clinical Privileges and Credentialing

"Clinical privilege" is "the process of authorizing a healthcare practitioner's specific scope and content of patient services" (Health Resources and Services Administration [HRSA], 2015, p. 83) and "credentialing is the process of assessing and confirming the license or certification, education, training and other qualifications of the licensed or certified healthcare practitioner" (HRSA, 2015, p. 88). The Joint Commission, formerly known as the Joint Commission on Accreditation of Healthcare Organizations (JCAHO), specifies characteristics of a process for the delineation of clinical privileges. The Joint Commission's 2012 accreditation manual for hospitals states that medical staff must credential and privilege all licensed independent practitioners (LIP; JCAHO, 2017). The process and procedural details must be outlined in medical staff bylaws. Non-LIPs, such as PAs and APRNs, may be privileged through an established medical staff process that reflects The Joint Commission's credentialing and privileging standards.

Clinical privileges have been successfully obtained for CNMs and CRNAs. Set standards are processes typically established through the appropriate medical departments (i.e., obstetrics or anesthesia). Clinical privileges for CNSs and NPs have been more difficult to obtain. The great diversity in qualifications for APRNs, including CRNAs and CNMs, makes it difficult for agencies to develop uniform clinical privileging guidelines for all APRNs.

Although there is some variability in the credentialing process, The JCAHO recommends a series of steps for medical staff. Credentialing is the first step in the process that leads to privileging. Typically, the credentialing process includes the application, verification of credentials, evaluation of applicant-specific information, and a recommendation to the governing medical board for appointment and privileges. The medical staff has the discretion to use the information provided to make the appropriate decision regarding privileges. The information that is required should include data on qualifications, such as licensure, education, experience, and clinical competence. A period of focused professional practice is implemented for all successful applicants who have requested privileges (JCAHO, 2017).

APRNs must go through a similar process of credentialing to obtain clinical privileges. Each institution has a specific process and form, although they all contain components required by the JCAHO. As a result, an APRN requesting clinical privileges at four different hospitals is likely to undergo four separate application procedures and reviews. The title given to the APRN will also likely vary, depending on each institution. Designations such as "allied health provider," "associate allied health provider," and "non-physician provider" are often used in granting clinical privileges for APRNs.

Institutions must have not only a credentialing process in place, but also a review process, including peer review every 2 years, for the renewal of clinical privileges. However, temporary privileges may be granted for a limited time. Most institutions use the same application forms and processes for LIPs and non-LIPs. These forms are medically focused and often difficult for providers who are not physicians to use. Some institutions tailor their credentialing process specifically for APRNs with appropriate terminology that reflects current regulations. State laws and hospital policies determine who can practice independently. The JCAHO defines an LIP as "any individual permitted by law and organization to provide care, treatment, and services, without direction or supervision" (JCAHO, 2017). In states that require a collaborating or supervising physician, practice agreements are required as part of the credentialing process.

As APRNs continue to practice within their full scope of practice in acute care facilities, clinical privileges become more important. There continues to be confusion among medical staff as to specific requirements for cosigning clinical documentation for PAs, APRNs, interns, residents, and fellows. Unfortunately, some institutions require physicians to cosign all clinical documentation, even if the law does not require it, to avoid any errors in documentation for billing purposes. There is also ongoing discussion regarding whether CNSs and NPs who are credentialed in acute care facilities should be certified as acute care NPs or CNSs.

The process for obtaining clinical privileges will be facilitated with a common language about advanced nursing practice among institutions and across states. The placement of nurses in high administrative posts in agencies as well as having APRNs on credentialing panels will also make it less difficult for APRNs to obtain clinical privileges. Educating staff, physicians, institutions, and communities regarding advanced nursing practice will be necessary before clinical privileges are granted without question for all APRNs.

LIABILITY

As APRNs assume more autonomy and independence, liability issues arise. APRNs must work within their scope of practice; maintain certification, including continuing education requirements; and retain adequate liability coverage.

To practice within their scope of practice, APRNs must comply with state and federal regulatory statutes/laws. The interpretation of law/statute through administrative rules will determine whether APRNs are practicing within their scope of practice. An example of the importance of administrative rules in interpreting state statutes is illustrated in the following case.

A pediatric NP became interested in pain management and was hired by a pain clinic. After working there for some time, it was requested that she obtain prescriptive authority to allow her to prescribe pain medication, including controlled substances for all age groups.

Based on the administrative rule that allows prescription orders appropriate to the APRN's area of competence as established by education, training, or experience, the board of nursing deemed the NP eligible to obtain prescriptive privileges because of her experience in the pain clinic. However, the NP believed that it was in her best interest to return to school and obtain postmaster's certification as an adult NP to expand her scope of practice to include all the populations to which she provided care.

There has been an increase in malpractice claims filed against APRNs in recent years, because more APRNs are employed more than ever before and often attorneys name anyone associated with the case to increase the award or recovery costs. Overall, however, APRNs—particularly NPs— have had fewer adverse claims against them compared with physicians. An annual analysis of the Healthcare Integrity and Protection Data Bank (HIPDB) of the number of accumulated malpractice reports or adverse actions submitted by NPs, PAs, and physicians, show in 2014 NPs have a lower percentage of malpractice claims than physicians, 41% versus 56%, respectively (Brock, Nicholson, & Hooker, 2017). From 2004 through 2010, 369 out of 2,664 anethesia-related malpractice payments associated with CRNAs. (Jordan, Ouraishi, & Liao, 2013). In a survey of nurse-midwives, 32% responded they had been named in a lawsuit (Guidera, McCool, Hanlon, Schulling, & Smith, 2012).

One question that many APRNs raise is whether they should carry their own malpractice insurance in addition to their employer's liability coverage. The simple answer is yes. As discussed previously, APRNs are not immune from malpractice claims. There exist a few myths surrounding malpractice claims such as the following:

• You are more likely to be sued if you carry your own insurance.
• You do not need insurance because you are covered by your employer.
• You get sued only if you do something wrong (Pohlman, 2012).

Not having insurance does not guarantee that you will not be sued nor is it protection against a lawsuit. You do not have to do something wrong, only the patient needs to believe you did something wrong and having insurance through place of employment does insure the employer will defend you.

Understanding the law may help dispel these misconceptions about malpractice. Medical malpractice is the failure of a medical professional to follow the accepted standards of practice of his or her profession, resulting in harm to the patient. "Vicarious liability" is a concept used when an employer is sued for an employee's actions or omissions. Although your employer may be sued, you still can be found liable and the employer can sue you for damages paid (Duncan & Turner, 2010).

APRNs must become familiar with legal terminology to avoid committing unintentional acts of negligence. Table 10.2 briefly outlines terms that are often unfamiliar. A "tort" or "civil wrong" occurs when professionals fail

TABLE 10.2 Legal Terminology

Tort	An injury or wrongdoing
Tort liability	The right of an injured individual to be made whole again
Intentional tort	An individual (APRN) commits an act with intent to bring about the result in question
Negligence	A failure to fulfill a responsibility that subsequently results in injury to an individual

to properly execute their duty to a client resulting in a breach, which is the actual and proximate cause of injury or harm (www.law.cornell.edu/wex/malpractice#). The term "intentional tort" means that an APRN commits an act that brings about an intended result or an act that has a substantial risk of the intended result. Intentional torts can include assault and battery (unwanted touch does not have to result in physical injury), false imprisonment (holding a patient against his or her will), intentional infliction of emotional distress (HIPAA violation), and fraud (misinformation; Duncan & Turner, 2010). Examples of malpractice (tort) claims fall under the following categories: failure, delayed or misdiagnosis, delayed or wrong treatment, improper consent, failure to monitor, and failure to instruct or communicate (Sweeney, La Mahieu, & Fryer, 2017).

During their careers, the majority of APRNs may confront the legal system via malpractice claims even if they did nothing wrong; therefore, being protected is imperative. Types of malpractice insurance are "occurrence policies" and "claims-made policies." Occurrence policies provide coverage for events occurring during the policy period regardless of when the claim is filed, while claims-made policies cover the claims if reported during the policy period. Malpractice litigation is here to stay until there is tort reform; APRNs should be proactive about insurance coverage.

APRNs can protect themselves from potential malpractice claims in several ways. First and foremost, APRNs must practice within their scope of practice and the legal scope as determined by their individual state. Second, APRNs should carry professional liability insurance either through their employer, through personal professional liability insurance, or both. APRNs can take several preventive measures to avoid legal or malpractice claims such as having thorough documentation and open communication with patient and family and other providers involved in the patient's care, following clinical practice guidelines and evidence-based practice, staying up-to-date with current practices, and knowing their limitations and when to refer.

Legal issues related to negligence and malpractice can be a cause of concern and stress for healthcare providers, including APRNs. APRNs should take preventive measures to limit the risk of having claims filed against them.

PRACTICE ISSUES

There are many practice issues that can be discussed; some have definitive answers, and some do not. Most practice issues have safety, legal, or ethical implications. Some practice issues may resolve as new legislation is passed or new policy is put in place, but other issues may persist, and new practice issues will emerge. This section discusses selected practice issues related to innovative technology, billing and reimbursement, blurred practice boundaries, and professional accountability. There are many gray areas in advanced nursing practice; therefore, knowing one's legal responsibility, scope of practice, and prescriptive authority is extremely important.

Innovative Health Technology

As healthcare technology grows exponentially, several issues arise. First, with advancement in treatment modalities, many patients are surviving beyond their prognostic time frames. As these patients survive longer, unanticipated consequences of their treatment may arise. For example, Zakak (2009) raises the possibility of fertility issues in childhood cancer survivors. Therapies used to treat the cancers may have been successful in terms of curing or remitting the cancer, but may have eliminated the patient's ability to conceive and later achieve the developmental milestone of parenthood. Anticipating consequences of therapies is essential in providing informed consent and in allowing patients to choose alternative treatments.

Another issue related to innovative technology is the choice of test that is needed to diagnose or follow up on a condition. Perhaps the clinical practice guideline suggests a CT scan for evaluation of a mass, but a newer technology is developed that may provide better diagnostic information. However, the new technology is much more expensive and puts the patient at a greater radiation risk. Elderly patients may choose not to undergo expensive diagnostic tests or treatment because they have lived a healthy, productive life and are prepared for death. APRNs will face many similar situations that conflict with personal ethical beliefs and must determine whether to support the patient's choice based on the ethical, regulatory, and legal boundaries of their practice.

Off-label use of pharmacologic agents is another example in which the original research submitted to the U.S. Food and Drug Administration (FDA) was for one indication but, through its use, another indication arose. The manufacturer often decides not to go through the process of gaining FDA approval for a second indication. If APRNs were to prescribe the medication for a use other than the approved indication, would prescribing that medication put them at risk for malpractice, even though the use of that medication for the nonapproved indication is common among healthcare providers?

Billing and Reimbursement Issues

Accurate billing and coding are difficult to learn, but it is extremely important to ensure that the APRN obtains the appropriate reimbursement

and does not overbill or underbill the patient. Although APRNs historically underbill for services provided, both underbilling and overbilling are
considered fraud. Chapter 11 provides an excellent overview of the reimbursement process, billing, and coding. Ongoing review and continuing education on reimbursement cannot be overemphasized. Some practice issues
related to billing and reimbursement arise from shared billing practices or
pressure from organizations to bill "incident-to" for higher reimbursement.

Along the lines of reimbursement is the choice of pharmacologic agents.
Pharmacy formularies adopted by insurance companies may insist on a certain pharmacologic agent for a certain diagnostic code. That drug may not
be the most beneficial for the patient. Prior authorizations can be requested,
but they are denied if the generic or formulary equivalent has not been
tried for a certain amount of time. If the medication is approved, it is often
approved at a higher copay for the patient. The time spent obtaining approval or the time the patient must spend trying and failing an alternative
agent diminishes the quality of care.

Blurred Boundaries

APRNs may be placed in situations in which there is not a clear delineation
of role. The APRN needs to feel comfortable when making any decision or
engaging in any procedure. For example, an NP whose practice is limited
to adults provides care for a 32-year-old mother. The mother asks the NP
to assume care for her 10-year-old daughter because she has confidence
in the NP and the closest provider for the daughter is 30 miles away. You
might argue that when adult-care NPs care for 10-year-olds, they are clearly
out of their scope of practice. However, if that 10-year-old were in a life-
threatening situation, would the NP be liable for not initiating care?

APRNs may encounter other situations that stretch the limits of educational preparation or that are not clearly defined within the regulatory
realm. Hudspeth (2007) discusses balancing the need for adequate educational preparation with the needs of behavioral health services. For example, an adult NP or a CNS may have a large percentage of patients with
behavioral health issues. APRNs will need to determine whether they have
adequate preparation to care for these patients or if more education and/or
certification is required. Brekken and Sheets (2008) address balancing the
need to provide adequate pain management with the following regulatory
guidelines for controlled substances. A recent random clinical trial demonstrated improved outcomes with providing vocational case management
services in primary care to support patients with musculoskeletal problems
(Bishop et al., 2014). The cost versus benefit of adding such services is often
a difficult decision for providers and managers.

Professional Accountability

The foundation of the APRN role is nursing and embedded in nursing professionalism is professional accountability. Professional accountability can
be a nebulous concept; however, one definition is taking responsibility for

one's judgments, actions, or omissions regarding patient care outcomes while maintaining competency and standards of nursing practice (Krautscheid, 2014). Closely aligned with accountability are the principles of ethics and legal aspects of healthcare. APRNs are responsible for maintaining clinical competence and this requires a commitment to lifelong learning. APRNs should embrace accountability as not a "blame game" but as an opportunity for learning and shared responsibility. Accountability transcends patient care but includes support and active participation in professional organizations (local, state, and/or national). Nursing organizations are a means to give a voice to APRNs and the profession.

APRNs, like every professional, will make an error in judgment at some point in their careers and will have to decide how to own the mistake and be accountable. Additionally, APRNs will be confronted with tough ethical decisions such as abortion and passive euthanasia. Regardless of the issue, APRNs must set the standard for professional accountability for protection and safety of the public.

SUMMARY

This chapter addresses professional issues that influence advanced nursing practice. APRNs may encounter situations that place them at risk for liability claims or regulatory misconduct. It is the responsibility of APRNs to have a full sense of their scope of practice, maintain adequate liability coverage, and practice within the legal authority for their state. Every APRN must understand his or her scope of practice, know the regulations in his or her state, and maintain appropriate certifications to demonstrate competence as an entry-level APRN. As the APRN regulatory model is implemented and titling of APRNs becomes more consistent, there will be less confusion regarding their roles in whatever settings they choose to practice. As more states implement full practice authority for APRNs, they will move from non-LIPs to LIPs within healthcare organizations.

REFERENCES

American Academy of Nurse Practitioner Certification Board. (2017). Values, mission and purpose. Retrieved from https://www.aanpcert.org/certs/purpose

American Association of Colleges of Nursing. (2006). The essentials of doctoral education for advanced practice nurses. Retrieved from http://www.aacnnursing.org/Education-Resources/AACN-Essentials

American Association of Colleges of Nursing. (2008). The essentials of baccalaureate education for professional nursing practice. Retrieved from http://www.aacnnursing.org/Education-Resources/AACN-Essentials

American Association of Colleges of Nursing. (2009). Update on the new comprehensive care certification exam. Retrieved from http://www.aacn.nche.edu/DNP/pdf/CCExamStatement.pdf

American Association of Colleges of Nursing. (2011). The essentials of master's education in nursing. Retrieved from http://www.aacnnursing.org/Education-Resources/AACN-Essentials.

American Association of Colleges of Nursing. (2015). The doctor of nursing practice: Current issues and clarifying recommendations. Retrieved from http://www.aacnnursing.org/Portals/42/DNP/DNP-Implementation.pdf

American Association of Critical Care Nurses Certification Corporation. (n.d.). About AACN Certification Corporation. Retrieved from https://www.aacn.org/about-aacn/about-aacn-cert-corp

American Association of Nurse Anesthetists. (2013). Guidelines for core clinical privileges for certified registered nurse anesthetists. Retrieved from https://www.aana.com/docs/default-source/practice-aana-com-web-documents-(all)/guidelines-for-core-clinical-privileges-for-crnas.pdf?sfvrsn=b20049b1_4

American College of Nurse-Midwives. (2012). Core competencies for basic midwifery. Retrieved from http://www.midwife.org/ACNM/files/ACNMLibraryData/UPLOADFILENAME/000000000050/Core%20Comptencies%20Dec%202012.pdf

American Midwifery Certification Board. (n.d.). Home page. Retrieved from http://www.amcbmidwife.org

American Nurses Association. (2013). Title "nurse" protection. Retrieved from http://www.nursingworld.org/MainMenuCategories/Policy-Advocacy/State/Legislative-Agenda-Reports/State-TitleNurse

American Nurses Credentialing Center. (2013). How to display your credentials. Retrieved from http://www.nursecredentialing.org/DisplayCredentials-Brochure.pdf

American Nurses Credentialing Center. (2014). Home page. Retrieved from http://www.nursecredentialing.org

APRN Consensus Workgroup and APRN Joint Dialogue Group. (2008). Consensus model for APRN regulation: Licensure, accreditation, certification and education. Retrieved from http://www.aacn.nche.edu/Education/pdl/APRNReport.pdf

Barton Associates. (2017). Nurse practitioner scope of practice laws. Retrieved from https://www.bartonassociates.com/locum-tenens-resources/nurse-practitioner-scope-of-practice-laws

Bishop, A., Wynne-Jones, G., Lawton, S. A., van der Windt, D., Main, C., Sowden, G., . . . Forster, N. C. (2014). Rationale, design and methods of the study of work and pain (SWAP): A cluster randomised controlled trial testing the addition of a vocational advice service to best current primary care for patients with musculoskeletal pain. *BMC Musculoskeletal Disorders, 15*(1), 232. doi:10.1186/1471-2474-15-232

Brekken, S. A., & Sheets, S. V. (2008). Pain management: A regulatory issue. *Nursing Administration Quarterly, 32*(4), 288–295. doi:10.1097/01.NAQ.0000336725.03065.44

Brock, D. M., Nicholson, J. G., & Hooker, R. S. (2017). Physician assistant and nurse practitioner malpractice trends. *Medical Care Research and Review, 74*(5), 613–624. doi:10.1177/1077558716659022

Council on Accreditation (n.d.). Homepage. Retrieved from http://home.coa.us.com/accredited-programs/Pages/CRNA-School-Search.aspx

Duncan, M. J., & Turner, R. E. (2010). *Torts a contemporary approach: Interactive casebook series* (2nd ed.). St. Paul, MN: Thomson-Reuters.

Federal Register. (1992). Definition and registration of mid-level practitioners 21 C.F.R. Parts 1301 and 1304. *Federal Register, 57*(146), 33465.

Guidera, M., McCool, W., Hanlon, A., Schulling, K., & Smith, A. (2012). Midwives and liability: Results from the 2009 nationwide survey of certified nurse midwives and certified midwives in the United States. *Journal of Midwifery & Women's Health, 57*(4), 345–352. doi:10.1111/j.1542-2011.2012.00201.x

Health Resources and Services Administration. (2015). Health center program compliance manual. Retrieved from https://bphc.hrsa.gov/programrequirements/pdf/healthcentercompliancemanual.pdf

Hudspeth, R. (2007). Balancing need, preparation and scope of practice: Issues impacting behavioral health services by advanced practice registered nurses. *Nursing Administration Quarterly, 31*(3), 264–265. doi:10.1097/01.NAQ.0000278940.34244.87

Institute of Medicine. (2011). *The future of nursing: Leading change, advancing health.* Washington, DC: National Academies Press.

Joint Commission on Accreditation of Healthcare Organizations. (2017). *Comprehensive accreditation manual for hospitals: The official handbook (CAMH).* Oakbrook Terrace, IL: Joint Commission Resources.

Jordan, L. M., Ouraishi, J. A., & Liao, J. (2013). The national practitioner data bank and CRNA anesthesia-related malpractice payments. *American Association of Nurse Anesthetists Journal, 81*(3), 178–182.

Krautscheid, L. C. (2014). Defining professional nursing accountability: A literature review. *Journal of Professional Nursing, 30,* 43–47. doi:10.1016/j.profnurs.2013.06.008

National Association of Clinical Nurse Specialists. (2009). *Core practice doctorate clinical nurse specialist (CNS) competencies.* Harrisburg, PA: Author.

National Board of Certification and Recertification for Nurse Anesthetists. (2017). Homepage. Retrieved from http://www.nbcrna.com/Pages/default.aspx

National Certification Corporation. (2015). Home page. Retrieved from https://www.nccwebsite.org

National Council of State Boards of Nursing. (2015). Nurse licensure compact Retrieved from https://www.ncsbn.org/nurse-licensure-compact.htm

National Council of State Boards of Nursing. (2017). Enhanced Nurse Licensure Compact (eNLC) enactment: A modern nurse licensure solution for the 21st Century. Retrieved from https://www.ncsbn.org/11070.htm

National Organization of Nurse Practitioner Faculties. (2016). *Criteria for evaluation of nurse practitioner programs* (5th ed.). Washington, DC: Author. Retrieved from http://c.ymcdn.com/sites/www.nonpf.org/resource/resmgr/Docs/EvalCriteria2016Final.pdf

National Organization of Nurse Practitioner Faculties. (2017). *Nurse practitioner core competencies with suggested curriculum content.* Washington, DC: Author. Retrieved from http://c.ymcdn.com/sites/www.nonpf.org/resource/resmgr/competencies/2017_NPCoreComps_with_Curric.pdf

Nurse Practitioner Roundtable. (2008). *Nurse practitioner DNP education, certification and titling: A unified statement.* Washington, DC: Author.

Oncology Nursing Certification Corporation. (2014). Home page. Retrieved from http://www.oncc.org

Orthopaedic Nurses Certification Board. (n.d.). ONC certification and NP certification. Retrieved from https://www.oncb.org/certifications/

Patient Protection and Affordable Care Act. (2010). PL 111-148. Retrieved from http://housedocs.house.gov/energycommerce/ppacacon.pdf

Pearson, L. J. (2009). The Pearson report. *The American Journal for Nurse Practitioners, 13*(2), 4–82.

Pediatric Nursing Certification Board. (2018). Pediatric primary care mental health specialist. Retrieved from https://www.pncb.org/pmhs

Phillips, S. (2018). 30th Annual APRN legislative update. *The Nurse Practitioner, 43*(1),27–54. doi:10.1097/01.NPR.0000527569.36428.ed

Pohlman, K. J. (2012). Why you need your own malpractice insurance. *American Nurse Today, 10*(11), 28–30.

Sonenberg, A., & Knepper, H. J. (2016). Considering disparities: How do nurse practitioner regulatory policies, access to care, and health outcomes vary across states? *Nursing Outlook, 65,* 143–153. doi:10.1016/j.outlook.2016.10.005

Stanley, J. M. (2012). Impact of new regulatory standards on advanced practice registered nursing: The APRN consensus model and LACE. *Nursing Clinics of North America, 47,* 241–250. doi:10.1016/j.cnur.2012.02.001

Strickland, D. (2018). Did you know? [Editorial]. *Colorado Nurse, 118*(1), 1–2.

Sweeney, C. F., LeMahieu, A., & Fryer, G. E. (2017) Nurse practitioner malpractice data: Informing education. *Journal of Professional Nursing, 33,* 271–275. doi:10.1111/j.1542-2011.2012.00201.x

Zakak, N. N. (2009). Fertility issues of childhood cancer survivors: The role of the pediatric nurse practitioner in fertility preservation. *Journal of Pediatric Oncology Nursing, 26*(1), 48–59. doi:10.1177/1043454208323617

Andra Fjone and Cheri Friedrich

REIMBURSEMENT REALITIES FOR THE APRN

Healthcare continues to change in new and growing ways. Meaningful use, burgeoning technology, financial capability, risk management, population health management, and data security are just a handful of those changes. It is thought that changes in policies around the Patient Protection and Affordable Care Act (ACA), new reimbursement programs such as the Medicare Access and CHIP Reauthorization Act of 2015 (MACRA) Quality Payment Program and Centers for Medicare and Medicaid Services (CMS), mergers and consolidation of healthcare plans, and finally, consumer changes and demands will all play roles in the upcoming healthcare changes (Appold, 2017). As a result of these many modifications, APRNs are poised for the changes as they continue to focus on leadership, system change, and best practice. APRNs of today are growing in numbers and playing meaningful roles in changing systems as they care for both individuals and populations. Among the many changes APRNs will encounter, meeting the Triple Aim continues to remain one of them. The Triple Aim is a framework from the Institute for Healthcare Improvement (IHI) to guide care delivery in which (a) costs are contained, (b) patient care experiences are improved, and (c) population health is addressed and improved (Berwick, Nolan, & Whittington, 2008). In 2014, this was updated to the Quadruple Aim as an expansion of the IHI's Triple Aim to include the concept that the work life of healthcare providers should be improved (Bodenheimer & Sinsky, 2014). New models of care are needed to achieve these goals. Interprofessional collaboration has been promoted as a means to achieving the Quadruple Aim, although it is unclear how billing within a team care model will occur and furthermore how team care will impact billing for APRNs. To date, the future of the ACA remains under question. Some suggest that legislative substitute proposals would create situations such as increases in premiums and loss of health insurance (Glied & Jackson, 2017).

Healthcare cost containment is critical yet hard to achieve without decreasing care quality. Factors such as the aging population's need for advanced treatment technologies, chronic diseases, obesity, and genetic advancements affect costs and are all areas where APRNs have practice and leadership opportunities if they understand reimbursement realities. It is well documented that APRNs provide high-quality, cost-effective care (Yox & Stanik-Hutt, 2016). To ensure that APRN care is recognized, APRN care must be visible through provider-specific coding and documentation. As reimbursement trends are expected to change from fee-for-service to outcome-based reimbursement, APRNs need to be informed and engaged in reimbursement processes and issues. This engagement should include negotiating contracts, lobbying insurance companies for direct reimbursement, and maintaining strong relationships with clinic administrators and coders. APRNs must understand the changing economics of healthcare. However, given the changing climate in healthcare today, APRNs also ought to work for significant healthcare reform to support cost-effectiveness for all (Martin-Misener et al., 2015).

ACCESS, QUALITY, AND COST

Healthcare costs are expected to rise as the population ages, expensive technologies develop, and the prevalence of chronic illness rises (Deloitte, 2014). Currently, the cost of one patient is 35% of provider income, compared to 5% in 2000 (Evans & Fleming, 2017). Employers continue to raise employees' cost sharing for healthcare by increasing the deductible amounts and copayments for care. Healthcare spending in 2012 rose more than 3% from 2009 to $2.8 trillion, or $8,233 per person in the United States (Martin, Hartman, Whittle, Catlin, & the National Health Expenditure Accounts Team, 2014). In 2017, those with employer-sponsored health insurance paid an average of $18,764 for family coverage, with additional out-of-pocket expenses for copayments, medications, and other health-related costs (Kaiser Family Foundation, 2017). This demonstrates a steady rise in healthcare costs over the past 6 years (Kaiser Family Foundation, 2017).

Although healthcare costs continue to increase worldwide, the American healthcare system remains the most expensive in the world. For example, healthcare spending grew to 17.2% of the U.S. gross domestic product (GDP) in 2016, far more than in any other developed country (Organization for Economic Co-operation and Development ([OECD], 2017b). This rate is in striking contrast to that of other countries providing a similar quality of healthcare. For instance, Canada spent 10.6% of its 2016 GDP on healthcare (OECD, 2017). Factors contributing to higher U.S. costs include a payment system that rewards doing more as opposed to being efficient, an aging U.S. population, and a focus on advancing technologies (Appleby, 2012).

Healthcare reform efforts are focusing on cost containment, disease prevention, and evidence-based practice as means to address the economic realities. However, there is no "quick fix" for long-standing issues related to healthcare access, quality, and cost-effectiveness. Healthcare is costing patients, employers, and payers more each year and has become a very closely watched economic indicator. APRNs must be well informed about the context and specifics of reimbursement to be successful in practice. Federal and state actions influence healthcare reimbursement in many ways, such as by regulating healthcare systems, by supporting research, and particularly by financing and delivering healthcare services. Reimbursement politics are played out in Congress, in state legislatures, and within county governments. Political processes may also take place at APRN work sites as employment agreements and organizational policies are negotiated. APRNs must understand the various healthcare forces and players, particularly issues related to access, quality, and cost.

Access to care is complex in the United States and is directly related to cost issues. Over the past 20 years, the peak for lack of health insurance was in 2010, when 48.6 million individuals (16%) in the United States lacked insurance coverage and access to healthcare compared to 9% or 28.6 million in 2016. (Clark, Norris, & Schiller, 2017). It is most likely that this improvement was the result of the ACA legislation passed in 2010. The primary goals of the ACA are to expand health coverage, lower healthcare costs, and shift focus from treatment to prevention (U.S. Department of Health and Human Services [DHHS], 2013). It is expected that with the implementation of the ACA, the numbers of those with insurance will increase unless there are changes in federal policies.

In 2016, approximately 67.5% of individuals with insurance were covered by private healthcare insurance, while 37.3% were covered by governmental insurance (Barnett & Berchick, 2017). Americans with insurance continue to have concerns because copayments are increasing and benefits are sometimes limited. Many health plans require referrals and prior authorizations for the more costly healthcare components. In addition, some health plans limit patients to seeing only the providers on their salaried staff (staff-model health maintenance organizations, or HMOs) or a contracted list of specialists and agencies (preferred provider organizations, or PPOs). Triage or tiering of clients according to the types and price of coverage offered by employer plans and insurance carriers is a way of limiting healthcare services. HMOs, self-insured companies, and small businesses may have high deductibles, copayments, and prior authorization procedures that limit choices of providers, procedures, and referrals. Another care model introduced along with the implementation of the ACA is that of accountable care organizations (ACOs). ACOs are groups of healthcare providers and hospitals that come together to give high-quality care to patients (CMS, 2017). The goal of this coordinated care is to reduce duplication of services, thereby reducing costs (CMS, 2017a).

Many programs attempt to monitor and improve healthcare quality. One example is the Agency for Healthcare Research and Quality (AHRQ), a federal agency devoted to tracking trends, providing model programs, and researching outcomes. Partnerships of public and private agencies, such as the program Consumer Assessment of Healthcare Providers and Systems (CAHPS), work together to assess care, report system performance, and recommend or fund improvement efforts. A myriad of reports of care outcomes of hospitals, nursing homes, and individual providers is available for comparison. The Commonwealth Fund, the Institute of Medicine (IOM), the Robert Wood Johnson Foundation, the National Committee for Quality Improvement, and National Quality Forum are just a few of the organizations very active in quality improvement efforts. Nurses working toward care improvement are active in all those entities as well as in many professional nursing organizations. APRNs can contribute to these efforts by membership and leadership in these organizations. This active engagement will ensure that APRNs stay abreast of current quality improvement efforts in healthcare, which can have a direct effect on reimbursement.

U.S. REIMBURSEMENT TRENDS

The U.S. healthcare delivery system hardly resembles the system in place just a decade ago, and a whole new language has developed that APRNs must understand (Table 11.1). The U.S. healthcare industry has adopted the bottom line–oriented, profit–loss mentality of the business world, now with the overlay of the law of the land (ACA) as it is being interpreted in each state. As this complexity pervades American healthcare, APRNs can offer ways of ensuring access and quality of care while keeping costs reasonable for consumers.

Capitated systems (that replace fee-for-service payments) are more commonly seen in the inpatient setting in most states. Hospital stays (regulated by federally administered diagnostic-related group [DRG] regulations) have been shortened because of the cost, and patients are discharged earlier and sicker than in the past. The amount of healthcare delivered in outpatient settings continues to grow, likely as a result of healthcare legislation (Premier, Inc., 2013). Although many outpatient services are still billed on a fee-for-service model, there is an increasing number of services where there is a contract with payers for coverage of outpatient client groups. In these models, payers contract with provider groups to pay a per-member amount to cover the cost of member healthcare services over a certain time period. Home care services may or may not be available on discharge, often putting burdens on families and communities to provide care that used to occur in hospitals. Medicare regulations have become more complex, and employer-paid healthcare benefits, not surprisingly, have become a very contentious issue in labor negotiations.

Prescription drug use has increased, partly due to direct-to-consumer advertising that urges patients to contact their healthcare providers for the latest "miracle" drug. In an attempt to provide medications while controlling costs, the federal government implemented a voluntary program called Part D of Medicare in 2006 to subsidize prescribed medications for those covered by Medicare who apply for this special program. Part D is a very complex program that is a public–private partnership; it offers the elderly many different plan choices, and the application process is very complex. Opinions are mixed regarding its effectiveness; prescription drug costs continue to be a large part of Medicare expenditures and much lobbying occurs from the pharmaceutical industry. Americans spend about 30% more on

TABLE 11.1   Reimbursement Vocabulary

Terminology	Definition
Actual charge	The amount of money a provider charges for a particular service, which may be more than the amount payers approve
Additional benefits	Healthcare services not covered by Medicare; additional benefits subject to cost sharing by plan enrollees
Adjusted community rating	Premium rates based on regional differences in healthcare costs; leads to great regional differences in Medicare payment rates to providers
ABN	A notice that a provider must have Medicare beneficiaries sign when providing a service that Medicare does not consider medically necessary; if the patient does not get an ABN to sign before the service is provided and Medicare does not pay for it, the patient does not have to pay for the service
Affiliated provider	A healthcare provider or facility that is paid by a health plan to give service to plan members (i.e., a credentialed provider)
Ancillary services	Professional services by a hospital or other inpatient facility (e.g., x-rays, drugs, laboratory services)
Appeal	A formal complaint made to a health plan
Approved amount (or approved charge)	The fee a payer sets as reasonable for a covered service (may be less than the amount charged by the provider)
Balance billing	A situation in which private fee-for-service providers can charge and bill Medicare patients 15% more than the plan's payment
Beneficiary	The name for a person who has health insurance through the Medicare or Medicaid program
Capitation	A per-member amount paid to providers to cover the cost of member healthcare services for a certain time period
Carrier	A private company that has a contract with Medicare to pay Medicare Part B bills
Catastrophic limit	The highest amount of money patients have to pay out of pocket during a certain time period for certain charges
CMS	Federal agency that runs Medicare and works with the states to run Medicaid programs
COBRA	A law that makes an employer continue to cover an employee for a period of time after spousal death, job loss, divorce, or hours/benefits reduction; typically requires payment of both employee and employer shares of the premium
Coordination of benefits	Process in which two or more health plans share costs of a claim
Cost sharing	The cost for medical care that patients pay (copayment, coinsurance, deductible)

(continued)

TABLE 11.1   Reimbursement Vocabulary *(continued)*

Terminology	Definition
Covered benefit	A service that is paid for (partially or fully) by a health plan
DRG	A payment system begun in 1983 to pay hospitals for healthcare based on patients' diagnosis, age, gender, and complications; DRGs affect length of hospital stay
Durable medical equipment/goods	Reusable equipment that is ordered for use in the home (e.g., walkers) and paid for under Medicare
Facilities charge	A charge billed to a health plan or provider for the facility in which the service was received; results in two bills (provider bill and facility bill)
Fiscal intermediary	A private company that contracts with Medicare to pay Part A and some Part B bills; located in various regions of the United States
Fraud and abuse	Fraud: to purposely bill for services that were never given or to bill for a service at a higher reimbursement rate than the service produced Abuse: payment for items or services that are billed by mistake
HMO/network	A health plan that contracts with group practices of providers to give services in one or more locations
Managed care plan with POS option	A managed care health plan that lets patients use providers and hospitals outside the plan for an additional cost
Medically necessary services	Services deemed by Medicare to be proper and needed for a medical diagnosis or specific treatment
MSA	A Medicare health plan option made up of two parts: (a) Medicare MSA Health Insurance Policy (has a high deductible) and (b) special savings account in which Medicare deposits money to help patients pay their own medical bills
PPO	A managed care plan in which hospitals and providers belong to a network and contract together with payers/employers to provide services at predetermined rates
Prior authorization	MCO approval that is necessary before receiving care from providers who are out of the PPO or not on the staff list (can be verbal or is a written form from the MCO)
Referral	A written document that must be received by a provider before giving care to a health plan beneficiary
RBRVS	A Medicare fee schedule established in 1989 to reimburse providers based on RVUs

ABN, advanced beneficiary notice; CMS, Centers for Medicare & Medicaid Services; COBRA, Consolidated Omnibus Budget Reconciliation Act; DRG, diagnosis-related group; HMO, health maintenance organization; MCO, managed care organization; MSA, medical savings account; POS, point-of-service; PPO, preferred provider organization; RBRVS, resource-based relative value scale; RVU, relative work value unit.

pharmaceuticals compared with Canada (OECD, 2017). Prescription drug use has now increased to 20% in the United States (Kessellheim, Avorn, & Sarpatwarik, 2016).

APRNs can now be directly reimbursed for their services and must be knowledgeable about trends, developments, and proposed payment systems and reimbursement schedules. APRNs will be successful in their practices to the extent that the value of their services is recognized by payers and employers and is equitably rewarded. APRNs must be cost-effective and must track their productivity within complex systems; however, the rapid pace of change in reimbursement legislation, policies, and procedures makes this a daunting task. APRNs can be cost-effective by offering high-quality care, working within healthcare home models, and managing chronic diseases.

APRNs were not always reimbursed for their services by public and private payers. A series of lobbying efforts at national and state levels occurred over time to make this possible. Federal and state legislation currently regulates APRN reimbursement. For example, the 1997 federal Balanced Budget Act (BBA; P.L. 105-33) provides direct Medicare reimbursement for nurse practitioners (NPs) and clinical nurse specialists (CNSs), effective January 1, 1998. Rules to implement this law were written by the CMS (formerly known as the Health Care Financing Administration [HCFA]) and were finalized in November 1998. These Medicare laws and rules influence the policies of nongovernmental payers, although there is a great deal of variability from state to state. APRNs must carefully monitor CMS activities to ensure that the policies continue to favor APRN reimbursement. The goal is to have provider-inclusive language, meaning that laws and policies do not specifically designate payment to physicians but use the term "providers," which is inclusive of NPs and CNSs. Terminology in policy and law is an extremely important issue for APRN practice. Since January 2011, nurse-midwives have been reimbursed by Medicare at 100% of the physician fee schedule, a major victory for that group of APRNs.

The Health Insurance Portability and Accountability Act (HIPAA), a law passed in 1996 (also sometimes called the "Kassebaum–Kennedy law"), began the practice of implementing provider-inclusive language in federal law and policy. It expanded healthcare coverage related to job loss or transfer and provided some patient protection by limiting ways that insurance companies could use preexisting medical conditions to deny health insurance coverage. Although HIPAA generally guarantees the right to renewal of health coverage, it did not supersede states' roles as the primary regulators of health insurance. It standardized healthcare billing and payment mechanisms across systems, a move that promised to reduce costs once it was fully implemented. As part of that standardization, stringent patient privacy regulations were also instituted. The anticipated cost and quality improvements from HIPAA have not yet been realized, although it has certainly had many positive results. Electronic health records (EHRs) have rapidly been introduced since HIPAA was passed, and there are predictions that in time EHRs will bring about cost savings and quality improvements.

There continues to be significant growth in retail-based healthcare, which debuted in the early 2000s. Retail-based clinics are called by many names, including convenient care clinics and in-store clinics. Their numbers increase yearly, and one study demonstrated a lower overall cost of healthcare (Sussman et al., 2014). Medical associations such as the American Academy of Pediatrics have openly stated that the use of retail-based clinics is an inappropriate choice for pediatric care (Laughlin, 2014). These clinics typically employ NPs and have given new visibility to APRN practice. They appear to offer consumers a good-quality alternative to care in ambulatory clinics and emergency departments for commonly occurring complaints.

Another model of care and reimbursement being introduced is termed "medical home," sometimes referred to as "healthcare home." This payment mechanism aims to reimburse designated practices for care coordination activities. The goal is to deliver community-based, continuous, comprehensive, culturally appropriate healthcare. Originally developed in pediatrics for children with chronic conditions, this model has been increasingly advocated for all primary care practices. NPs are in a perfect position for leading medical homes with their knowledge of care coordination, chronic illness management, and patient education (Stokowski, 2012). It has also been shown that this model of care will help meet the expected primary care physician shortage (Auerbach et al., 2013). It is essential that APRNs track medical/healthcare home models of care and reimbursement policies to ensure that they all contain provider-inclusive language. If not, this model of care will benefit physician practices and either exclude or make invisible the work of APRNs. The cost–benefit of the model is a matter of controversy (Friedberg, Schneider, Rosenthal, Volpp, & Werner, 2014).

Pay-for-performance (also called P4P) is another healthcare trend that APRNs must carefully track and use to their best advantage. Reimbursement is linked to outcome measures by public and private payers, including the CMS. The goal is to provide incentives for quality care, a worthy aim. However, clinical performance is not easily measured, given multifactorial patient outcomes, and P4P has had mixed reviews as a strategy to decrease costs and increase care quality (Chien, Eastman, Li, & Rosenthal, 2012).

REIMBURSEMENT STRUCTURES

Third-Party Payers

APRNs must understand many issues about healthcare regulation (Figure 11.1), including the relationships among entities that pay for and provide services. For example:

1. For-profit insurance companies known as "indemnity providers" (e.g., Aetna, Prudential)
2. Government payment programs (e.g., Medicare, Medicaid, Tricare/ CHAMPUS, the military health system)

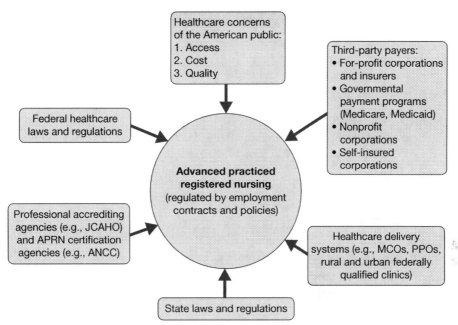

FIGURE 11.1 Reimbursement regulations for APRNs.

3. Nonprofit corporations (e.g., BlueCross/BlueShield)
4. Self-insuring corporations or coalitions (e.g., union healthcare plans)

Although payer policies and procedures differ greatly, most are influenced by the CMS Medicare regulations that enact federal legislation. Payers pay fee-for-service bills, the traditional way that healthcare has been funded. More recently, they pay for healthcare delivered under service contracts with HMOs and PPOs; provider systems must compete and bid for those contracts, unions participate in the negotiations, and contracts are rebid every few years. Employers typically offer their employees a choice of approved health system plans with which they can contract. Other employers self-insure by directly contracting with provider networks for their employees' care. These competitive contracts are frequently renegotiated in response to rising healthcare costs. The federal and state interpretations of the ACA through state insurance exchanges are dynamic, political, and an area of rapid change. Thus, healthcare finance is complex and volatile, and provider system costs are under constant review by payers, regulators, and the general public.

APRNs must be individually identified through payer credentialing to obtain reimbursement under their own names. Payer credentialing makes APRNs visible because their contributions can be specifically identified. Although many payers allow APRNs to bill individually, others refuse to reimburse APRN services, even in states with laws that mandate third-party APRN reimbursement. Medicare and Medicaid have moved many clients from fee-for-service payment systems into managed care reimbursement systems, in which case managed care organization (MCO) policies overlay CMS regulations. Therefore, APRNs must be cognizant of the many layers of reimbursement policies and procedures in their state, region, and organization.

Provider Systems

U.S. healthcare is delivered by many types of providers, each with its own policies, regulations, and practices affecting APRN reimbursement (Table 11.1). These types of providers include:

1. MCOs
2. Managed care networks
3. HMOs
4. PPOs
5. Nurse-managed centers (NMCs)
6. Fee-for-service private practices
7. Home healthcare agencies
8. Public health agencies
9. Community health centers
10. Federally qualified health centers (FQHCs)
11. Migrant health clinics
12. Indian Health Board (IHB) clinics and hospitals
13. Rural health clinics (RHCs)
14. Retail-based clinics

Some types of FQHCs have policies that mandate APRNs be employed in order for the clinic to receive funding dollars. These regulations were passed based on federal studies that demonstrated APRN safety and cost-effectiveness (Yox & Stanik-Hutt, 2016). FQHCs credential APRNs for reimbursement and hospital privileges, provide them membership on provider panels, and validate their scope of practice. In most other systems, however, APRNs must negotiate for their place and power. APRNs must strive to obtain leadership positions in provider systems so that their contributions to patient outcomes are identified and valued by administrators and payers. Examples of leadership roles include performing administrative functions, participating on policy committees, and conducting research projects.

One way that APRNs have shown leadership and have achieved some level of autonomous practice is through the creation of nurse-managed health clinics (NMHCs). Often serving underinsured and uninsured populations with the associated limitations in funding, NMHCs have new visibility because of their being included in the ACA. Key to their success is the National Nursing Centers Consortium that promotes nurse-led care delivery. Successful NMHCs must have low administrative overhead costs, low fixed costs, and the ability to generate sufficient patient volume. There is increasing evidence that NMHCs offer quality, cost-effective care (Ely, 2015). These outcomes have enabled NMHCs to obtain further grants to expand.

SELECTED ENTITIES AND PROVIDER SYSTEMS
Medicare

Medicare was established in 1965 as part of President Lyndon Johnson's Great Society initiative; its programs are oriented primarily to acute care for the elderly. The goal was to create a safety net for the nation's elderly, who had endured hardships in the World Wars and the Depression during the 1930s. Medicare is a two-part, federally funded healthcare program; approximately 95% of the nation's elderly are enrolled in Medicare Part A. Part A provides hospital insurance that covers inpatient services, up to 100 days in a skilled nursing facility (SNF) following hospitalization, and some home healthcare. Although there are no premiums for Part A Medicare, patient cost sharing is required. Cost sharing consists of an annual deductible as well as a payment percentage. Medicare does not cover eye examinations, medications, or long-term nursing care. Medicare Part B pays for physician visits, services and supplies, outpatient services, and home healthcare, all at rates set by the federal government.

The 1997 BBA (P.L. 105-33) allows Medicare reimbursement of services provided by NPs and CNSs if the services are reimbursable when provided by a physician and if the services are within the APRN scope of practice. The law removed all restrictions on the practice setting and permitted NPs and CNSs to submit fees for services rendered in hospitals, SNFs, nursing homes, comprehensive outpatient rehabilitation facilities, community mental health centers, and rural health centers. Payments for NP and CNS services are discounted, compared with physician reimbursement, to 80% of the lesser of either the actual charge or 85% of the physician fee schedule amount.

NPs and CNSs billing under their own names must complete claim forms (called "Form 1500") using their unique national provider identifier (NPI) numbers. These numbers are obtained from the CMS. Established as part of the 1997 legislation, this provider-specific tracking number is used by all systems for administrative and financial transactions.

Some APRNs do not submit claims under their own names, although this practice is typically discouraged by nursing leaders and professional organizations because it implements a system of physician supervision of APRN practice. Currently, 23 states have full practice authority for NPs, with only 15 states having full practice authority for all APRN roles (certified registered nurse anesthetists [CRNA], NP, midwifery, and CNS; American Association of Nurse Practitioners, 2017; National Council of State Boards of Nursing, 2017). Many additional states are continuing to actively seek independent practice.

Medicare has a payment system for nursing and physician assistant services rendered under physician supervision called "incident-to" billing. Incident-to billing allows APRNs to bill under physician names for services that are provided as incident-to physician services. Payment then equals 100% of the physician fee schedule, as opposed to the 85% rate for most NPs. Although incident-to billing increases the revenue that APRNs can generate under current reimbursement rates, this billing practice raises red flags for fraud and abuse because it is governed by a tangle of federal regulations. APRN-billable activities must be integrated into daily physician practice. Incident-to billing is typically interpreted as implying direct supervision of APRNs by physicians. Supervising physicians must be physically present (although not in the patient examination room) at all times when APRNs are providing billable services, and physicians must perform all the initial patient visits and must establish the plans of care that APRNs then follow. Incident-to billing limits APRN autonomy and may also be very impractical. For example, if the physician leaves the building for lunch or vacation, the APRN could not bill incident-to for patients seen during that time frame. (*Note*: APRNs could, however, bill for this care under their own names if they were individually credentialed as providers with the payer; the practice would receive 85% of the physician fee if they did so, rather than the 100% incident-to payment.) Incident-to billing makes the contribution of APRNs to the fiscal output of organizations invisible. Billing under their own provider numbers (NPIs) is now strongly encouraged to avoid the potential for billing fraud and to permit full utilization of the legal APRN scope of practice.

Another Medicare billing practice incorporates a system that reimburses providers based on relative work value units (RVUs). Established in 1989, the Resource-Based Relative Value Scale (RBRVS) is a system aligned with Current Procedural Terminology (CPT) codes. Each CPT code is assigned a relative dollar value by the CMS based on practice research about work and practice expenses and professional liability insurance costs. Allowable service charges are determined annually by multiplying this RVU by a standard dollar amount conversion factor established by the CMS, based on the CMS's determination of regional cost variations (the geographical adjustment factor, GAF). The CMS publishes its RBRVS annually in the *Federal Register*, and practices then use the RBRVS to determine their fees.

The 1997 BBA (P.L. 105-33) provided both access and barriers to Medicare reimbursement for APRNs. During the rule-writing process for this act, the definition of "collaboration" was debated. The primary debate was about the impact of regulatory collaboration language on APRN practice in states where physician collaboration is not required and APRNs practice independently. This contentious issue continues to be closely monitored federally and in each state by APRN professional groups. Because state APRN practice laws by and large determine APRN practice, collaboration is a continuing and important issue for all APRNs. Most contentious was the language in the 1997 BBA that set APRN reimbursement at 85% of the physician rate; this was a compromise, and the bill would not have passed had APRNs not agreed to this requirement. This law still stands today and some believe this keeps healthcare costs down.

P.L. 105-33 regulations require that to be credentialed as Medicare providers NPs or CNSs must be master's-prepared registered nurses authorized to practice as NPs or CNSs by the state in which the services are furnished and be certified as NPs or CNSs by recognized national certifying bodies that have established standards. In the past, these requirements had been problematic for many CNSs because national certification had not been highly pursued, but today most employers require CNSs to be nationally certified and for the CNSs whose practice includes direct patient care their services are reimbursable. CNSs in psychiatry and mental health have set the stage for this path as they have pursued reimbursement since the early 1970s and typically are nationally certified.

The rules also contained a time-limited "grandfather" clause to allow certified NPs without master's degrees to obtain provider numbers if they applied before January 1, 1999. In general, P.L. 105-33 was a victory for NPs and CNSs and met the intent of the law, which was to increase greater consumer access to NPs and CNSs. The legislation lifted some of the barriers to APRN reimbursement.

Medicaid

Medicaid expanded the 1965 federal Medicare system by providing funds for states to pay for healthcare of low-income groups. Federally supported and state administered, Medicaid covers costs of care for vulnerable groups through programs such as Aid to Families with Dependent Children (AFDC). Low-income elderly persons and some individuals with disabilities are also covered under this program. Medicaid is different from Medicare in that it is a vendor program, meaning that providers offering services to these individuals or families must accept the Medicaid reimbursement as full payment and cannot request copayments from patients. Because Medicaid payments are low (typically less than 50% of submitted bills), many providers (including dentists) restrict the number of Medicaid clients whom they serve. Some states enroll Medicaid patients in MCOs by establishing contracts with MCOs in programs called "prepaid medical assistance programs" (PMAPs).

Section 6405 of the Omnibus Budget Reconciliation Act of 1989 (H.R. 3299) authorizes Medicaid payment for services of certified pediatric NPs and certified family NPs. Requirements necessary for reimbursement include possession of a current RN license in the state in which services are provided, and compliance with state APRN Medicaid reimbursement rates, which vary between 70% and 100% of physician fees, depending on the state.

Indemnity Insurers

Indemnity insurers are traditional insurance companies that pay for but do not deliver healthcare. They typically require an annual deductible that members self-pay; once this deductible is reached, the company will pay 80% of their members' healthcare costs on a per person, per procedure basis. Reimbursement rates are based on "usual and customary charges," which vary between regions and companies. If provider charges are more than the indemnity insurer allows, patients are responsible to pay the balance.

Some indemnity insurance companies will pay for APRN services. APRNs can contact these companies to negotiate for recognition as reimbursable providers.

Managed Care Organizations

Capitated managed care developed rapidly in the 1990s in response to many economic and political forces. One factor was that the U.S. post–World War II baby boom generation began transitioning into middle age, increasing the number of healthcare consumers. This trend is projected to greatly increase costs, particularly for expensive, emerging technologies. MCOs sell health service packages to employers, individuals, or governmental agencies. Services are provided by the MCO panel of healthcare providers, who may or may not be MCO employees. APRNs can apply to become primary care providers (PCPs) on MCO provider panels, but this recognition has been slow in coming. MCOs reimburse PCPs using a fee-for-service, a capitated, or a fee-per-member basis, or by using a combination of fee-for-service and capitation.

MCOs are continuing to grow in the United States and are typically large, complex organizations. They stress the importance of health promotion, chronic care management, and patient education, and they typically provide their members with preventive services. They have so far been unable to demonstrate the expected cost savings. Some managed care strategies, such as employing economies of scale in purchasing, centralizing services such as emergency care, and developing systems for referrals and after-hours care have been cost-effective. However, administrative costs are very high.

Managed care is frequently interpreted as "managed costs." Efforts by CMS to uncover fraud in Medicare/Medicaid billing have added to the negative light in which many providers and consumers view MCOs. APRNs are also voicing their discomfort with MCO policies, particularly about the expectations that limit the length of patient visits to 10 to 15 minutes. RVU billing in MCOs is also a system that concerns APRNs who value time and care continuity with their clients. In high-production managed care models, APRNs may not be able to fulfill their responsibilities to prevent illness, coordinate care, and teach patients about their treatment plans.

CNM and CRNA Reimbursement

Certified nurse-midwives (CNMs) successfully obtain third-party reimbursement for their services based on their cost-effectiveness and high level of consumer satisfaction. Excellent research about CNM outcomes is compelling to payers seeking safe care at reasonable cost. In 1973, Washington was the first state to enact laws permitting CNM reimbursement by private and public benefit plans, which opened the door for other states to follow. The American College of Nurse-Midwives (ACNM) provides its members with excellent resources for billing, coding, and reimbursement through its website and publications. State laws and regulations must be in place to support CNM activities, including reimbursement. CNMs and all APRNs must be active in public policy formulation in order to establish favorable legal and regulatory practice climates.

Although few of their clients qualify for Medicare, CMS Medicare regulations achieved equitable midwifery payments from 65% to 100% of the physician fee schedule, as of January 2011. This is important in part because Medicare regulations affect all payers in setting this precedent of establishing a widely used payment process. Another important change occurred for CNMs in 2010 when the ACA recognized freestanding birth center facilities as mandated covered services (Cole & Avery, 2017). In some systems, CNMs work in incident-to relationships with physicians, which raises the potential for fraudulent claims, if all the aspects of incident-to regulations are not strictly followed. Billing under their own names is strongly recommended for all APRNs, including CNMs, so that autonomous practice can provide the best possible care to clients and families.

Despite many difficulties, CRNAs have been successful in obtaining third-party reimbursement. OBRA granted CRNAs the right to be directly reimbursed for their services to Medicare recipients. CRNA services are also reimbursed directly by Medicaid and a number of commercial carriers. When both a CRNA and an anesthesiologist participate in the same case, the services of both anesthesia providers can be billed according to the extent of their involvement in the case. Independently billing CRNAs provide savings for governmental programs and for private payers because they typically charge less than their physician counterparts. However, it is interesting to note that in 2016 the U.S. Department of Veterans Affairs (VA) Care system granted full practice authority for all APRNs except CRNAs (VA, 2016) This highlights the many complex issues regarding CRNA working relationships with physicians (including anesthesiologists) affecting their work environments and billing practices. The American Association of Nurse Anesthetists offers CRNAs many reimbursement resources.

DOCUMENTATION AND CODING TO GAIN REIMBURSEMENT

Documentation is the key to reimbursement and must be sufficient to support the level of charge being requested. In addition, APRNs must understand their billing process and be able to use several types of diagnostic and procedure codes. One type of code is called the "Healthcare Common Procedure Coding System" (HCPCS), which assigns a dollar amount to patient care activities. For example, there are HCPCS codes for immunization and wound suturing. Each patient visit is also coded using CPT codes, another part of the uniform coding language. The CPT coding directory covers all possible types of patient–provider interactions. It is owned and updated annually by the American Medical Association (AMA) and has been adopted by Medicare and other third-party payers (AMA, 2017).

A subgroup of CPT codes includes the Evaluation and Management Codes (E&M Codes), the CPT codes most used by APRNs (typically CPT codes 99201 through 99456). These five-digit codes are based on the levels of history taking and physical examination, complexity of decision making, counseling, and minutes of face-to-face time in each patient encounter. APRNs must distinguish between new patients and established patients in their choice of codes because new patients are reimbursed at a higher rate than established patients. A new patient is a patient who has not received professional services within the past 3 years from a provider in the same specialty in the same practice. Telephone communication, however, is considered a professional service.

In addition to assigning a CPT code on the standard claim forms (Form 1500), APRNs must select appropriate diagnostic codes from the *International Classification of Diseases, 10th Revision, Clinical Modification (ICD-10)*. *ICD-10* is based on the World Health Organization (WHO) disease classification. The 43rd World Health Assembly endorsed the *ICD-10* in May 1990. *ICD-10* took effect in the United States in October 2015 and is currently under revision, with an expected release date for *ICD-11* in 2018 (WHO, 2017). ICD codes assign symptoms and diseases numeric codes: characters 1 to 3, categories 4 to 6 (etiology, anatomical site, and severity, respectively), and 7 extensions (injuries, fractures, etc.; CMS, 2017).

Documentation begins with a concise statement of the chief complaint, usually stated in the patient's own words in the medical history (Table 11.2). The classic eight variables should be used to document the chief complaint: location, quality, severity, duration, timing, context, modifying factors, and signs/symptoms. For billing purposes, there are four categories of history taking: problem-focused, expanded problem-focused, detailed, and comprehensive. Each level expands the history according to the level of history taking required to investigate the chief complaint. A problem-focused history consists of the chief complaint and brief history of the present illness (HPI) or problem. An expanded problem-focused history adds a problem-pertinent review of systems (ROS). The ROS has data categories including constitutional, ear/eye/nose/throat, cardiac, respiratory, gastrointestinal, genitourinary, musculoskeletal, skin, breast, neurologic, psychiatric, endocrine, hematology/lymphatic, and allergic/ immune. The detailed level extends the HPI and ROS and adds a pertinent past/family/ social history (PFSH). The PFSH consists of three components: past history with illnesses, operations, injuries, and treatments; family history of relevant diseases; and an age-appropriate review of past and current social activities. If a PFSH is on the chart from an earlier encounter, it does not need to be restated, but it must be documented that the PFSH was reviewed with the patient and updated. The comprehensive history involves an extended HPI, complete ROS, and complete PFSH.

The physical examination follows a similar pattern with the same names for the four levels. The problem-focused examination is limited to the affected body area or organ system. The expanded problem-focused examination adds examination of other symptomatic or related systems. The detailed examination is similar but more detailed, and the comprehensive examination is a complete single-system or multisystem examination.

TABLE 11.2 Documentation for Reimbursement

Component	Level 1	Level 2	Level 3	Level 4	Level 5
History	Minimal	Problem-focused; 1–3 elements in HPI; no ROS; no PFSH	Expanded problem-focused; 1–3 HPI elements; ROS for 1 related system; no PFSH	Detailed; 4+ HPI elements; 3+ chronic conditions; ROS for 2–9 systems; 1+ items of PFSH	Comprehensive; 4+ HPI elements; 3+ chronic conditions; ROS for 10+ systems; 1+ items from 2+ of 3 PFSH areas
Examination	Minimal	Problem-focused; 1–5 elements of body or organ system examination	Expanded problem-focused; 6–12 examination elements of body or systems	Detailed; 12–18 examination elements of body or systems	Comprehensive; 18+ examination elements in at least nine systems of body areas
Decision-making examples	Minimal	Straightforward	Low complexity (e.g., routine medications; occupational/ physical therapy; IV lines)	Prescribed medications; MRI; closed reduction of fracture	Medications; monitor medications; resuscitate; refer for major surgery
Risk	Minimal	Minimal	Low	Moderate	High
Time	5 minutes	10 minutes	15 minutes	25 minutes	40 minutes

HPI, history of present illness; IV, intravenous; PFSH, patient/family/social history; ROS, review of systems.

The levels of decision making refer to the complexity of establishing the diagnosis or treatment plan and are influenced by the number of possible diagnoses or management options; the size and complexity of the medical record; tests or other information that must be reviewed and analyzed during the visit; the risk of significant complications, morbidity or mortality; and the diagnostic procedures and management options.

There are four categories of decision making: straightforward, low complexity, moderate complexity, and high complexity. Straightforward decision making, the first level, involves a minimal number of diagnoses or options, minimally complex data, and a minimal risk of complications. Low complexity increases those components to a limited level from the minimal level. The moderately complex level involves multiple diagnoses or options, moderate complexity of data, and a moderate risk of complications. The high complexity level is an encounter that deals with an extensive number of diagnoses or options, extensive complexity of data, and a high risk of complications.

Four additional components can be used to alter the coding, which include counseling, coordination of care, complexity of the presenting problem, and amount of time spent with the patient. To use those elements, careful documentation is necessary. The time category can include face-to-face time, plus review of the patient chart, writing of notes, and communicating with other professionals and patient family members. Time is the key billing factor to use if counseling and coordination of care exceed 50% of the total visit time.

APRNs can bill for services rendered in nursing homes and SNFs. They can also bill for hospital services as long as they are not employees of the hospital. There are three levels of encounters in those settings: detailed, detailed-comprehensive, and comprehensive, each with corresponding required components. Another way to bill is using three categories of subsequent nursing facility care (one-problem history, expanded focus, and detailed). Physicians are mandated to visit nursing home clients a minimum of 12 visits per year; half of these mandated visits can be covered by APRNs. These visits are billable by the APRN as are additional visits that are medically necessary. In addition to skilled nursing home visits, APRNs also can bill for their services in emergency departments using special codes that are appropriate to that setting.

Some specific pointers regarding documentation are important. When a diagnosis is uncertain, coding the presenting symptom is advisable, such as "pain" or "fever." Listing "rule out" differential diagnoses on the encounter form is not acceptable, nor are the terms "possible" or "suspected." "Abnormal" is not an acceptable term without further description; however, "normal" and "negative" are allowed. A checklist with positive items further explained is also acceptable. All laboratory test and radiographic requests must be justified to Medicare in terms of the medical necessity of their charges.

An example of a satisfactory way to document with billing based on time would be: "Total time, 25 minutes; counseling, 15 minutes; discussed results of tests, provided three options for treatment; follow-up in

3 months." To document care coordination, chart notes might say: "Spent 25 minutes reviewing medications with family and explaining laboratory tests; appointments coordinated for return visit in 3 months; public health nurse contacted regarding need for medication supervision." An APRN can list multiple codes for a single visit and can bill for both an evaluation and management (E&M) visit and a procedure (e.g., examination with suture removal). In complex patients, APRNs can bill for two services in one visit (e.g., a general well examination and an acute asthma visit) if a special modifier is used in addition to the two sets of coding and documentation; patients might have to pay two copayments in that circumstance.

Organizations must submit bills quickly because there is typically a 3-month turnaround time from the payers, which affects revenue flow. It is important to remember that the amounts billed out may be very different from the amounts collected from payers. For example, in many states, Medicaid pays less than 50% of typical billed amounts.

Healthcare organizations employ coding specialists and hire consultants to conduct audits and teach staff about these important issues. Consultants often find that organizations are undercoding for their services. Coding too high (called "upcoding") can trigger Medicare fraud investigations. Medicare carriers expect to see a bell-shaped curve with most visits at the CPT code 99213 level (problem-focused history, expanded problem-focused examination, low-complexity decision making). However, this is problematic for practices that provide a great deal of care to patients with complex or chronic illnesses.

Most organizations design a superbill for processing claims that incorporates all of the coding information in one place, including procedures, facility charges, vaccines, E&M codes, *ICD-10* codes, and any other relevant information. The document trail must be available for internal and external audit purposes. APRNs must communicate regularly with billing, coding, and audit staff and must participate in regular revision of the superbill. The increasing use of computer-based charting is leading to more standardization of these processes and forms.

Inadequate documentation and coding result in loss of revenue to organizations (and therefore to providers), inability to track outcomes of care, and possible penalties if audits turn up discrepancies. Inadequate documentation also leaves APRNs vulnerable in legal investigations. Thorough, accurate documentation provides an auditable evidence trail for reimbursement.

Documentation also is used to audit care quality. Some MCOs and PPOs reward practices and providers for complying with established practice protocols and standards as part of their quest to implement best-practice, evidence-based care. APRNs must be cognizant of coding requirements and provide documentation that reflects the excellence of their care.

SUMMARY

U.S. healthcare has undergone tremendous changes during recent decades. For example, DRGs were put in place to control costs as part of a prospective payment system. DRGs decreased hospital stays, causing an explosion in the need for SNFs, home healthcare programs, and increased patient visits to outpatient clinics. With healthcare costs burgeoning, APRNs are cost-effective providers of quality patient care. To prove the affordability and quality of their care, however, APRNs must be visible to payers and consumers. Visibility is enhanced when APRNs obtain their own provider numbers, lobby for direct reimbursement from insurance companies, document appropriately, and accurately speak the language of coding and billing. Furthermore, APRNs become visible as they develop strong relationships with administrators and billing staff and track their billing and collections outcomes. APRNs must share their reimbursement expertise with each other in order to raise the performance of all APRNs. APRNs who are not well informed about their practice revenue generation are at a great disadvantage in determining their fiscal impact on systems.

APRNs typically individually negotiate their own employment contracts, a process greatly strengthened by having productivity and financial data. In addition, tracking APRN cost-effectiveness, productivity, and fiscal outcomes is essential to the entire nursing profession as it makes nurses' work visible in the bottom line of organizations. The American Nurses Association (ANA) and other nursing professional organizations have long lobbied for direct reimbursement for healthcare and continue to pursue the goal of making nursing's contribution visible in overall cost analyses. Measuring care outcomes is one of nursing's highest priorities.

APRNs were traditionally educated to provide care closely aligned to specific settings. Now they face the additional challenge of understanding multiple systems that change rapidly and reimbursement policies that constantly evolve. APRNs must not only practice competently but also must understand healthcare economics. Therefore, basic and continuing education of APRNs is essential, and nurse educators and administrators must understand and teach about APRN reimbursement. Educational content on leadership, financial management, politics, and health policy is essential to keep APRNs' place at the table where decisions are made, policies are developed, and systems are designed.

Lobbying at various legislative levels is also crucial for APRN reimbursement. There is a pressing need for consistent payment policies across states that are reflected in federal laws and regulations. Legislative and regulatory goals include the following:

- Legislation requiring APRN payments that are on par with physicians (the "equal pay for equal work" principle)
- Laws that ensure public access to APRN care (e.g., changes to the Employee Retirement Income Security Act of 1974 [ERISA] that exempts self-insured organizations from state regulation and allows them to be more restrictive than regulated organizations)
- Laws requiring payers to credential and list APRNs as licensed independent providers (LIPs), thus placing APRNs on MCO provider panels

as specialty and PCPs (Research must continue to examine the characteristics, quality, and cost/benefit ratio of APRN care. APRN care that
is evidence-based should be carefully studied to document its specific
components and outcomes, including fiscal outcomes.)
- Study of regulatory compliance as well as the effectiveness of various
methods of educating APRNs about these vital issues

In conclusion, APRNs must understand the realities of healthcare reimbursement to be effective providers and leaders in healthcare.

REFERENCES

American Association of Nurse Practitioners. (2017). State practice environ-
ment. Retrieved from https://www.aanp.org/legislation-regulation/
state-legislation/state-practice-environment/66-legislation-regulation/
state-practice-environment/1380-state-practice-by-type
American Medical Association. (2017). *CPT® 2017 professional edition.* Chicago,
IL: Author.
Appleby, J. (2012). Seven factors driving up your health care costs. *Kaiser Health
News.* Retrieved from http://www.kaiserhealthnews.org/stories/2012/
october/25/health-care-costs.aspx
Appold, K. (2017). Top four healthcare industry changes to watch in 2017.
Retrieved from http://managedhealthcareexecutive.modernmedicine
.com/managed-healthcare-executive/news/top-four-healthcare-industry
-changes-watch-2017
Auerbach, D. I., Chen, P. G., Friedberg, M. W., Reid, R., Lau, C., Buerhaus, P. I.,
& Mehrotra, A. (2013). Nurse-managed health centers and patient-centered
medical homes could mitigate expected primary care physician shortage.
Health Affairs, 32(11), 1933–1941. doi:10.1377/hlthaff.2013.0596
Barnett, J. C., & Berchick, E. R. (2017). *Health insurance coverage in the United
States: 2016 current population reports.* Retrieved from https://www.census
.gov/content/dam/Census/library/publications/2017/demo/p60-260.pdf
Berwick, D. M., Nolan, T. W., & Whittington, J. (2008). The triple aim: Care, health
and cost. *Health Affairs, 27,* 759–769. doi:10.1377/hlthaff.27.3.759
Bodenheimer, T., & Sinsky, C. (2014). From triple to quadruple aim: Care of the
patient requires care of the provider. *Annals of Family Medicine, 12*(6), 573–576.
doi:10.1370/afm.1713
Centers for Medicare & Medicaid Services. (2017a). Accountable care organizations. Retrieved from https://www.cms.gov/Medicare/Medicare-Fee-for
-Service-Payment/ACO
Centers for Medicare & Medicaid Services. (2017b). ICD-10: Official CMS industry resources for the ICD-10 transition. Retrieved from https://www.cms
.gov/Medicare/Coding/ICD10
Chien, A., Eastman, D., Li, Z., & Rosenthal, M. (2012). Impact of a pay for performance program to improve diabetes care in the safety net. *Preventive
Medicine, 55,* S80–S85. doi:10.1016/j.ypmed.2012.05.004
Clark, T., Norris, T., & Schiller, J. (2017). *Early release of selected estimates based on
release of the 2016 National Health Interview Survey.* Hyatsville, MD: National
Center for Health Statistics. Retrieved from https://www.cdc.gov/nchs/
data/nhis/earlyrelease/earlyrelease201705.pdf

Cole, L. J., & Avery, M. D. (Eds.). (2017). *Freestanding birth centers: Innovation, evidence, optimal outcomes*. New York, NY: Springer Publishing.

Deloitte. (2014). 2014 Global health care outlook: Shared challenges, shared opportunities. Retrieved from https://www2.deloitte.com/content/dam/Deloitte/global/Documents/Life-Sciences-Health-Care/dttl-lshc-2014-global-health-care-sector-report.pdf

Ely, L. (2015). Nurse-managed health centers: Barriers and benefits toward financial stability when integrating primary care and mental health. *Nursing Economic$, 33*(4), 193–202.

Evans, M., & Fleming, K. (2017). What we can all do about rising healthcare costs. Retrieved from https://www.forbes.com/sites/allbusiness/2017/06/28/what-we-can-all-do-about-rising-healthcare-costs/#7caff90d2f37

Friedberg, M., Schneider, E., Rosenthal, M., Volpp, K., & Werner, R. (2014). Association between participation in a multipayer medical home intervention and changes in quality, utilization and cost of care. *Journal of the American Medical Association, 311*(8), 815–825. doi:10.1001/jama.2014.353

Glied, S., & Jackson, A. (2017). The Affordable Care Act and insurance coverage. *American Journal of Public Health (AJPH) Policy, 107*(4), 538–540. doi:10.2105/AJPH.2017.303665

H.R. 3299-Omnibus Budget Reconciliation Act of 1989, PL-101-239. Retrieved from https://www.congress.gov/bill/101st-congress/house-bill/3299/text

Kaiser Family Foundation. (2017). Premiums for employer-sponsored family health coverage rise slowly for sixth straight year, up 3% but averaging $18,764 in 2017. Retrieved from https://www.kff.org/private-insurance/press-release/premiums-for-employer-sponsored-family-health-coverage-rise-slowly-for-sixth-straight-year-up-3-but-averaging-18764-in-2017

Kessellheim, S., Avorn, J, & Sarpatwarik, A. (2016). The high cost of prescription drugs in the United States: Origins and prospects for reform. *Journal of the American Medical Association, 316*(8), 858–871. doi:10.1001/jama.2016.11237

Laughlin, J. (2014). AAP principles concerning retail-based clinics. *Pediatrics*. Retrieved from http://pediatrics.aappublications.org/content/133/3/e794

Martin, A., Hartman, M., Whittle, L., Catlin, A., & the National Health Expenditure Accounts Team. (2014). National health spending in 2012: Rate of health spending growth remained low for the fourth consecutive year. *Health Affairs, 33*(1), 67–77. doi:10.1377/hlthaff.2013.1254

Martin-Misener, R., Harbman, P., Donald, F., Reid, K., Kilpatrick, K., Carter, N., . . . DiCenso, A. (2015). Cost-effectiveness of nurse practitioners in primary and specialised ambulatory care: Systematic review. *BMJ Open, 5*(6), e007167. doi:10.1136/bmjopen-2014-007167

National Council of State Boards of Nursing. (2017). Implementation status map. Retrieved from https://www.ncsbn.org/5397.htm

Organization for Economic Co-operation and Development. (2017a). Pharmaceutical spending. doi:10.1787/998febf6-en

Organization for Economic Co-operation and Development. (2017b). Health spending. Retrieved from https://data.oecd.org/healthres/health-spending.htm#indicator-chart

Premier, Inc. (2013). Providers projecting significant inpatient to outpatient admission shift in 2013. Retrieved from http://issuu.com/premiercs/docs/eo_spring2013

Stokowski, L. (2012). Nurse practitioners and medical homes: A natural fit. *Medscape*. Retrieved from https://www.medscape.com/viewarticle/772300_2

Sussman, A., Dunham, L., Snower, K., Hu, M., Matlin, O., Shrank, W., . . . Brennan, T. (2014). Retail clinic utilization associated with lower total cost of care. *The American Journal of Managed Care, 19*(4), 148–158.

U.S. Department of Health and Human Services. (2013). Key features of the Affordable Care Act. Retrieved from http://www.hhs.gov/healthcare/facts/timeline/index.html

U.S. Department of Veterans Affairs. (2016). VA grants full practice authority to advanced practice registered nurses. Retrieved from https://www.va.gov/opa/pressrel/pressrelease.cfm?id=2847

World Health Organization. (2017). International classification of diseases. Retrieved from http://www.who.int/classifications/icd/revision/en

Yox, S., & Stanik-Hutt, J. (2016, July 12). APRNs vs physicians: Outcomes, quality, and effectiveness of care according to the evidence. *Medscape*. Retrieved from https://www.medscape.com/viewarticle/865779

Deborah J. Kenny

ETHICAL ISSUES IN ADVANCED PRACTICE NURSING

APRNs make ethical decisions on a daily basis, such as, "Even though a certain treatment is better for Mr. Smith, but he cannot afford it because his insurance will not pay for it, should I prescribe him a less effective treatment that he can afford?" Or, "What does Ms. Thompson, who has terminal ovarian cancer, want regarding her end-of-life wishes? Should I refer her to Dr. Jones, as she has indicated, who is willing to provide her with medication to aid her in dying?" These same nurses also make multiple practical and clinical decisions every day, such as, "Which medication would be best for this clinical scenario?" or, "What would be the way to present lifestyle changes in such a manner that it motivates Billy to handle his own diabetes?" APRNs must be able to distinguish between practical and ethical issues. However, it is not always clear-cut, nor is it easy. Many different theories and perspectives exist, making the field of ethics extremely complex and difficult to apply. Additionally, there is no universal definition of ethics that one can turn to for guidance, but rather numerous theories, philosophies, and methods of making decisions. Ethics and its practical application require a basic knowledge of some of these underpinnings as well as a reflection of personal and cultural values. The ability for ethical decision making is central to the provision of healthcare and is essential to healthcare organizations (Kotalik et al., 2014).

According to Pellegrino (2001), "Cure may be futile, but care is never futile" (p. 568). Nursing is a caring profession and this means that APRNs may sometimes find themselves in situations where their professional mandate is to treat their patients, but not always in a manner in which they would want to be treated. Roach and Canadian Hospital Association (1987) defined the five "Cs" of caring: compassion, competence, confidence, conscience, and commitment. These require the APRNs to engage in self-reflection and self-awareness when dealing with what might seem like ethical issues.

This chapter focuses on attempting to define ethical issues and provides some philosophical background, offering some of the more recent frameworks inherent to the practice of medical ethics. It also offers a number of practical models for ethical decision making. It ties ethical decision making into professional models of care and, finally, it discusses some examples of more common ethical issues seen in advanced practice and provides case studies for consideration.

DEFINITIONS AND THEORY

The word "ethics" is derived from the Greek word *ethos*, which literally means "character." The term, though it seems simple on the surface, has been notoriously difficult to define, as it is very context dependent (Beauchamp & Childress, 2013; Field, 1931–1932; Ostman, Nasman, Eriksson, & Nystrom, 2017; van Hooft, 1996). Numerous conceptions of the term developed, depending on which basic philosophical foundation one happened to espouse. Even recent literature will use older philosophical foundations to define ethics.

Utilitarianism is generally thought of as the notion of "the greatest good for the greatest number of people." By nature, it is consequentialist in that it offers an explanation of the consequences of action. Both John Stuart Mill and Jeremy Bentham wrote about utilitarianism as their foundation, but their objective was primarily external and sought to inform public policy and social justice (Beauchamp & Childress, 2013). Deontological or Kantian ethics is "rule-based" and describes a "duty" or obligation to act in a way that is prudent or right, because it is what everyone would do under the same circumstances. Immanuel Kant first described the "Categorical Imperative," which states, "I ought never to act except in such a way that I also will that my maxim become a universal law." (Beauchamp & Childress, 2013, p. 363). However, the fallacy there would be that we have no way of knowing what others would actually do under those circumstances (as cited in Broad, 1916). The older and mostly traditional European philosophical models may or may not work in a complex and global world.

Some of the more recent theories include Virtue Ethics Theory, in which it is assumed that an individual who possesses good moral strength will act in ways that reflect on his or her virtue (Sellman, 2017). Sellman (2017) does compare this theory with some of the more universal theories, such as utilitarianism and deontology. He postulates that virtue ethics offers an attribute of humanity that utilitarianism and deontology may not. However, there are several arguments that this theory, in and of itself, does not lend itself toward consistent and specific decision making, as it does not allow for contextual differences in situations. Holland (2012) argues that virtue ethics is too narrow in scope to have a prominent place in nursing because there are times when nurses must make decisions that are incongruent with their personal values, such as truth telling when there may be questionable practices, aid in dying, and whistleblowing against colleagues engaging in workplace violence.

Pollard (2015) describes a relational ethic framework, in which there is joint respect and engagement between the patient and the APRN. Interaction is required, but it also demands knowledge of ethical principles by the APRN and reasoning ability by the patient to assist in mutual decision making. The important point in relational ethics is that decision making includes all the stakeholders. Decisions within this framework are not one sided. Pollard provides a framework for decision making that is described later in this chapter. Another contemporary theory is that of Caring Ethics. This is based on the work of Gilligan (1977) and Noddings (1988), who contended that there are gender differences in moral development and that caring decisions are made differently. They advocated a feminist approach to ethics and education on caring. Watson furthered this work in the 1970s and 1980s in the development of her Theory of Human Caring. Watson (1997) described caring as an ethic and the basis for the evolution of the art of nursing practice. Both Watson (1997) and van Hooft (1996) discussed ethics from an ontological point of view. That is, ethics in a complex world cannot be completely based on external rules and principles, but rather is an expression of what we care about most from an internal viewpoint. Later, Pellegrino (2001) and Ostman et al. (2017) argue that ethics in the health professions must be based on both internal and external models. Ostman et al. (2017) further reason that internal philosophies are personal and individualized, but they must intertwine with the external, more rules-based models in order to create what is termed as an ethos of both "freedom and responsibility" (p. 8).

Truog et al. (2015) have introduced a new term, "microethics," in which they characterize this as an internal view. They contend that this approach is very context dependent and often not directly visible, or always amenable to some of the more traditional theories. They further describe microethics as including the struggles of both patient and clinician in making complex decisions (Truog et al., 2015). For example, consider a clinician having to offer and patients having to choose between equally undesirable options such as moving a frail elderly patient from his or her home into an assisted living facility where he or she can be looked after, or leaving him or her in an unsafe home situation with family members who are neglectful. In this case, both patient and family must consider all the complexities and consequences of either decision, and neither is desired by the patient.

In 1977, Beauchamp and Childress, considered by many to be the authorities of modern ethics in the United States, wrote one of the first texts on biomedical ethics (now in its seventh edition). In the book, they described four moral principles by which all biomedical ethical decisions should be made. They go into a great deal of detail in their work and have continually updated throughout the years, but the four principles remain the same. These are based primarily on the Belmont Report Principles (Department of Health, Education and Welfare, 1979), which guide the protection of research involving human subjects. Application of these principles is practical, though not always straightforward. The following is a brief discussion of each of these four principles and how they might apply to advanced nursing practice.

The first principle is that of respect for autonomy. Beauchamp and Childress (2013) contend that autonomy has three conditions: (a) that one act intentionally, (b) with a full understanding of the situation and context, and (c) without outside influences that might determine one's action. This is much more than simply allowing patients to make choices or indicate preferences. It would not include someone with a diminished capacity who might be influenced or controlled by others. Theories of autonomy are plentiful and, like trying to define ethics, attempting to define autonomy is difficult because there are varying degrees and nuances. It is incumbent on the APRN to ensure an autonomous person or their surrogate has all the information necessary to make informed and reasoned choices. The APRN should also realize that acting against ones' values does not mean they are not acting autonomously. Sometimes an autonomous person will act quite differently in one circumstance than he or she would in another. For example, a patient who is nearing the end of his or her life might suddenly become fearful and want as much treatment as possible, even though he or she might fully understand its futility. Beauchamp and Childress (2013) provide concrete examples of some of the rules of respect for autonomy. These include truth telling, respect for privacy, confidentiality, consent for interventions, and assisting in decision making when asked.

The second of the four principles is nonmaleficence. This is the only principle not specifically contained in the Belmont Report (U.S. Department of Health, Education, and Welfare, 1979), but is subsumed under beneficence. Essentially, nonmaleficence means that one has a duty not to cause harm. This is and has been a debated part of the Hippocratic Oath. For example, when a physician orders a medication for a patient with a terminal disease who wishes to end his or her life, is he or she causing harm? Some might say that prescribing a life-ending medication would be doing harm on multiple levels, harming the patient, and going against the values our society, in which saving or prolonging life is the norm. Others would say that allowing a terminal patient to end their life and potential suffering is respecting their right to self-determination. Perhaps, a clinic is chronically understaffed because of resources and access is difficult for patients. Is it harming those who need, but cannot get care? These are only some of the ethical questions APRNs may need to tackle.

The third of the four principles is beneficence. As opposed to nonmaleficence, this entails direct action to promote welfare and help others, or more simply, to benefit others. Beauchamp and Childress (2013) explain that we are not morally obliged to help others, but that we should do so, even if there is no relationship to another. As APRNs, we have a duty, by virtue of our professional responsibility, to benefit those for whom we care. They provide five conditions under which health professionals have a duty to provide benefits. Primarily this duty consists of an action to prevent harm and an action in which the benefits outweigh the risks of providing care or treatment.

The final of the four principles is justice. As with the other principles, justice is difficult to define, but its essence is that individuals are treated equitably or according to what they are owed. Benefits and burdens are allocated according to social norms. There are numerous theories of justice according to these norms. A deeper explanation of justice is beyond the scope of this chapter. Most APRNs recognize that there are disparities in treatment, particularly among vulnerable individuals or groups. The evolution of justice in medical ethics was born out of particular research involving these vulnerable groups, for example, prisoners. Beauchamp and Childress (2013) discuss allocation of resources based on priority setting and rationing of scarce treatment. This alone creates ethical dilemmas as APRNs try to determine who has what right to which care.

A recent dilemma that touches all four of the principles of bioethics and gained worldwide attention was the Charlie Gard case (Hammond-Browning, 2017; Truog, 2017; Wilkinson & Savulesco, 2018), in which a national healthcare system decided further treatment of this infant with a severe and debilitating genetic neurological disorder was futile and harming the child. Charlie's parents could afford and wanted to continue treatment in the United States with a treatment that had little scientific basis. National leaders became involved and the world responded. The National Health System believed further treatment to be harmful and futile. After numerous appeals by the parents to continue treatment, the courts sided with the healthcare system, and Charlie was subsequently taken off life support and died. In the end, even his death in a hospice was not what the parents wanted. What were some of the ethical issues in this case? Whose rights dictated the level of care in this case? Was it the patient's right, the parents' right, or the healthcare system's right? How did the healthcare system determine a comatose child was being harmed by further treatment? The patient could not speak for himself. Did the world have the right to become involved and side with the parents? Should the parents' rights have been overridden in the way the healthcare system allowed Charlie to die? Whose interests were served in this case? Who was harmed? What about the direct caregivers in this case? Were their needs considered? This entire case was a quagmire of ethical issues that are highly contentious and will continue to serve as a model case for ethicists and APRNs alike. Advanced practice nurses will face many questions such as these on a daily basis, having to grapple with a crippling disease, futile treatments, stakeholders, scarce resources, and inequities in healthcare access.

MODELS FOR ETHICAL DECISION MAKING

The first step in providing frameworks to ethical decision making is to differentiate between an ethical "problem" and an ethical "dilemma." Tschudin (1992) defines the former as an issue that can be solved and further defines a dilemma as one in which there is an issue where there are two opposing solutions, both of which can be equally detrimental. Most issues that present themselves in patient care are ethical problems. Beauchamp and Childress (2013) describe practical ethics as the norms and other moral means by which the practitioner makes decisions within his or her practice.

Numerous ethical decision-making frameworks exist that can aid the APRN in making decisions with regard to ethical issues. Several models are described as follows. Ediger (2015) provides a "Four Topics" approach to ethical decision making based on Beauchamp and Childress's (2013) principles. The APRN asks a series of questions based on four identified topics. The first topic of "Medical Indications" includes asking questions regarding the indications for or against a treatment, its appropriateness, the evidence supporting it, and medical facts of the particular case. The APRN then moves on to the second topic of "Patient Preferences." Here the nurse actually asks the patient his or her preferences, providing autonomy and input into his or her care. Internal and external barriers to decision making on the part of both the patient and the APRN are considered. For example, what are the capacities of the patient for making a reasoned decision; how can coercion be avoided in a potentially paternalistic environment? The third topic examines the "Patient's Quality of life." What things need to be considered when addressing long- and short-term risks with the patient? What does the patient consider to be the quality of life? For example, you have a patient whom you have seen numerous times for injury associated with a chosen lifestyle, say skiing. What conversation needs to take place around the risk of skiing and what does the patient say about the quality of life should he or she be required to give up skiing. This is important because patients may prefer to risk injury to maintain what might be a risky lifestyle, but are willing to make that trade-off. In this case, risks and benefits should be carefully weighed and discussed between provider and patient. Finally, the fourth topic to be considered in Ediger's (2015) model is that of "Contextual Features." Who are the stakeholders in the decision? What factors, such as religious preference or finances, may impact the decision? Systematically moving through each of these four topics can provide a thorough view of the issue and may help all stakeholders come to a satisfactory resolution.

Pollard (2015) described a model using relational ethics. Her premise is that ethical decision making is done so within the setting of a relationship between patient and clinician. She believes this relationship to be interdependent and tied together. However, it changes and may create more questions than answers at times. Both the APRN and the patient must consider the humanness and culture of the other. What the patient desires is not always self-evident, but working sensitively with both humanity and culture in mind can help the APRN to move closer to a decision that is mutually favorable to both the APRN and the patient. She contends this humanism diminishes the chance that there is more equity of one over the other (paternalism). The relationship begins with mutual respect, then engagement from the perspective of trying to understand the others' wants and desires, but not from the standpoint of putting themselves in the others' shoes. Then the APRN uses his or her knowledge and skills from this perspective, using universal ethical principles to reason out a solution with the patient. Both environment and uncertainty will play into the decisions, but provide the need to dig deeper by asking questions that will contribute to the understanding of the other. Pollard (2015) explains that it is this questioning and self-reflection that will lead to an answer to ethical quandaries.

Kotalik et al. (2014) provide a framework of ethics based on the mission, vision, and values of an organization. They contend ethics are contained within the values of an organization and, therefore, provide a framework from which ethical questions may be asked reflecting those values, and that it may differ from organization to organization. For example, if an organization values respect, then the framework questions would reflect this. They further state that care must be taken to ensure that the ethical framework based on mission, vision, and values actually matches actual practice within the organization, or it would not be useful.

Crossan, Mazutis, and Seijts (2013) provide a model in which a provider's values, virtues, and character strengths all contribute to ethical decision making. They present this model, not as linear, but rather circular in that self-reflection plays a pivotal role in deepening moral development. This reflection would then lead to awareness and enhanced ability to make judgments that would lead to ethical behavior in the clinical arena. This would lead one back to self-reflection and an assessment of the decision made.

Magelssen, Pedersen, and Førde (2016) provide guidance to using ethical theory when making clinical ethical decisions. They divide the process into four roles when facing moral encounters. Individuals become aware of and identify a decision as a moral challenge. Next, they use ethical theories to make and present a logical argument. Then they use their perspective to shape the dialogue with regard to the challenge. Finally, they reflect on and interpret the problem from multiple angles. However, they contend that knowledge of basic ethical theory is needed in order to form valid conclusions.

There are numerous other ethical decision-making frameworks available and all provide a backdrop of how one should go about making decisions in the face of ethical dilemma. What all these models have in common is the need to reflect on both internal and external values. The APRN must be able to examine critical issues from many perspectives, to include organizational, patient, and personal values, and be able to weave these together to come to a resolution that is acceptable to all stakeholders.

PROFESSIONAL CONDUCT
Advanced Practice Nursing

As professionals, all nurses, regardless of their practice levels, must abide by professional standards. It is naturally assumed that APRNs not only follow the common morality of their own society, but also the moral standards for their profession. Most professionals (healthcare or not) have their own set of ethical standards by which they should practice. These standards generally contain or subsume ethical statements within them. At the most basic nursing level, the American Nurses Association (ANA, 2015) has defined nine provisions of a *Code of Ethics* that it is incumbent on the nurse to follow (Exhibit 12.1).

All of the provisions presuppose ethical practice in the care of patients in their requirement to maintain the four principles of medical ethics. Only

Exhibit 12.1 ANA *CODE OF ETHICS*

1. The nurse practices with compassion and respect for the inherent dignity, worth, and unique attributes of every person.

2. The nurse's primary commitment is to the patient, whether an individual, family, group, or community.

3. The nurse promotes; advocates for; and protects rights, health, and safety of the patient.

4. The nurse has the authority, accountability, and responsibility for nursing practice; makes decisions; and takes action consistent with the obligation to promote health and to provide optimal care.

5. The nurse owes the same duties to self as to others, including the responsibility to promote health and safety, preserve wholeness of character and integrity, maintain competence, and continue personal and professional growth.

6. The nurse, through individual and collective effort, establishes, maintains, and improves the ethical environment of work setting and conditions of employment that are conducive to safe, quality healthcare.

7. The nurse, in roles and settings, advances the profession through research and scholarly inquiry, professional standards development, and the generation of both nursing and health policy.

8. The nurse collaborates with other health professionals and the public to protect human rights, promote health diplomacy, and reduce health disparities.

9. The profession of nursing, collectively through its professional organizations, must articulate nursing values, maintain integrity of the profession, and integrate principles of social justice into nursing and health policy.

ANA, American Nurses Association.

Source: From American Nurses Association. (2015). Code of ethics for nurses with interpretive statement. Retrieved from http://nursingworld.org/DocumentVault/Ethics-1/Code-of-Ethics-for-Nurses.html

one (Provision 6) specifically mentions ethics and that is in the environment of care. However, Provision 8 states that the nurse should collaborate with both other practitioners and the public to protect human rights, and Provision 9 calls for the integration of social justice into nursing and also into nursing policy. At the master's level, APRNs are expected to "use a variety of theories and frameworks, including nursing and ethical theories in the analysis of clinical problems, illness prevention, and health promotion strategies . . . " (American Association of Colleges of Nursing [AACN], 2011, p. 9). Advanced Doctorate of Nursing Practice nurses are expected to "Integrate nursing science with knowledge from ethics, the biophysical, psychosocial, analytical, and organizational sciences as the basis for the highest level of nursing practice" (AACN, 2006, p. 9).

Interprofessional Conduct

Because caring for patients is interdisciplinary, APRNs must also work with other professionals to provide ethical and competent care for patients. The Interprofessional Education Collaborative (IPEC, 2016) has developed four core competencies that shape this care. They include mutual respect with other professions, using one's own role as a collaborative team member, communicating with other professionals as well as patients, and relationship building as part of a collaborative team. The first competency is built on values and ethics for practice. There are numerous subcompetencies that include health equity, social justice, respect between patients and other professionals, and management of ethical dilemmas (IPEC, 2016).

MORAL DISTRESS AND ETHICS MODELS FOR DECISION MAKING

There are times when conflict in the workplace or between professions or between nurses and the organizational system can be a cause of moral distress. It was first described by Jameton (1984) as the distress that occurs when an individual identifies an appropriate ethical action, yet is constrained by external forces. Holly (1993) began to explore moral distress and ethical predicaments in acute care nurses in the context of the hospital environment. What she found was that nurses believed that patients were sometimes exploited and not treated as rational humans, that nurses felt excluded from ethical decision making, and that they experienced anguish over perceived powerlessness to act on what they perceived to be the best interest of the patients. One recent and very public example of this is when a nurse (Alex Wubbels) was arrested in an emergency room as she was attempting to follow hospital procedure and respect an unconscious patient's rights not to have blood drawn without his consent, but was being ordered to do so by law enforcement. Of course, this nurse was personally conflicted over hospital policies; what she was being asked to do; and attempting to protect the rights of an unconscious patient.

Based on previous work in this area, Corley, Elswick, Gorman, and Clor (2001) went on to develop and test the Moral Distress Scale. A factor analysis of the scale revealed three factors: (a) there is a strong individual responsibility to act in the ethical best interest of the patient, (b) this results in tension caused by not acting in the patient's best interest, and (c) stress can also be caused by deception in the care of the patient, for example, performing a partial or slow code. Interestingly, they found that demographics (age or gender) did not predict the level of moral distress.

Moral distress has had a continued and increased interest as this has been found to be negatively correlated with job satisfaction, burnout, and retention (Fourie, 2015; Pauly, Varcoe, & Storch, 2012; Trautmann, Epstein, Rovnyak, & Snyder, 2015). Although this has been extensively researched, little has been done to examine moral distress in APRNs and what particular ethical issues they face in the primary care environment. Johnstone and Hutchinson (2015) provide a different light on moral distress in that they believe there will inevitably be disagreements in moral judgment and that research should focus on linking moral distress to patient care quality and creating evidence-based methods to prevent conflicts and to assist nurses with cogent ways to resolve issues that cause moral distress.

DIFFERING ETHICAL ISSUES

Sometimes ethical issues will cross other boundaries and the APRN must be mindful of this. Bioethical issues should not be considered in isolation, but rather are rooted in the lives of individuals (Sodeke, 2012). For example, cultural, legal, socioeconomic, and professional boundaries exist. At times, they may appear to be very clear-cut, such as when a supervisor asks one to order a lab test or do a procedure that is unnecessary in order to allow billing for a higher level of service for the patient. However, sometimes they are not as clear, such as disparities in healthcare related to one's socioeconomic status and resource use. Garland-Thompson (2017) suggests specific cultural and disability ethical issues can arise from a person having a debility and having to live in a body that is somehow disabled or disfigured. Although bioethics in America has evolved in a more secular context of morality, religious questions often arise within the context of bioethics. These include questions regarding both the beginning and end of life and their definitions according to one's religion (Messikomer, Fox, & Swazey, 2001). Kotalik and Martin (2016), in speaking of the Canadian indigenous population, emphasize the importance of adapting ethical decisions to the culture of the individual. They explain that there are times when the traditional principle-based approach is not congruent with the culture and decision-making logic of an individual and this must be considered.

SUMMARY

The study and application of ethical principles in the care and treatment of patients are extremely complex. Often there are no correct answers or definitive algorithms to guide the APRN. There are differing views, principles, theories, and guidelines, all within the context of complicated human beings who have the ability to change their minds and determine what they want and/or do not want. The application of ethical principles in care requires both external guidelines and internal values. In a global and interprofessional environment, these can be difficult to tease out. Much of the time case examples come from the acute and/or hospital environments, and it can be difficult to find exemplars from the primary care arena. However, this does not mean that these issues do not arise in primary care. Many do, and the practitioner applies ethical principles on a daily basis.

ACKNOWLEDGMENT

The author acknowledges the contributions of Karen Feldt to this chapter in the previous edition.

REFERENCES

American Association of Colleges of Nursing. (2006). The essentials of doctoral education for advanced nursing practice. Retrieved from http://www.aacnnursing.org/Portals/42/Publications/DNPEssentials.pdf

American Association of Colleges of Nursing. (2011). The essentials of master's education in nursing. Retrieved from http://www.aacnnursing.org/Portals/42/Publications/MastersEssentials11.pdf

American Nurses Association. (2015). Code of ethics for nurses with interpretive statements. Retrieved from http://nursingworld.org/DocumentVault/Ethics-1/Code-of-Ethics-for-Nurses.html

Beauchamp, T. L., & Childress, J. F. (2013). *Principles of biomedical ethics* (7th ed.). New York, NY: Oxford University Press.

Broad, C. D. (1916). On the function of false hypotheses in ethics. *International Journal of Ethics, 26,* 377–397. doi:10.1086/intejethi.26.3.2377052

Corley, M. C., Elswick, R. K., Gorman, M., & Clor, T. (2001). Development and evaluation of a moral distress scale. *Journal of Advanced Nursing, 33*(2), 250–256. doi:10.1046/j.1365-2648.2001.01658.x

Crossan, M., Mazutis, D., & Seijts, G. (2013). The role of virtues, values, and character strength in ethical decision making. *Journal of Business Ethics, 113*(4), 567–581. doi:10.1007/s10551-013-1680-8

Ediger, M. J. (2015). Teaching clinical ethics using the four topic method. *International Journal of Athletic Therapy and Training, 20*(6), 10–13. doi:10.1123/ijatt.2014-0118

Field, G. C. (1931–1932). The place of definition in ethics. *Proceedings of the Aristotelian Society, 32,* 79–94. doi:10.1093/aristotelian/32.1.79

Fourie, C. (2015). Moral distress and moral conflict in clinical ethics. *Bioethics, 29*(2), 91–97. doi:10.1111/bioe.12064

Garland-Thomson, R. (2017). Disability bioethics: From theory to practice. *Kennedy Institute of Ethics Journal, 27*(2), 323–339. doi:10.1353/ken.2017.0020

Gilligan, C. (1977). In a different voice: Women's conception of self and morality. *Harvard Educational Review, 47,* 481–517. doi:10.17763/haer.47.4.g6167429416hg5l0

Hammond-Browning, N. (2017). When doctors and parents don't agree: The story of Charlie Gard. *Journal of Bioethical Inquiry, 14*(4), 461–468. doi:10.1007/s11673-017-9814-9

Holland, S. (2012). Furthering the sceptical case against virtue ethics in nursing ethics. *Nursing Philosophy, 13*(4), 266–275. doi:10.1111/j.1466-769X.2012.00541.x

Holly, C. M. (1993). The ethical quandaries of acute care nursing practice. *Journal of Professional Nursing, 9*(2), 110–115. doi:10.1016/8755-7223(93)90027-A

Interprofessional Education Collaborative. (2016). *Core competencies for interprofessional collaborative practice: 2016 update.* Washington, DC: Interprofessional Education Collaborative.

Jameton, A. (1984). *Nursing practice: The ethical issues.* Englewood Cliffs, NJ: Prentice Hall.

Johnstone, M. J., & Hutchinson, A. (2015). "Moral distress"—Time to abandon a flawed nursing construct? *Nursing Ethics, 22*(1), 5–14. doi:10.1177/0969733013505312

Kotalik, J., Covino, C., Doucette, N., Henderson, S., Langlois, M., McDaid, K., & Pedri, L. M. (2014). Framework for ethical decision-making based on mission, vision and values of the institution. *HEC Forum, 26*(2), 125–133. doi:10.1007/s10730-014-9235-7

Kotalik, J., & Martin, G. (2016). Aboriginal healthcare and bioethics: A reflection on the teaching of the Seven Grandfathers. *American Journal of BioEthics, 16*(5), 38–43. doi:10.1080/15265161.2016.1159749

Magelssen, M., Pedersen, R., & Førde, R. (2016). Four roles of ethical theory in clinical ethics consultation. *The American Journal of Bioethics, 16*(9), 26–33. doi:10.1080/15265161.2016.1196254

Messikomer, C. M., Fox, R. R., & Swazey, J. P. (2001). The presence and influence of religion in American bioethics. *Perspectives in Biology and Medicine, 44*(4), 485–508. doi:10.1353/pbm.2001.0069

Noddings, N. (1988). An ethic of caring and its implications for instructional arrangements. *American Journal of Education, 96,* 215–230. doi:10.1086/443894

Ostman, L., Nasman, Y., Eriksson, K., & Nystrom, L. (2017). Ethos: The heart of ethics and health. *Nursing Ethics.* doi:10.1177/0969733017695655

Pauly, B. M., Varcoe, C., & Storch, J. (2012). Framing the issues: Moral distress in health care. *HEC Forum, 24*(1), 1–11. doi:10.1007/s10730-012-9176-y

Pellegrino, E. D. (2001). The internal morality of clinical medicine: A paradigm for the ethics of the helping and healing professions. *The Journal of Medicine and Philosophy, 26*(6), 559–579. doi:10.1076/jmep.26.6.559.2998

Pollard, C. L. (2015). What is the right thing to do: Use of a relational ethic framework to guide clinical decision-making. *International Journal of Caring Sciences, 8,* 362–368.

Roach, M. S., & Canadian Hospital Association. (1987). *The human act of caring: A blueprint for the health professions.* Ottawa, ON, Canada: Canadian Healthcare Association Press.

Sellman, D. (2017). Virtue ethics and nursing practice. In P. A. Scott (ed.), *Key concepts and issues in nursing ethics.* Cham, Switzerland: Springer International Publishing AG. doi:10.1007/978-3-319-49250-6_4

Sodeke, S. O. (2012). Tuskegee University experience challenges conventional wisdom: Is integrative bioethics practice the new ethics for the public's health? *Journal of Health Care for the Poor and Underserved, 23*(4 Suppl.), 15–33. doi:10.1353/hpu.2012.0169

Trautmann, J., Epstein, E., Rovnyak, V., & Snyder, A. (2015). Relationships among moral distress, level of practice independence, and intent to leave of nurse practitioners in emergency departments: Results from a national survey. *Advanced Emergency Nursing Journal, 37*(2), 134–145. doi:10.1097/TME.0000000000000060

Truog, R. D. (2017). The United Kingdom sets limits on experimental treatments: The case of Charlie Gard. *The Journal of the American Medical Association, 318*(11), 1001–1002. doi:10.1001/jama.2017.10410

Truog, R. D., Brown, S. D., Browning, D., Hundert, E. M., Rider, E. A., Bell, S. K., & Meyer, E. C. (2015). Microethics: The ethics of everyday clinical practice. *The Hastings Center Report, 45*(1), 11–17. doi:10.1002/hast.413

Tschudin, V. (1992). *Ethics in nursing.* Oxford, UK: Butterworth-Heinemann, Ltd.

U.S. Department of Health, Education, and Welfare. (1979). *The Belmont report: Ethical principles and guidelines for the protection of human subjects of research.* Washington, DC: OPRR Reports.

van Hooft, S. (1996). Bioethics and caring. *Journal of Medical Ethics, 22*(2), 83–89. doi:10.1136/jme.22.2.83

Watson, J. (1997). The theory of human caring: Retrospective and prospective. *Nursing Science Quarterly, 10*(1), 49–52. doi:10.1177/089431849701000114

Wilkinson, D., & Savulescu, J. (2018). Hard lessons: Learning from the Charlie Gard case. *Journal of Medical Ethics, 44,* 438–442. doi:10.1136/medethics-2017-104492

Patricia Biller Krauskopf

13

EVIDENCE-BASED PRACTICE: STAYING INFORMED AND TRANSLATING RESEARCH INTO PRACTICE AND POLICY

Nearly two decades ago, the Institute of Medicine (IOM) recommended evidence-based practice (EBP) as a core competency (IOM, 2001). EBP is the process of using current research to guide patient care while incorporating patient values and clinical decision making. With the initiation of the Patient Protection and Affordable Care Act (ACA) and the realization of Patient-Centered Outcomes Research Institute, APRNs are critical in the transformation of healthcare delivery systems. As members of the healthcare team, APRNs play important roles in patient care, community engagement, and policy development. If an APRN is going to be a competent clinician and participate in redesigning the healthcare system, then he or she must become a consumer of and/or participant in research. The APRN not only has to be familiar with current research but also must be able to translate the research into practice.

When examining published research, clinicians need to be aware that there is, on average, a 15- to 24-month lag time from completed research outcomes to publication and a 6- to 13-year delay for inclusion in databases and systematic reviews (e.g., Cochrane Community, 2018; Green, 2014; Ross, Mocanu, Lampropulos, Tse, & Krumholz, 2013; Toroser et al., 2017). It has been reported that the typical time from bench research to implementation into practice is 15 to 20 years (Carpenter et al., 2012), culminating in only 14% of research actually reaching clinical practice (Green, 2014). In an effort to increase dissemination and utilization of research, the World Health Organization recently published a position paper calling for the timely submission within 12 months and publication of results within 24 months after the close of a study (Moorthy, Karam, Vannice, & Kieny, 2015).

TABLE 13.1   Examples of Email Updates

Healthcare Update News Service	admin@healthcareupdatenewsservice.com
MDLinx Family Med	newsletter@newsthree.mdlinx.com
Medscape Special Report	Medscape_Special_Report@mail.medscape.com
Consultant360	newsletters@consultant360.com
MedPage Today	daily.headlines@medpagetoday.com
Merck Medicus	MerckMedicus@1merck.com
DocGuide	webmaster3@docguide.com
Total E-Clips	totaleclips@fbresearch.org
Physician's First Watch	FirstWatch@jwatch.org
ADVANCE for Nurses	advancefornurses@emedia.advanceweb.com
Food and Drug Administration	www.fda.gov/AboutFDA/ContactFDA/StayInformed/GetEmailUpdates/default.htm
Agency for Healthcare Research and Quality	www.ahrq.gov
Centers for Disease Control and Prevention	www.cdc.gov/Other/emailupdates/
Practice-Based Research Networks	PBRNLIST@list.ahrq.gov

Staying up to date with current research can be challenging for the busy clinician. Although not a perfect solution, email updates can assist the APRN in addressing this complex problem. Table 13.1 provides examples of email updates that provide weekly or daily clinical updates.

In addition to email updates, there are online subscriptions such as *UpToDate* that are updated frequently and provide clinicians with latest evidence-based treatment recommendations. APRNs can also enlist the support of a medical or health sciences librarian to assist in finding topics of interest. Developing collaborative relationships with health sciences, librarians can enhance the literature-searching process (Gerberi & Marienau, 2017) so that retrieval of evidence is easy and the accumulation of useless information and wasted time are avoided. Other strategies to manage the overwhelming amount of new evidence include access to evidence-based journals, which typically scan multiple journals for relevant research or organizing interprofessional journal clubs where recent research can be discussed.

TRANSLATING RESEARCH INTO PRACTICE

The translation of research into practice requires the integration of three processes: disseminating research evidence to the clinician, critically analyzing such evidence, and applying such evidence to practice. The latter two steps are embedded in EBP and are discussed later in this chapter.

Historically, there have been several models (diffusion, systematic reviews, industrial commodity, system engineering, and social innovation) that were developed to explain how research evidence reaches the clinician and to identify how this evidence translates into practice (Scott, 2007). The early *diffusion model* depicts information from journals and conferences as being transferred by "osmosis." The stronger the evidence, the more likely it was that research would filter down to the practitioner and find its way into practice. Unfortunately, this method did not assist the clinician in applying the evidence to the clinical arena.

Systematic reviews, meta-analyses, and clinical guidelines were developed to simplify the process. Experts would analyze and summarize the research and make recommendations, thus facilitating the application of the evidence into practice. Some practitioners resisted the application of guidelines because there was not always consensus among experts and some clinicians believed the guidelines were prescriptive and did not allow for patient variability.

The *industrial commodity* approach, like clinical practice guidelines, was an effort to distribute information and improve its use in clinical practice. Healthcare industry stakeholders (e.g., regulatory and insurance agencies) used case reviews, audits, and educational outreach programs to change clinical practice. Change was sometimes avoided because providers thought they were no longer in control of healthcare decisions.

Systems engineering, the utilization of early electronic information systems to improve access to information, did not interface well with clinical practices; their reliability came into question, and individual adoption of this methodology was limited. Recently, this model has been used in nursing as a framework for clinical reasoning and applying EBP (Simpson, McComb, & Kirkpatrick, 2017). In addition, the Systems Engineering Initiative for Patient Safety (SEIPS) model has been useful in guiding several recent nursing research studies (Doyle Settle, 2017; Ngam et al., 2017; Steege & Rainbow, 2017).

Social innovation examines the motivators of behavioral change within social systems, utilizing the characteristics of change and social learning to distribute new information and facilitate its application to practice. In essence, this model assesses the provider's readiness for change and tailors an educational program and materials with this variable in mind. In addition, opinion leaders, peer networks, and key players in social networks (e.g., patients, insurers, administrators) are used to influence provider behavior. Interestingly, there is strong evidence that patient-mediated intervention or patient/consumer education is a powerful motivator for change.

In general, the failure of these models to change practice may be related to the "disconnect" between research and implementation into practice. Some research is not clinically relevant, and other research is preliminary or done with unsound methodology (Dogherty, Harrison, Graham, Vandyk, & Keeping-Burke, 2013). When the research is clinically relevant and methodologically sound, there can still be separation between research and practice. Several variables such as sample characteristics, the lack of comparisons, and the feasibility of the interventions contribute to the failure of adopting and applying research evidence to practice. From a clinician's viewpoint, "the right patients," or representative patients (e.g., ethnic and racial minorities, low income, and women), are either not included in clinical trials or not reported in the results (Charrow, Xia, Joyce, & Mostaghini, 2017; Ratto et al., 2017) and most intervention trials are all or none (e.g., treatment vs. placebo) rather than comparisons of less expensive alternatives. The use of nontraditional research methods such as mixed methods research also must be evaluated carefully as unrepresented small samples may be used requiring skill in interpretation (Bressan et al., 2017).

One missing component in the aforementioned models is "knowledge translation," which is described as a "dynamic and iterative process that includes synthesis, dissemination, exchange, and ethically-sound application of knowledge to improve the health" (Menear, Grindrod, Clouston, Norton, & Légaré, 2012, p. 623). Knowledge translation enables the clinician to view the research from a socioeconomic and cultural perspective rather than from a disease state. Furthermore, it facilitates the application of research to practice.

Another factor that may be absent is the flow of information. Typically, research flows from the researcher to the clinician when it should be bidirectional (Carpenter et al., 2012). Practitioners should be active in identifying salient issues found in clinical practice that researchers should address. Researchers should seek input from clinicians to design research studies to examine relevant questions and models for implementation.

Another component is the disconnect between the community-based physician and academic research centers. However, in 2000, Congress charged the Agency for Healthcare Research and Quality (AHRQ) with assisting in the development of primary care practice-based research networks (PBRNs) to close the "reality gap" between the clinical evidence and what clinicians and patients want to know (AHRQ, 2012; Carpenter et al., 2012). PBRNs are collaborative relationships between academic centers and community-based practitioners. Although PBRNs comprise primarily physician networks, APRN networks also exist (American Academy of Nurse Practitioner Network for Research, Advanced Practice Nurse-Ambulatory Research Consortium, and Advanced Practice Nurse Research Network, www.ahrq.gov). PBRNs are a source for ongoing health services research, clinical research, and prevention research that is specific to a community or state. These forums for research improve its relevance to patients and clinicians and ease the transfer of clinical data into clinical practice.

Finally, with a refinement and resurgence in the use of information, technology systems may facilitate the transfer of research and guide implementation into practice. Expansion of the utilization of electronic medical records and Web 2.0 (a term used to portray interactive Internet use) applications can be tools for the transfer of research to practice to providers and consumers (Brossard, 2013). Web 2.0 technologies have the capability to share information through electronic messaging, video conferencing, YouTube, and blogs. Social networking (Twitter, wikis, Facebook, LinkedIn, etc.), another Web 2.0 application, can connect clinical researchers, clinicians, consumers, and policy makers (Brossard, 2013; Curtis, Fryh, Shaban, & Considine, 2017), and the use of Facebook and Twitter has been shown to facilitate translating evidence into practice (Maloney et al., 2015).

EVIDENCE-BASED PRACTICE

EBP is the integration of research and clinical judgment that is used to evaluate and manage patient issues (Sackett, Rosenberg, Gray, Haynes, & Richardson, 1996). The key elements of EBP are clinically relevant research that is patient-centered and clinical judgment that includes clinical expertise and incorporates the patient-specific characteristics and preferences.

EBP is not a "cookbook" approach to care, nor was it designed as a healthcare cost-cutting tool (Sackett et al., 1996). EBP does not replace clinical judgment; however, EBP can direct healthcare policy.

EBP has been reviewed and discussed in healthcare delivery systems for several decades, yet it is still shrouded in controversy. Some argue that the best evidence is not always relevant to a given patient or practice and that it cannot replace clinical decision making (Ubbink, Guyatt, & Vermeulen, 2013). This argument is flawed: EBP is the template for making clinical decisions, not a prescription for patient care. Clinical experience is not usurped by research; rather, the research evidence serves as a complement or adjunct to the clinician's judgment.

Assimilating EBP into healthcare, the practitioner incorporates six steps: (a) ask the question, (b) collect data from literature review, (c) critically assess the research, (d) integrate the findings into practice, (e) evaluate the outcomes of the decision that was made, and (f) disseminate the results (Fencl & Matthews, 2017). The healthcare provider does not have to follow each step. For example, the clinician identifies the question, but systematic reviews or practice guidelines have completed the synthesis of the literature. An essential role for today's APRN is the implementation of the research findings into practice.

Characteristics of the Question or Clinical Problem

Identifying the problem or defining the question is the beginning of the exploratory process. Although several models exist to formulate the question with clarity, the simplest approach is PICO (population/problem, intervention, comparison interventions, and outcomes; Fencl & Matthews, 2017). *Population/problem* refers to the patient or condition of interest. As clinicians begin to formulate the question, they must identify the most important characteristics of the patient (e.g., age, race, gender) or the attributes of the condition that will be examined in the research. *Intervention* searches for the answers to what the clinician desires to do, such as identifying prognostic indicators, drug therapy, or diagnostic tests to be performed. *Comparison interventions* addresses alternative therapies (e.g., differences between two drugs) or approaches (e.g., diagnostic test options), although in some cases there is no need for comparisons or alternative options. *Outcomes* answers what is to be accomplished and what the effect (positive or negative) of the intervention will be.

Sources of Answers

When the practitioner has clearly articulated the question, the next step is to look for answers. Several electronic databases, such as the Cumulative Index of Nursing and Allied Health Literature (CINAHL), MEDLINE, Database of Abstracts of Review of Effects (DARE), the Cochrane Library, and others, can be useful tools in searching for information.

The value of the Internet cannot be overstated. There are several reliable sources of clinical guidelines and systematic reviews. Refer to Table 13.2 for a listing of these resources and web addresses.

Evaluation of Research

After locating the answers or the evidence that addresses the question as defined by the clinician, the final step is a critical assessment of the research. This step is probably the most difficult element of the process.

TABLE 13.2 Systematic Reviews and Clinical Guidelines

AHRQ	www.ahrq.gov/clinic/epcix.htm
Bandolier	/www.bandolier.org.uk
Clinical evidence	www.clinicalevidence.bmj.com/ceweb/index.jsp
Cochrane Database of Systematic Reviews	www.cochranelibrary.com/
DARE	www.crd.york.ac.uk/crdweb
TRIP	www.tripdatabase.com/index.html
U.S. National Guideline Clearinghouse	www.guideline.gov
USPSTF	www.ahrq.gov/clinic/uspstfix.htm
Health Evidence/McMaster University	www.health-evidence.ca
Bibliomap and DoPHER, Evidence for Policy and Practice Information Centre	www.eppi.ioe.ac.uk/cms/Databases/tabid/185/Default.aspx

AHRQ, Agency for Healthcare Research and Quality; DARE, Database of Abstracts of Review of Effects; DoPHER, Database of Promoting Health Effectiveness Reviews; TRIP, Turning Research into Practice; USPSTF, U.S. Preventive Services Task Force.

To understand the relevance and validity of research, the practitioner must be familiar with the levels of research studies. The hierarchy of research for interventions has its foundation in the randomized controlled trials (RCTs), traditionally known to provide the best evidence. Although some variation in the level of evidence hierarchy exists, most agree that meta-analyses of RCTs are highest and expert opinions are lowest in providing evidence (Mick, 2016; Peterson et al., 2014). Exhibit 13.1 illustrates the hierarchy of intervention studies.

The top level includes integrative studies and meta-analyses (Levin & Chang, 2014), which summarize and draw conclusions from multiple RCTs as if they were one study. Internationally these are recognized as the highest level in EBP (Cochrane Community, 2018). Next, more precise systematic reviews focus on a specific clinical topic and answer a particular question. The next level includes well-developed RCTs conducted at multiple (preferred) or single centers. RCTs are rigorously planned experimental studies that evaluate the effect of an intervention on patients. Nonexperimental studies are below this and include cohort, case-controlled, cross-sectional, and longitudinal studies. Cohort studies are observational and include large populations that are followed over time and compared with another group that does not have the therapy or condition being studied. Case–control studies retrospectively compare patients who have a condition with those who do not. Cross-sectional studies frequently used to determine prevalence, observe a population at a specific point in time. The final level of evidence is made up of case reports, case series, and expert opinion. They relate to a single patient and have no control group (Ingham-Broomfield, 2016: Singh, 2015).

Although RCTs are viewed by many as the gold standard in clinical decision making, the contributions of qualitative studies should not be devalued. Qualitative data are needed to answer questions of why, how,

---

Exhibit 13.1 HIERARCHY OF INTERVENTION STUDIES

Integrative studies meta-analysis   Highest

Systematic reviews

RCTs[a] multicenter, one-site RCT

  Cohort studies (longitudinal)[b]

  Case–control studies (retrospective)

  Cross-sectional studies (prevalence)

  Qualitative studies

Case reports/series

Expert opinion   Lowest

[a] Randomized controlled trials.
[b] Cohort studies can also be prospective or retrospective.

and when, and are seldom included in RCTs in enough detail to apply an intervention consistently (Lutzen, 2017).

This hierarchy may not be appropriate for certain questions or evidence might not be available at the higher levels in the hierarchy. If this occurs, then one would need to consider the next best available level of evidence (Singh, 2015).

The internal validity of the research depends on a critical analysis of the intent of the research and the methodology used to examine the results; external validity, in contrast, is assessed by answering the question of generalizability to a larger population (Medina McKeon & McKeon, 2016). From this analysis, the clinician can then discern the relevance of the evidence as it relates to a specific patient, population, or problem.

BARRIERS TO TRANSLATING RESEARCH INTO PRACTICE AND POLICY

The obstacles that prevent the translation of research into practice are many and complex. These barriers can be summarized into two categories: individual characteristics and systems or organizational factors.

Individual barriers that have been reported include insufficient knowledge about the research process, lack of competence in reading and evaluating research or scientific articles and reports, lack of time, lack of knowledge of statistical analyses, and sometimes lack of authority to change practice (Ubbink et al., 2013; Weng et al., 2013). Organizational or system barriers that have been described are lack of access to research, inadequate resources to implement change, and lack of support from staff and colleagues (Ubbink et al., 2013; Weng et al., 2013).

Individual Characteristics

APRNs prepared at the master's level and doctorate of nursing practice (DNP) level are taught to critique research, initiate EBP initiatives, and translate findings into practice; however, educational preparation alone does not seem to be sufficient to result in the application of research into practice. Some studies suggest that attitudes toward EBP may be as important as educational preparation in the implementation of research into practice (Stokkel, Olsen, Espehaug, & Nortvedt, 2014; Ubbink et al., 2013).

Clinical information must filter down to individual clinicians and cross disciplines (Curtis et al., 2017). The lack of interprofessional collaboration compromises research efforts between disciplines (e.g., biological sciences and physical sciences) and prevents the transmission of research data from one discipline to another. Although the different interests among various healthcare disciplines are justified, the artificial boundaries and turf issues created by different professions impede the flow of information and obscure the one commonality or unifying factor that should be improving patient care.

System/Organizational Barriers

Many healthcare institutions, whether they are hospitals or primary care clinics, frequently spend resources on acquiring and using new and innovative medical equipment and developing new procedures to improve patient care. Failure to invest in human technology such as the development of behavioral interventions, prevention strategies, or quality improvement programs or the failure to develop processes that support nurses and others in the evaluation of interventions and policy development are examples of implementation failure (Rangachari, Rissing, & Rethemeyer, 2013). Without infrastructure support, nurses, particularly APRNs, may perceive that they do not have the authority or organizational support to develop or evaluate new models of care.

Although many institutions have adopted electronic technology in their medical records with the intent of consolidating patient information and reducing errors, little technology is incorporated into the systems that directly access the clinical research or clinical practice guidelines that may improve patient care. Computer information systems (CISs) that are integrated into electronic medical records are often underused, in part because practicing clinicians are often not engaged in the development of these systems.

SOLUTIONS: A ROLE FOR APRNS

The solutions for translating research into practice and policy are as diverse and multifaceted as the barriers. Proposed solutions can be examined at three levels: the micro level (individual clinician and patient), the meso-level (systems or organizations), and the macro level (economic and political; Solvang, Hanisch, & Reinhardt, 2017).

Micro-Level Solutions

Possible solutions for addressing the barriers to translating research into practice on the micro level require an examination of patient and clinician perspectives. Although much of the previous discussion has focused on the practitioner, a brief discussion of the patient's interface with the clinician's decision making is in order.

Patient Perspective

From the patient's perspective, the clinician is a repository of information, and the underlying assumption is that the clinician's expertise is based on current and accurate information. The role of the clinician is to present the relevant information, risks, and benefits of interventions so that the patient can make an informed decision. Often, this information is complex and is presented in a way that does not empower the patient to participate in the decision-making process (Taber, Warren, & Day, 2016). Ultimately, the result of this type of interaction leads to miscommunication and withdrawal of the patient from active participation.

APRNs are skilled in the art of communication and have a fundamental understanding of adult learning principles. With this skill set, APRNs can reduce the flow of misinformation by serving as interpreters of information from lay media sources or other healthcare professionals. Informed patients can make appropriate healthcare decisions and can become participants in their own healthcare.

Practitioner Perspective

From a practitioner's perspective, the failure to use research to guide practice is governed by attitudes about research and its relevance to clinical practice. To increase the relevance of research, the patient population's needs should be the driving force for the research agenda. As articulated earlier, the flow of information should be bidirectional between the researcher and clinician. APRNs should be the link between the researcher and the patient population. They should assist the researcher design studies that answer clinical questions that are relevant to patients and clinicians. APRNs play a vital role in implementing new interventions or guidelines and they should be active participants in constructing and testing implementation models and delivery systems. Furthermore, the APRN needs to recognize that when there are gaps in the evidence, the patient's exposure to unnecessary risks and expenditures increases. Doctor of nursing practice–prepared APRNs were found to have increased capability in implementation of EBP (Hellier & Cline, 2016).

Clinical faculty can have a profound influence on students' opinions about research and its relationship to practice (McLean et al., 2013). When EBP is incorporated into curriculum and educational experiences, attitudes are changed, and the APRN students' skills in research translation and utilization are increased (Singleton, 2017).

Translating research into practice requires changes not only in attitudes but also in behavior. Most models for clinical practice change, such as Advancing Research and Clinical Practice Through Collaboration, Promoting Action on Research Implementation in Health Services, Johns Hopkins Nursing Evidence-Based Practice Model, or the Iowa Model of Evidence-Based Practice (Schaffer, Sandau, & Diedrick, 2013), advocate the development of collaborative interprofessional teams to promote changes in practice. The members of these teams are variable and dependent on the practice site, the expertise of the individual members, and the current problem or patient issue being examined.

For many years, APRNs have been the bridge between nursing, medicine, and other healthcare professionals and patients. APRNs should assume a major role in interprofessional collaborative teams. They can serve as mentors for nursing staff and allied healthcare professionals in the implementation of EBP and can function as the translators or interpreters of research in these teams.

Meso-Level Solutions

Application of evidence into nursing or clinical practice is more achievable when it becomes a habitual practice (Nilsen, Neher, Ellstrom, & Gardner, 2017), such as being integrated into workflow. Institutional support for the integration of research into practice can come through the development of CISs. Information systems that provide immediate access to databases with synopses of best evidence that is relevant and has undergone critical review are necessary for practitioners to make informed or evidence-based choices. CIS with embedded guidelines can prompt the clinicians to integrate EBP into clinical decision making.

The development of CIS should be a collaborative effort between the clinicians and the institution rather than the institution purchasing a system that may or may not meet the needs of the practitioner. APRNs who have been prepared at the DNP level or who have expertise in informatics have the skills necessary to be members of the CIS design team. If they are not directly involved in CIS design, APRNs should work with institutions when decisions are being made to purchase or design informatics systems for enhancing clinical services.

Institutional investment in human capital is important if research is to be translated into clinical services. This investment includes activities such as training staff, cultivating and supporting research implementation, mentoring, and providing resources (time and fiscal support) for developing a research agenda.

Armed with the knowledge of healthcare systems, APRNs can function as change agents within organizations. They have the leadership skills to garner institutional support, engage the stakeholders, and institute changes that support EBP at all levels of care delivery.

As CISs develop, best practices are becoming integrated into some of these systems. As clinical doctoral programs develop, APRNs will be more knowledgeable about information systems and can participate in their development.

Macro-Level Solutions

Healthcare providers do not function in a vacuum. Practitioners must function within an economic and political system. Healthcare is governed by the "cost of doing business." When they are considering the adoption of new practices, clinicians are forced to consider the cost to the patient. Obviously, if the cost exceeds the patient's resources, often the intervention will not be followed or will be unsuccessful. Even if the evidence supports a new technology or drug, the feasibility is determined by the economic impact.

The issue of cost transcends the individual patient and permeates all healthcare delivery systems. On a systems level, administrators have to evaluate the fiscal impact of new interventions. Administrators must weigh the new method against the old and determine the added value of the new treatment plan. If APRNs believe that a new intervention is in the best interest of patient care, these clinicians must be prepared to evaluate the cost–benefit ratio of new practice.

APRNs should also become astute fiscal managers. They must appreciate that EBP does not suggest that all new evidence can or should be the standard of care. Most APRNs have been trained to focus on the delivery of care to the individual patient; however, in the current health system, with its limited resources, the emphasis must shift to a population perspective and cost containment.

Politicians are not healthcare experts and rely on multiple sources for information regarding EBP. In general, the goals of the politician are to allocate limited resources to accomplish the greatest good and to regulate healthcare systems and providers to protect the public from harm.

As members of the nursing profession and as part of the largest healthcare provider network, APRNs have considerable political clout and should use this power to influence politicians. When advocating for the adoption of new evidence, the APRN must be mindful of the goals of the policy makers.

SUMMARY

Becoming competent practitioners requires not only the acquisition of clinical skills but also the ability to use research to guide practice. With the proliferation of new evidence, APRNs must be able to critically analyze and evaluate the evidence and appraise its utility. Applying the skills acquired during their educational experience, APRNs can and should become the translators of research into practice and policy.

APRNs have the skill set to understand the research process, and they are effective change agents. Therefore, they are in the position to identify the determinants of the clinician's and patient's behaviors and to design models that will not only facilitate the transfer of knowledge into clinical practice but also assist in the implementation process. APRNs, particularly those prepared at the clinical doctorate level, are leaders in implementing EBP and mentoring others as well in this transition (Singleton, 2017). This role consists of applying new interventions designed in academic research centers to primary care clinics.

Even when research is adapted to the primary care setting, there is no guarantee that this will facilitate implementation. As discussed earlier, the models that currently exist to promote adoption and implementation of research into practice are inadequate. The evidence is clear that provider education, computerized clinical support, and financial incentives have minimal or modest effect on increasing the use of EBP. The answer may be in using the best of all models and formulating a new paradigm to bridge the gap between research and practice.

The DNP expands the APRN's skill set to include becoming a change agent, understanding and developing informatics systems, and appreciating the operations of healthcare systems. Therefore, APRNs prepared at the doctoral level are in the position to expand and put into operation the previously discussed systems engineering and social innovation models for the dissemination and application of research. In this way, they can further elaborate the translation of research into practice.

As APRNs assume leadership roles in healthcare, they should become proactive in removing the barriers to translating research into practice. Now and in the future, APRNs can and should be the innovators in healthcare delivery systems through research.

REFERENCES

Agency for Healthcare Research and Quality. (2012). Primary care practice-based research networks: An AHRQ initiative. Retrieved from http://www.ahrq.gov/research/findings/factsheets/primary/pbrn/index.html

Bressan, V., Bagnasco, A., Aleo, G., Timmins, F., Barisone, M., Bianchi, M., . . . Sasso, L. (2017). Mixed-methods research in nursing: A critical review. *Journal of Clinical Nursing, 26*, 2878–2890. doi:10.1111/jocn.13631

Brossard, D. (2013). New media landscapes and the science information consumer. *Proceedings of the National Academy of Sciences of the United States, 110*(Suppl. 3), 14096–14101. doi:10.1073/pnas.1212744110

Carpenter, W. R., Meyer, A., Wu, Y., Qaqish, B., Sanoff, H. A., Goldberg, R. M., & Weiner, B. J. (2012). Translating research into practice: The role of provider-based research networks in the diffusion of an evidence-based colon cancer treatment innovation. *Medical Care, 50*(8), 737–748. doi:10.1097/MLR.0b013e31824ebe13

Charrow, A., Xia, F. D., Joyce, C., & Mostaghimi, A. (2017). Diversity in dermatology clinical trials: A systematic review. *Journal of the American Medical Association Dermatology, 153*(2), 193–198. doi:10.1001/jamadermatolo.2016.4129

Cochrane Community. (2018). Registering new reviews. Retrieved from https://community.cochrane.org/review-production/production-resources/proposing-and-registering-new-cochrane-reviews.

Curtis, K., Fryh, M., Shaban, R. A., & Considine. J. (2017). Translating research findings to clinical practice. *Journal of Clinical Nursing, 26*(5/6), 862–872. doi:10.1111/jocn.13586

Dogherty, E. J., Harrison, M. B., Graham, I. D., Vandyk, A. D., & Keeping-Burke, A. (2013). Turning knowledge into action at the point-of-care: The collective experience of nurses facilitating the implementation of evidence-based practice. *Worldviews on Evidence-Based Nursing, 10*(3), 129–139. doi:10.1111/wvn.12009

Doyle Settle, M. (2017). Human milk management redesign: Improving quality and safety and reducing neonatal intensive care unit nurse stress. *Creative Nursing, 23*(1), 47–52. doi:10.1891/1078-4535.23.1.47

Fencl, J. L., & Matthews, C. (2017). Translating evidence into practice: How advanced practice RNs can guide nurses in challenging established practice to arrive at best practice. *Association of periOperative Nurses Journal, 105*(5), 378–392. doi:10.1016/j.aorn.2017.09.002

Gerberi, D., & Marienau, M. S. (2017). Literature searching for practice research. *American Association of Nurse Anesthetists Journal, 85*(3), 194–204.

Green, L. (2014). Closing the chasm between research and practice: Evidence of and for change *Health Promotion Journal of Australia, 25*, 25–29. doi:10.1071/HE13101

Hellier, S., & Cline, T. (2016). Factors that affect nurse practitioners' implementation of evidence-based practice. *Journal of the American Association of Nurse Practitioners, 28*(11), 612–621. doi:10.1002/2327-6924.12394

Ingham-Broomfield, R. (2016). A nurses' guide to the hierarchy of research designs and evidence. *Australian Journal of Advanced Nursing, 33*(3), 38–43.

Institute of Medicine. (2001). *Crossing the quality chasm: A new health system for the 21st century.* Washington, DC: National Academies Press.

Levin, R. F., & Chang, A. (2014). Tactics for teaching evidence-based practice: Determining the level of evidence of a study. *Worldviews of Evidence-Based Nursing, 11*(1), 75–78. doi:10.1111/wvn.12023

Lutzen, K. (2017). The value of qualitative methods in prioritized healthcare research. *Nordic Journal of Nursing Research, 37*(4), 175–176. doi:10.1177/2057158517745474

Maloney, S., Tunnecliff, J., Morgan, P., Gaida, J. E., Clearihan, L., Sadasivan S., . . . Ilic, D. (2015). Translating evidence into practice via social media: A mixed-methods study. *Journal of Medical Internet Research, 17*(10), e242. doi:10.2196/jmir.4763

McLean, A. L., Saunders, C., Velu, P. P., Iredale, J., Hor, K., & Russell, C. D. (2013). Twelve tips for teachers to encourage student engagement in academic medicine. *Medical Teacher, 35,* 549–554. doi:10.3109/0142159X.2013.775412

Medina McKeon, J. M., & McKeon, P. O. (2016). A balancing act between control and generalizability. *Human Kinetics, 21*(2), 1–3. doi:10.1123/ijatt.2016-0010

Menear, M., Grindrod, K., Clouston, K., Norton, P., & Légaré, F. (2012). Advancing knowledge translation in primary care [commentary]. *Canadian Family Physician, 58,* 623–627.

Mick, J. (2016). Teaching EBP column: The appraising evidence game. *Worldviews on Evidence-Based Nursing, 13*(2), 176–179. doi:10:1111/wvn.12139

Moorthy, V. S., Karam, G., Vannice, K. S., & Kieny, M. (2015). Rationale for WHO's new position calling for prompt reporting and public disclosure of international clinical trial results. *PLOS Medicine, 12,* e1001819. doi:10.1371/journal.pmed.1001819

Ngam, C., Hundt, A. S., Haun, H., Carayon, P., Stevens, L., & Safdar, N. (2017). Barriers and facilitators to *Clostridium dificile* infection prevention: A nursing perspective. *American Journal of Infection Control, 45*(12), 1363–1368. doi:10.1016/j.ajic.2017.07.009

Nilsen, P., Neher, M., Ellstrom, P., & Gardner, B. (2017). Implementation of evidence-based practice from a learning perspective. *Worldviews on Evidence-Based Nursing, 14*(3), 192–199. doi:10.1111/wvn.12212

Peterson, M. H., Barnason, S., Donnelly, B., Hill, K., Miley, H., Riggs, L., & Whiteman, K. (2014). Choosing best evidence to guide clinical practice: Application of AACN levels of evidence. *Critical Care Nurse, 34*(2), 58–68. doi:10.4037/ccn2014411

Rangachari, P., Rissing, P., & Rethemeyer, K. (2013). Awareness of evidence-based practices alone does not translate to implementation: Insights from implementation research. *Quality Management in Health Care, 22*(2), 117–125. doi:10.1097/QMH.0b013e31828bc21d

Ratto, A. B., Anthony, B. J., Pugliese, C., Mendez, R., Safer-Lichtenstein, J., Dudley, K. M., . . . Anthony, L. G. (2017). Lessons learned: Engaging culturally diverse families in neurodevelopmental disorders interventional research. *Autism, 21*(5), 622–634. doi:10.1177/1362361316650394

Ross, J. S., Mocanu, M., Lampropulos, J. F., Tse, T., & Krumholz, H. M. (2013). Time to publication among clinical trials. *Journal of the American Medical Association Internal Medicine, 173*(9), 825–828. doi:10.1001/jamainternmed.2013.136

Sackett, D. L., Rosenberg, M., Gray, J. A., Haynes, R. B., & Richardson, W. S. (1996). Evidence-based medicine: What it is and what it isn't. *British Medical Journal, 312*, 71–72. doi:10.1097/00007632-199805150-00001

Schaffer, M. A., Sandau, K. E., & Diedrick, L. (2013). Evidence-based practice models for organizational change: Overview and practical applications. *Journal of Advanced Nursing, 69*(5), 1197–1209. doi:10.1111/j.1365-2648.2012.06122.x

Scott, I. A. (2007). The evolving science of translating research evidence into practice. *Evidence Based Medicine, 12*(1) 4–7. doi:10.1136/ebm.12.1.4

Simpson, V., McComb, S. A., & Kirkpatrick, J. M. (2017). Enhancing critical thinking via a clinical scholar approach. *Journal of Nursing Education, 56*(11), 679–682. doi:10.3928/01484834-20171020-08

Singh, A. P. (2015). What is hierarchy of evidence? *Bone and Spine*. Retrieved from http://boneandspine.com/what-is-hierarchy-of-evidence

Singleton, J. K. (2017). Evidence-based practice beliefs and implementation in doctor of nursing practice students. *Worldviews on Evidence-Based Nursing, 14*(5), 412–418. doi:10.1111/wvn.12228

Solvang, P. K., Hanisch, H., & Reinhardt, J. D. (2017). The rehabilitation research matrix: Producing knowledge at micro, meso and macro levels. *Journal of Disability and Rehabilitation, 39*(19), 1983–1989. doi:10.1080/09638288.2016.1212115

Steege, L. M., & Rainbow, J. G. (2017). Fatigue in hospital nurses—"Supernurse" culture is a barrier to addressing problems: A qualitative interview study. *International Journal of Nursing Studies, 67*, 20–28. doi:10.1016/j.ijnurstu.2016.11.014

Stokkel, K., Olsen, N. R., Espehaug, B., & Nortvedt, M. W. (2014). Evidence-based practice beliefs and implementation among nurses: A cross-sectional study. *BioMed Central Nursing, 13*(8). Retrieved from http://www.biomedcentral.com/1472-6955/13/8. doi:10.1186/1472-6955-13-8

Taber, C., Warren, J., & Day, K. (2016). Improving the quality of informed consent in clinical research with information technology. *Studies in Health Technology & Informatics, 231*, 135–142. doi:10.3233/978-1-61499-712-2-135

Toroser, D., Carlson, J., Robinson, M., Gegner, J., Girard, V., Smette, L., . . . O'Kelly, J. (2017). Factors impacting time to acceptance and publication for peer-reviewed publications. *Current Medical Research and Opinion, 33*(7), 1183–1189. doi:10.1080/03007995.2016.1271778

Ubbink, D. T., Guyatt, G. H., & Vermeulen, H. (2013). Framework of policy recommendations for implementation of evidence-based practice: A systematic scoping review. *British Medical Journal Open, 3*, pii: e001881. doi:10.1136/bmjopen-2012-001881

Weng, Y. H., Kuo, K. N., Yang, C. Y., Lo, H. L., Chen, C., & Chiu, Y. W. (2013). Implementation of evidence-based practice across medical, nursing, pharmacological and allied healthcare professionals: A questionnaire survey in nationwide hospital settings. *Implementation Science, 8*(112). doi:10.1186/1748-5908-8-112

Vicki J. Brownrigg

HEALTH INFORMATION TECHNOLOGY FOR THE APRN

APRNs must be knowledgeable users of health information technology (HIT) to ensure high-quality, efficient care, and be familiar with the terms "health information technology," "certified electronic health records" (EHRs), "meaningful use," and "telehealth" (Curtis, 2010). However, many APRNs and other providers remain uncertain about what HIT means for them, their practices, and their patients (Rathert, Porter, Mittler, & Fleig-Palmer, 2017).

Although HIT can be traced to the 1960s, when computers were initially introduced into healthcare (Saba & Westra, 2011), it did not receive widespread attention until the release of the Institute of Medicine (IOM) Quality Series in 2000 (IOM, 2000). Subsequent IOM reports concluded that increased use of technology is essential to ensure high-quality, safe patient care (IOM, 2001, 2011).

Propelled by the publication of the early IOM reports, HIT entered the national healthcare dialogue in 2004 when President George W. Bush signed an executive order mandating electronic health records (EHRs) for most Americans by 2014. Congress strengthened this directive with passage of the Health Information Technology for Economic and Clinical Health (HITECH) Act in 2009 as part of the American Recovery and Reinvestment Act (ARRA). HITECH provided $27 billion in incentives during a 10-year period for providers and hospitals to adopt EHRs and use them meaningfully (Blumenthal & Tavenner, 2010). However, the meaningful use incentive program was discontinued in January 2016 due to its emphasis on process instead of outcomes as well as difficulties encountered by healthcare providers and organizations to meet Stage 3 requirements (American Health Information Management Association [AHIMA], 2016). There was a shift in policy to pay providers based on quality outcomes as opposed to payment based on how technology was instituted (AHIMA, 2016).

Although a number of definitions of HIT exist (see Exhibit 14.1), the element common to each definition is an explicit or implicit reference to information. The term "informatics" refers to the discipline of study concerned

Exhibit 14.1 HIT DEFINITIONS

Term	Abbreviation	Description
Analytics	—	"The systematic use of data combined with quantitative as well as qualitative analysis to make decisions" (Simpao, Ahumada, Gálvez, & Rehman, 2014, p. 44).
Clinical decision support	CDS	"(1) An application that uses preestablished rules and guidelines that can be created and edited by the health care organization and integrates clinical data from several sources to generate alerts and treatment suggestions. (2) Computer system designed to help health professionals make clinical decisions" (HiMSS, 2010, p. 21).
Electronic health record	EHR	"A longitudinal electronic record of patient health information produced by encounters in one or more care settings. Included in this information are patient demographics, progress notes, problems, medications, vital signs, past medical history, immunizations, laboratory data, and radiology reports. The EHR automates and streamlines the clinician's workflow. The EHR has the ability to generate a complete record of a clinical patient encounter, as well as supporting other care-related activities such as decision support, quality management, and outcomes reporting" (HiMSS, 2010, p. 119).
Health information exchange	HIE	"The sharing action between any two or more organizations with an executed business/legal arrangement that have deployed commonly agreed-upon technology with applied standards, for the purpose of electronically exchanging health-related data between the organizations" (HiMSS, 2010, p. 57).
Health information technology	HIT, Health IT	*Health information technology* is an all-encompassing term referring to any technology that captures, processes, and stores health information" (Marcotte et al., 2012, p. 11). "HIT makes it possible for healthcare providers to better manage patient care through secure use and sharing of health information. HIT includes the use of electronic health records (EHRs) instead of paper medical records to maintain people's health information" (ONC, 2018).

(continued)

Informatics	—	"The discipline concerned with the study of information and manipulation of information via computer-based tools" (HiMSS, 2010, p. 62).
Interoperability	—	"The ability of different operating and software systems, applications, and services to communicate and exchange data in an accurate, effective, and consistent manner" (HiMSS, 2010, p. 201).
Mobile health	mHealth	"Application of mobile technology either by consumers or providers, for monitoring health status or improving health outcomes, including wire-less diagnostic and clinical decision support" (Kumar et al., 2013, p. 228).
Patient portal	—	"Provider-tethered applications that allow patients to electronically access health information that is documented and managed by a health care institution" (Ammenwerth, Schnell-Inderst, & Hoerbst, 2012, p. 1).
Personal health records	—	"Electronic application(s) through which individuals can maintain and manage their health information (and that of others for whom they are authorized) in a private, secure, and confidential environment" (HiMSS, 2010, p. 104).
Security	—	"Measures and controls that ensure confidentiality, integrity, availability, and accountability of the information processed and stored by a computer" (HIMSS, 2010, p. 119).
Store and forward	—	"Transmission of static images or audio–video clips to a remote data storage device from which they can be retrieved by a medical practitioner for review and consultation at any time" (HIMSS, 2010, p. 126).
Telehealth	—	"Using communications networks to provide health services including, but not limited to, direct care, health prevention, consulting, and home visits to patients in a geographical location different than the provider of these services" (HiMSS, 2010, p. 130).

with electronic information (Healthcare Information and Management Systems Society Government Relations [HiMSS], 2010), and HIT is the operationalization of this discipline. It is the documentation, storage, utilization, sharing, and analysis of health information for the benefit of those entrusted to the care of healthcare providers. Information technology provides the mechanism that allows healthcare providers to effectively and efficiently store and access needed information when caring for a single patient, groups of patients, or entire populations.

HIT is not simply the entry of patient information into an EHR. The importance of HIT lies in how the information is used after it has been entered into the patient record. If the information is used only to record a single patient's health status and treatment, a paper document serves the purpose. However, as the IOM quality reports conclude, simply documenting the information is no longer sufficient (Blumenthal & Tavenner, 2010; IOM, 2001, 2011). For example, the APRN can access real-time information to systematically track patient progress over time, compare the effectiveness of different treatment modalities across a group of patients, or analyze the outcomes of treatments provided by healthcare providers across multiple disciplines. The ability to obtain this level of information from paper charts or EHRs without interoperability capabilities is at best cumbersome and, at worst, impossible.

This chapter discusses common information management resources that APRNs are using or are likely to encounter in the near future HIT controversies and failures. HIT-related terms are introduced throughout the chapter with initial reference to these terms presented in italics. Definitions of terms are presented in Exhibit 14.1.

INFORMATION MANAGEMENT RESOURCES

Electronic Health Record (EHR)

The EHR is a specific application within the broader category of HIT. EHR is a data repository that allows healthcare providers to access a complete collection of patient information using a single resource (see Exhibit 14.1). The EHR often provides the healthcare provider access to other HIT functions that are designed to improve patient safety and outcomes such as computerized practitioner order entry (CPOE), clinical decision support (CDS), *interoperability, health information exchanges* (HIE), and quality improvement (QI).

The 2004 mandate for widespread adoption of EHRs was based on the premise that using the technology would "improve health outcomes by improving quality and efficiency of care, enhancing patients' engagement in their care, and building an infrastructure to digitally exchange health information" (Marcotte et al., 2012, p. 731). Although some evidence exists to support this premise of improved health outcomes (Kern, Edwards, & Kaushal, 2016; King, Patel, Jamoom, & Furukawa, 2014; Lammers & McLaughlin, 2017), other studies suggest the adoption of EHRs and HIT alone is not sufficient to improve patient outcomes (Bowman, 2013; Cohen & Adler-Milstein, 2016).

Consumer Engagement and Personal Health Record (PHR)

Consumer engagement and shared decision making (SDM) are increasingly becoming a national priority for changing the healthcare landscape.

It is asserted that improved patient engagement and SDM will result in improved patient outcomes and enhancement of the health of the nation (Ammenwerth et al., 2012; Goldzweig et al., 2013; Shay & Lafata, 2015). Moreover, it is reported that PHRs provide a mechanism with potential to drive SDM (Davis, Roudsari, Rawourth, Courtney, & MacKay, 2017; Irizarry, Dabbs, & Curran, 2015).

Although the exact definition of PHRs continues to evolve (Jordan-Marsh, 2011), they are generally described as repositories for health data contributed by the consumer and providers. PHRs include tools that allow consumers to become more engaged in their own healthcare decisions (Koeniger-Donohue, Kumar, Hawkins, & Stowell, 2014).

PHRs can be divided into those that are "tethered" or linked to an EHR maintained by healthcare providers with the provider determining the extent of the information that is included in the record. Tethered PHRs are commonly referred to as "patient portals" (Irizarry et al., 2015). These web-based programs enable the consumer to carry out simple tasks, including ordering prescription refills, requesting an appointment, and sending questions to a healthcare provider. Patient portals allow consumers to view parts of their records under certain circumstances. For example, some laboratory values may be shown to the consumer immediately, primarily those that require little interpretation and are familiar to consumers, such as cholesterol level. Other laboratory results might be revealed to the patient after review and interpretation by the provider. Still others might never be available through the web-based application due to privacy concerns, such as the results of an HIV test or genetic screening result. Overall, consumer response to patient portals has been positive although there is little evidence at this time to support the assertion that patient portals affect patient outcomes (Ammenwerth et al., 2012; Davis et al., 2017).

Untethered PHRs are controlled and maintained by the consumer who enters personal information into the record. Information contained in the untethered PHR is determined by the consumer and only persons approved by the consumer have access to the information (Irizarry et al., 2017). Little research has been done to determine the value of the untethered PHR (Irizarry et al., 2017).

Clinical Decision Support Systems (CDSSs)

CDSSs integrate information about a particular patient with a knowledge base from a variety of sources to generate patient-specific alerts and recommendations designed to aid the provider or patient in making health-related decisions (Blum et al., 2015; Bright et al., 2012; HiMSS, 2010; Hunt, Haynes, Hanna, & Smith, 1998). Bright et al. (2012) classified CDSSs into three categories: classic, information retrieval tools, and knowledge sources.

Classic CDSSs are those systems that automatically provide patient-specific alerts and treatment recommendations based on preprogrammed criteria (Bright et al., 2012). The classic CDSSs are often an element of

EHRs and are commonly related to drug dosages; treatment interactions; and alerts related to patient diagnoses, age, allergies, and potential drug duplications. The second type of CDSSs described by Bright et al. (2012) is "information retrieval tools," the prototype of which is the *infobutton.* Infobuttons are often embedded within EHRs or clinical information systems to assist providers in retrieving online information based on the context of specific patient and/or provider attributes (Del Fiol et al., 2012; Teixeira, Cook, Heale, & Del Fiol, 2017). A commonly used infobutton imbedded in EHRs is the HL7 infobutton standard (Teixeira et al., 2017). Another application that has been studied, but is not commercially available, is an infobutton linked directly to the "UpToDate" CDSS (Dragan, Newman, Stark, Steffensen, & Karimbux, 2015). "Knowledge resources," the third type of CDSSs, are point-of-care products that allow the healthcare provider to obtain pertinent information related to the care of the patient. Knowledge resources differ from the other CDSS categories in that the healthcare provider, not the CDSS, must apply the information accessed from the CDSS to the specific attributes of the patient. Examples of knowledge resources include proprietary products such as UpToDate, Epocrates, and Lexicomp, as well as numerous low-cost and free apps developed by governmental agencies and professional healthcare organizations. These resources are designed to be accessed quickly and used at the point of care. They are often available online or by using wireless mobile devices (mHealth CDSS).

The IOM report *Crossing the Quality Chasm* (IOM, 2001) identified CDSSs as a key approach to enhancing the quality of patient safety and improving patient outcomes by providing access to evidence-based recommendations at the point of care. There is some evidence that the projection made in the IOM reports was correct and CDSSs can be effective in improving the quality of either provider processes and/or patient outcomes (Bright et al., 2012; Jaspers, Smuelers, Vermeulen, & Peute, 2011; Robbins et al., 2012; Roshanov et al., 2011). However, recent systematic reviews of CDSSs indicate the results of randomized controlled trials investigating CDSSs are mixed, demonstrating some improvement in provider processes with limited evidence of improved patient outcomes (Blum et al., 2015; Bright et al., 2012; Jaspers et al., 2011; Jia, Zhang, Chen, Zhao, & Zhang, 2016, Roshanov et al., 2011).

Telehealth

The terms *telemedicine* and *telehealth* are often differentiated into whether healthcare providers use the technology as a means of interaction with patients (telemedicine) or consumers use the technology to access health information (telehealth; Kvedar, Coye, & Everett, 2014; Sprague, 2014). However, because this differentiation between telemedicine and telehealth is not universally defined, for the purposes of this chapter, the more encompassing term of *telehealth* will be used in reference to the use of telecommunications in healthcare (see Exhibit 14.1).

Telehealth can be divided into three categories: interactive videocon-ferencing, store and forward (asynchronous) technology, and remote pa-tient monitoring. Interactive videoconferencing uses live video between providers and patients, most often for specialty consultations. The tech-nology brings the expert to the patient and primary care provider, elimi-nating distance as a barrier to accessing specialty medical care. Psychiatry, dermatology, and cardiology are examples of specialty consultations rou-tinely conducted via telehealth. Project ECHO (Extension for Community Healthcare Outcomes) is an acclaimed telehealth project that was adopted in New Mexico to provide specialty care to patients with chronic hepatitis C in remote areas of the state. It has now spread to other regions of the United States and abroad and encompasses a multitude of chronic illnesses (Zhou, Crawford, Serhal, Kurdyak, & Sockalingam, 2016). This program uses videoconferencing to provide a venue for specialists and primary care providers to meet virtually to discuss specific patient cases. The interaction provides two advantages by simultaneously providing remote specialty consultations and primary care provider education on specialty care of patients with chronic illness.

Other examples of telehealth videoconferencing include its use in emer-gency departments (EDs) and intensive care units (ICUs) for direct access to specialist care. The Veterans Administration (VA) and Department of Defense have extensive telehealth videoconferencing programs throughout the United States and abroad. Videoconferencing for delivery of specialty healthcare is increasingly being used by Departments of Corrections.

Store and forward telehealth is used for consultations in which simulta-neous participation of two or more healthcare providers is not required. Radiology is currently the most common store and forward telemedicine specialty practice. Radiographs are digitized, transmitted, and read at a dis-tance. The practice is often used when a radiologist is not on site in health-care facilities that use outside specialty radiologists (Center for Connected Health Policy, n.d.). Other store and forward telemedicine specialties in-clude ophthalmology, dermatology, and wound care.

The third common type of telehealth is *remote monitoring*, which allows remote observation of patient status using technology. Telemonitoring equipment available for use in the home includes scales, blood pressure monitors, pulse oximeters, glucose monitoring equipment, electrocardio-graph monitoring equipment, and peak flow meters, all used to monitor patients from a distance.

The VA and home health agencies have been using remote moni-toring successfully for many years and have demonstrated the value of telemonitoring in the home. Patients are instructed in the use of a va-riety of devices that connect to a central system to monitor their health conditions. For example, measurements taken using the remote monitoring equipment automatically transmit through a phone line to a central server, which is then accessed by a nurse monitoring a patient caseload. The ad-vantage of the system is that the nurse monitors the patient daily, allowing recognition of subtle changes in the patient's condition from the uploaded data. The nurse can then contact the patient and other healthcare providers as needed. Telehealth remote monitoring studies investigating hospitalization rates show promising results (Bashi, Karunanithi, Fatehl, Dine, & Walters, 2017; Kitsiou, Pare, & Jaana, 2015).

Mobile Health (mHealth)

Mobile Health (mHealth), a subset of telehealth, is the use of mobile or wireless devices by healthcare providers and/or healthcare consumers (see Exhibit 14.1). Mobile technology provides a system to continuously monitor patient health status, provides communication between two or more healthcare providers, provides communication between patients and healthcare providers, promotes healthy lifestyles, and enhances management of chronic disease (Klonoff, 2013; Kumar et al., 2013). Examples of mHealth devices include smartphones, tablets, patient monitoring devices, wearable health devices, and laptop computers. Stand-alone patient monitoring devices, such as wearable appliances that continuously track specific health parameters (e.g., pulse, blood pressure, and blood glucose) and transmit this information to healthcare providers, are becoming widely available (Klonoff, 2013). Similar commercial technology for download to smartphones and tablets is being developed and marketed at exponential rates with the reported number of health and medical apps increasing from 1,000 to 20,000 between 2011 and 2013 (HiMSS, 2013).

Health Professional mHealth CDSSs

Healthcare providers are increasingly using mobile devices to access CDSSs. Popular proprietary CDSS programs such as UpToDate, Epocrates, and Lexicomp were discussed previously. These programs provide a thorough review of the most recent information on disease processes, diagnostics, and treatment choices. Other mobile CDSS apps provide easy access to patient-specific recommendations simply by entering a few quick keystrokes, eliminating the need to search through pages of algorithms and clinical practice guidelines. One such program is the AHRQ electronic preventive services selector (ePSS) software that is available for download to Android, iOS, BlackBerry, and Windows devices at no cost. The software provides instant access to U.S. Preventive Services Task Force (USPSTF) recommendations for specific patients based on provider input into drop-down boxes of patient age, sex, pregnancy status, tobacco use, and sexual activity status. Similar free apps are available from the Centers for Disease Control for selection of contraceptive methods based on patient health conditions. Other apps are available for a small price from reputable healthcare associations such as one from the Society for Lower Genital Tract Disorders that provides immediate access to the Updated Consensus Guidelines for Managing Abnormal Cervical Cancer Screening Tests and Cancer Precursors. A full discussion of available mHealth CDSS apps is beyond the scope of this chapter. The reader is encouraged to search governmental and professional healthcare websites if interested in mHealth apps that provide quick access to treatment guidelines.

Consumer mHealth CDSSs

Continuous patient monitoring devices with embedded decision support that automatically analyzes patient data and provides immediate treatment advice to the patient are rapidly being implemented in the care of patients with diabetes and other chronic illnesses. Using mHealth technology, the healthcare provider can preprogram these devices with decision support advice individualized to the patient.

Like all HIT applications, rigorous research is needed to determine the safety and efficacy of mHealth CDSSs (Klonoff, 2013; Kumar et al., 2013; Silberman & Clark, 2012; van Heerden, Tomlinson, & Swartz, 2012). This is especially important in the use of consumer mHealth CDSSs, where it is essential that the reliability of the monitoring devices is established before widespread use to ensure patient safety. Rigorous investigation of mHealth has been met with unique challenges, however, because the devices and apps quickly become obsolete as newer technology is developed and marketed (Kumar et al., 2013).

Analysis of Health Information

According to data from the Office of the National Coordinator of Health Information Technology (ONC, 2016), 86.9% of all office-based physicians in the United States were using EHRs in 2015 and 96% of all nonfederal hospitals in the United States have certified EHR technology (Henry, Pylypchuk, Searcy, & Patel, 2016). This widespread adoption of EHRs has resulted in a massive accumulation of complex patient data that are collectively referred to as "big data" (Simpao et al., 2014). Because of the enormous amount of available data, traditional analytic programs are insufficient, resulting in a need for new, advanced data analysis methods. To meet this new demand, analytics programs (see Exhibit 14.1) are being deployed to systematically integrate data from various different, seemingly incongruent, sources to guide decision making across healthcare (Simpao et al., 2014).

Predictive analytics is the technology that promises to accomplish the goals of improved patient outcomes at lower costs. *Predictive analytics* is defined as "the use of electronic algorithms that forecast future events in real time" (Cohen, Amarasingham, Shah, Xie, & Lo, 2014, p. 1139). Although widely used in other industries such as business, finance, and retail, predictive analytics is relatively new to healthcare. Early applications in large inpatient settings include analytics for predicting patients at high risk for adverse and/or high-cost events such as cardiopulmonary arrest or readmissions. These predictions assist in allocating or reallocating resources to patients at greatest risk for adverse events (Cohen et al., 2014). Suggested future applications of predictive analytics in the hospital setting include patient triage and prediction of patients at risk for rapid deterioration in their condition (Bates, Saria, Ohno-Machado, Shah, & Escobar, 2014).

As the field of predictive analytics evolves, the APRN can expect to see its use in primary care settings in addition to the acute care hospitals. This will lead to greater accuracy in making diagnostic and treatment decisions based on data from millions of patients throughout the world (Hernandez & Zhang, 2017). Decisions on when it is safe to follow the patient in the primary care setting and when patients should be referred to specialists can be guided by the information obtained through predictive analytics. It is likely that as the use of predictive analytics matures, new and unforeseen uses will also emerge.

Current HIT Controversies and Failures

Despite the rapid growth in HIT, controversies remain in the adoption rates and outcomes associated with the technology. On the short list of these controversies are problems with interoperability and privacy and security concerns. These issues must be addressed and solutions found before the APRN can fully experience the long-term benefits of HIT.

Interoperability

Sharing of information across healthcare systems is paramount to the transformation of U.S. healthcare into a system with improved outcomes and decreased costs (Le, 2013). Interoperability provides a mechanism for sharing of patient information among providers, healthcare systems, third-party payers, and consumers. The ONC has contended that interoperability is the foundation necessary for realization of the HIT benefits that have long been espoused. Interoperability and sharing of patient information have been slow to start, but are rapidly improving. Recent surveys found the rate of physicians electronically sharing data with other providers reached 42% in 2014, showing a 7% increase over 2013 (ONC, 2015). Another survey found that a majority of physician respondents indicated that HIE will positively affect patient care, care coordination, and cost of care (Bipartisan Policy Center, 2012). Lack of interface between EHRs, cost, and financial sustainability are among primary concerns cited by providers regarding their participation and ability to share health information. These concerns must be addressed to ensure full-scale interoperability and realization of the projected benefits of HIT.

Patient Privacy

Patient privacy and security of healthcare information are an area of concern increasingly being voiced among HIT experts. According to 2017 data from the Protenus Breach Arometer Annual Report, healthcare data breaches totaled 477 and impacted 5,579,348 patient records (Proteus, 2018). Thirty-seven percent of the 2017 breaches were from insider incidents (i.e., insider error or insider wrongdoing) and involved 30% of the breached records. Hacking breaches (i.e., ransomware and malware attacks) were responsible for 37% of all breaching incidents, affecting 3,437,742 patient records (Protenus Inc., 2018). Although the number of hacking incidents increased from 2016, the overall number of patient records that were affected decreased from 23,695,069 in 2016 (Protenus, Inc., 2018).

To protect electronic information from security breaches, the U.S. Department of Health and Human Services (DHHS) requires an authorized testing and certification body (ATCB) to certify all EHRs. Before granting certification, the ATCB attests that the EHR meets security requirements in seven areas: access control, emergency access, automatic log-off, audit log, integrity, authentication, and general encryption (Office of Inspector General [OIG], 2014). However, in a 2014 audit, the OIG found that EHR certification does not necessarily ensure security and protection of patient information. This finding is underscored by the increase in the number of security breaches as well as the total number of consumers who are impacted.

SUMMARY

HIT resources and tools are available to help healthcare providers and consumers locate and manage information, support decision making, and improve safety. Recognizing the need for information and knowing about resources that can help to provide relevant information are vital skills for APRNs. By keeping abreast of technology, APRNs will be able to benefit from HIT tools, resources, and innovations.

HIT is being developed at an unprecedented pace; the resources described in this chapter should be viewed only as a representative sample of the informatics tools available to APRNs, not as an exhaustive list. New resources are constantly being developed, and the reader is encouraged to use this chapter as a starting point for considering HIT resources for practice. Many mechanisms for staying abreast of current technology, such as professional development and APRN journals, provide opportunities to learn about and evaluate new innovations as they become available.

REFERENCES

American Health Information Management Association. (2016, January 13). CMS to end meaningful use in 2016. Retrieved from http://journal.ahima.org/2016/01/13/cms-to-end-meaningful-use-in-2016

Ammenwerth, E., Schnell-Inderst, P., & Hoerbst, A. (2012). The impact of electronic patient portals on patient care: A systematic review of controlled trials. *Journal of Medical Internet Research, 14*(6), e162. doi:10.2196/jmir.2238

Bashi, N., Karunanithi, M., Fatehi, F., Ding, H., & Walters, D. (2017). Remote monitoring of patients with heart failure: An overview of systematic reviews. *Journal of Medical Internet Research, 19*(1), e18. doi:10.2196/jmir.6571

Bates, D., Saria, S., Ohno-Machado, L., Shah, A., & Escobar, G. (2014). Big data in health care: Using analytics to identify and manage high-risk and high-cost patients. *Health Affairs, 33*(7), 1123–1131. doi:10.1377/hlthaff.2014.0041

Bipartisan Policy Center. (2012). *Clinician perspectives on electronic health information sharing for transitions of care.* Washington, DC: Author.

Blum, D., Raj, S. X., Oberholzer, R., Riphagen, I. I., Strasser, F., & Kaasa, S. (2015). Computer-based clinical decision support systems and patient-reported outcomes: A systematic review. *The Patient*, 8(5), 397–409. doi:10.1007/s40271-014-0100-1

Blumenthal, D., & Tavenner, M. (2010). The "meaningful use" regulation for electronic health records. *New England Journal of Medicine, 363*(6), 501–504. doi:10.1056/NEJMp1006114

Bowman, S. (2013). Impact of electronic health record systems on information integrity: Quality and safety implications. *Perspectives in Health Information Management, 101c*, 1–19.

Bright, T., Wong, A., Dhurjati, R., Bristow, E., Bastian, L., Coeytaux, R., . . . Lobach, D. (2012). Effect of clinical decision-support systems: A systematic review. *Annals of Internal Medicine, 157*(1), 29–43. doi:10.7326/0003-4819-157-1-201207030-00450

Center for Connected Health Policy. (n.d.). Store and forward. Retrieved from http://www.cchpca.org/store-and-forward

Cohen, G. R., & Adler-Milstein, J. (2016) Meaning use care coordination criteria: Perceived barriers and benefits among primary care providers. *Journal of the American Medical Informatics Association, 23*, e147–e151. doi:10.1093/jamia/ocv147

Cohen, I., Amarasingham, R., Shah, A., Xie, B., & Lo, B. (2014). The legal and ethical concerns that arise from using complex predictive analytics in health care. *Health Affairs, 33*(7), 1139–1147. doi:10.1377/hlthaff.2014.0048

Curtis, J. (2010). Implementation of health information technology. *Journal for Nurse Practitioners, 6*(3), 228–229.

Davis, S., Roudsari, A., Raworth, R., Courtney, K. L., & MacKay, L. (2017). Shared decision-making using personal health record technology: A scoping review at the crossroads. *Journal of the American Medical Informatics Association, 24*(4), 857–866. doi:10.1093/jamia/ocw172

Del Fiol, G., Huser, V., Strasberg, H., Maviglia, S., Curtis, C., & Cimino, J. (2012). Implementations of the HL7 context-aware knowledge retrieval ("Infobutton") standard: Challenges, strengths, limitations, and uptake. *Journal of Biomedical Informatics, 45*(4), 726–735. doi:10.1016/j.jbi.2011.12.006

Dragan, I. F., Newman, M., Stark, P., Steffensen, B., & Karimbux, N. (2015). Using a simulated infobutton linked to an evidence-based resource to research drug-drug interactions: A pilot study with third-year dental students. *Journal of Dental Education, 79*(11), 1349–1355.

Goldzweig, C., Orshansky, G., Paige, N., Towfigh, A., Haggstrom, D., Miake-Lye, I., . . . Shekelle, P. (2013). Electronic patient portals: Evidence on health outcomes, satisfaction, efficiency, and attitudes: A systematic review. *Annals of Internal Medicine, 159*(10), 677–687. doi:10.7326/0003-4819-159-10-201311190-00006

Healthcare Information and Management Systems Society. (2010). *HiMSS dictionary of healthcare information technology terms, acronyms and organizations* (2nd ed.). Chicago, IL: Author.

Healthcare Information and Management Systems Society. (2013). Personal health information: Paradigm for providers and patients to transform healthcare through patient engagement. Retrieved from https://s3.amazonaws.com/rdcms-himss/files/production/public/FileDownloads/FINAL%20PAPER%20Personal%20Health%20IT%20-%20Paradigm%20for%20Providers-Patients%20to%20Transform%20Healthcare%20through%20Patient%20Engagement_FINAL%20(3)vk.pdf

Henry, J., Pylypchuk, Y., Searcy, T., & Patel, V. (2016, May). *Adoption of electronic health record systems among U.S. non-federal acute hospitals: 2008-2015.* ONC Data Brief, no. 35. Washington, DC: Office of the National Coordinator for Health Information Technology.

Hernandez, I., & Zhang, Y. (2017). Using predictive analytics and big data to optimize pharmaceutical outcomes. *American Journal of Health-System Pharmacy, 74*(18), 1494–1500. doi:10.2146/ajhp161011

Hunt, D. L., Haynes, R. B., Hanna, S. E., & Smith, K. (1998). Effects of computer-based clinical decision support systems on physician performance and patient outcomes: A systematic review. *Journal of American Medical Association, 280*(15), 1339–1346. doi:10.1001/jama.280.15.1339

Institute of Medicine Committee on Quality of Health Care in America. (2001). *Crossing the quality chasm: A new health system for the 21st century.* Washington, DC: National Academies Press.

Institute of Medicine Committee on Quality of Health Care in America. (2011). *Health IT and patient safety: Building safer systems for better care.* Washington, DC: National Academies Press.

Irizarry, T., DeVito Dabbs, A., & Curran, C. R. (2015). Patient portals and patient engagement: A state of the science review. *Journal of Medical Internet Research, 17*(6), e148. doi:10.2196/jmir.4255

Irizarry, T., Shoemake, J., Nisen, M.L., Czaja, S., Beach, S., & Devito Dabbs, A. (2017). Patient portals as a tool for health care engagement: A mixed-method study of older adults with varying levels of health literacy and prior patient portal use. *Journal of Medical Internet Research,19*(3), e99. doi:10.2196/jmir.7099

Jaspers, M., Smuelers, M., Vermeulen, H., & Peute, L. (2011). Effects of clinical decision-support systems on practitioner performance and patient outcomes: A synthesis of high-quality systematic review findings. *Journal of the American Medical Informatics Association, 18*(3), 327–334. doi:10.1136/amiajnl-2011-000094

Jia, P., Zhang, L., Chen, J., Zhao, P., & Zhang, M. (2016). The effects of clinical decision support systems on medication safety: An overview. *Plos One, 11*(12), e0167683. doi:10.1371/journal.pone.0167683

Jordan-Marsh, M. (2011). *Health technology literacy: A transdisciplinary framework for consumer-oriented practice.* Sudbury, MA: Jones & Bartlett.

Kern, L. M., Edwards, A., & Kaushal, R. (2016). The meaningful use of electronic health records and health care utilization. *American Journal of Medical Quality, 31*(4), 301–307. doi:10.1177/1062860615572439

King, J., Patel, F., Jamoom, E., & Furukawa, M. (2014). Clinical benefits of electronic health record use: National findings. *Health Services Research, 49*(1, pt. 2), 392–404. doi:10.1111/1475-6773.12135

Kitsiou, S., Paré, G., & Jaana, M. (2015). Effects of home telemonitoring interventions on patients with chronic heart failure: An overview of systematic reviews. *Journal of Medical Internet Research, 17*(3), e63. doi:10.2196/jmir.4174

Klonoff, D. (2013). The current status of mHealth for diabetes: Will it be the next big thing? *Journal of Diabetes Science and Technology, 7*(3), 749–758. doi:10.1177/193229681300700321

Koeniger-Donohue, R., Kumar Agarwal, N., Hawkins, J. W., & Stowell, S. (2014). Role of nurse practitioners in encouraging use of personal health records. *Nurse Practitioner, 39*(7), 1–8. doi:10.1097/01.NPR.0000450743.39981.93

Kohn, L. T., Corrigan, J. M., & Donaldson, M. S. (Eds.). (2000). *To err is human: Building a safer health system*. Washington, DC: National Academies Press.

Kumar, S., Nilsen, W., Abernethy, A., Atienza, A., Patrick, K., Pavel, M.,…Swendeman, D. (2013). Mobile health technology evaluation: The mHealth evidence workshop. *American Journal of Preventive Medicine, 45*(2), 228–236. doi:10.1016/j.amepre.2013.03.017

Kvedar, J., Coye, M., & Everett, W. (2014). Connected health: A review of technologies and strategies to improve patient care with telemedicine and telehealth. *Health Affairs, 33*(2), 194–199. doi:10.1377/hlthaff.2013.0992

Lammers, E., & McLaughlin, C. (2017). Meaningful use of electronic health records and medicare expenditures: Evidence from a panel data analysis of U.S. health care markets, 2010-2013. *Health Services Research, 52*(4), 1364–1386. doi:10.1111/1475-6773.12550

Le, P. (2013). Strategic interoperability unleashing the full potential of EHRs. *Health Management Technology, 34*(10), 16.

Marcotte, L., Seidman, J., Trudel, K., Berwick, D., Blumenthal, D., Mostashari, F., & Jain, S. (2012). Achieving meaningful use of health information technology: A guide for physicians to the EHR incentive programs. *Archives of Internal Medicine, 172*(9), 731–736. doi:10.1001/archinternmed.2012.872

Office of Inspector General, Department of Health and Human Services. (2014). The Office of the National Coordinator for Health Information Technology's oversight of the testing and certification of electronic health records. Retrieved from https://oig.hhs.gov/oas/reports/region6/61100063.pdf

Office of National Coordinator for Health Information Technology (n.d.). Interoperability. Retrieved from https://www.healthit.gov/topic/interoperability

Office of the National Coordinator for Health Information Technology. (2015). ONC Data Brief, No 31. Retrieved from https://www.healthit.gov/sites/default/files/briefs/oncdatabrief31_physician_e_exchange.pdf

Office of the National Coordinator for Health Information Technology. (2016). Office-based physician electronic health record adoption. Health IT Quick-Stat #50. Retrieved from http://dashboard.healthit.gov/quickstats/pages/physician-ehr-adoption-trends.php

Office of the National Coordinator for Health Information Technology (2018). What are the advantages of of electronic health records. Retrieved from https://www.healthit.gov/faq/what-are-advantages-electronic-health-records

Protenus, Inc. (2018). 1.13M patient records breached in Q1 2018, proprietary data shows disclosed breaches are just the tip of the iceberg. Retrieved from https://cdn2.hubspot.net/hubfs/2331613/Breach_Barometer/2018/Q1%202018/Q1%202018%20Protenus%20Breach%20Barometer.pdf?utm_campaign=June%20Forbes%20article%20-%20GDPR&utm_source=Forbes%20article

Rathert, C., Porter, T. H., Mittler, J. N., & Fleig-Palmer, M. (2017). Seven years after meaningful use: Physicians' and nurses' experiences with electronic health records. *Health Care Management Review*. (ePub ahead of print.) doi:10.1097/HMR.0000000000000168

Robbins, G., Lester, W., Johnson, K., Chang, Y., Estey, G., Surrao, D., . . . Freedberg, K. (2012). Efficacy of a clinical decision-support system in an HIV practice: A randomized trial. *Annals of Internal Medicine, 157*(11), 757–766. doi:10.7326/0003-4819-157-11-201212040-00003

Roshanov, P., Misra, S., Gerstein, H., Garg, A., Sebaldt, R., Mackay, J., ... Haynes, R. (2011). Computerized clinical decision support systems for chronic disease management: A decision-maker-researcher partnership systematic review. *Implementation Science, 6*, 92. doi:10.1186/1748-5908-6-92

Saba, K., & Westra, B. (2011). Historical perspectives of nursing informatics. In V. K. Saba & K. A. McCormick (Eds.), *Essentials of nursing informatics* (5th ed., pp. 11–29). New York, NY: McGraw-Hill.

Shay, L. A., & Lafata, J. E. (2015). Where is the evidence? A systematic review of shared decision making and patient outcomes. *Medical Decision Making, 35*(1), 114–131. doi:10.1177/0272989X14551638

Silberman, M. J., & Clark, L. (2012). M-health: The union of technology and health care regulation. *Journal of Medical Practice Management, 28*(2), 118–120.

Simpao, A., Ahumada, L., Gálvez, J., & Rehman, M. (2014). A review of analytics and clinical informatics in health care. *Journal of Medical Systems, 38*(4), 45. doi:10.1007/s10916-014-0045-x

Sprague, N. (2014, April 11). Telehealth: Into the mainstream? *National Policy Forum.* Retrieved from http://www.nhpf.org/library/details.cfm/2960

Teixeira, M., Cook, D. A., Heale, B. E., & Del Fiol, G. (2017). Optimization of infobutton design and implementation: A systematic review. *Journal of Biomedical Informatics, 74*, 10–19. doi:10.1016/j.jbi.2017.08.010

van Heerden, A., Tomlinson, M., & Swartz, L. (2012). Point of care in your pocket: A research agenda for the field on m-health. *Bulletin of the World Health Organization, 90*(5), 393–394. doi:10.2471/BLT.11.099788

Zhou, C., Crawford, A., Serhal, E., Kurdyak, P., & Sockalingam, S. (2016). The impact of project ECHO on participant and patient outcomes: A systematic review. *Academic Medicine, 91*(10), 1439–1461. doi:10.1097/ACM.0000000000001328

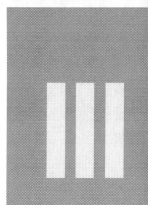

TRANSITIONS TO THE ADVANCED PRACTICE ROLE

15

Patricia A. White and Kathryn A. Blair

SCHOLARSHIP OF PRACTICE

An ongoing dialogue in the field of clinical nursing is focusing on the importance of scholarly nursing research (Limoges & Acorn, 2016; Riley & Beal, 2013; Sigma Theta Tau International Clinical Scholarship Task Force, 1999; Wilkes, Mannix, & Jackson, 2013). This emerging dialogue is often characterized by its clarion call for nursing scholarship to move the study of clinical practice into systematic, academic, and rigorous research (Limoges & Acorn, 2016). This growing movement in clinical nursing scholarship also seeks to transform the practice of nursing in the clinical realm into rigorously investigated inquiries, discovery, and knowledge that is informed by evidence-based practice, applied and shared beyond this context (Limoges & Acorn, 2016; Riley & Beal, 2013; Sigma Theta Tau International Clinical Scholarship Task Force, 1999; Wilkes et al., 2013).

A major development in this movement occurred recently as a result of the position statement issued by the American Association of Colleges of Nursing (AACN) on defining nursing scholarship. In 2016, the AACN put forth its position on nursing scholarship which stated that:

> Scholarship in nursing can be defined as those activities that systematically advance the teaching, research, and practice of nursing through rigorous inquiry that; 1) is significant to the profession, 2) is creative, 3) can be documented, 4) can be replicated or elaborated, and 5) can be peer-reviewed through various methods.

Citing the shifting academic landscape in many disciplines across colleges and universities nationwide, the AACN's Task Force on Defining Standards for the Scholarship of Nursing concluded that, "Nowhere is this dialogue more pertinent than in nursing, where rigorous scholarly inquiry must be applied in the realities and demands of practice" (AACN, 2016). The AACN also provided standards that correspond to Boyer's model of scholarship by which nursing scholarship is to be conducted. These include the scholarship of discovery, the scholarship of teaching, the scholarship of application, and the scholarship of integration (AACN, 2016; Boyer, 1990). In addition to the statement on nursing scholarship, its definition, and standards issued by the AACN, significant voices in the current nursing literature theorize that clinical nursing scholarship should be built on the foundations of Boyer's model for scholarly inquiry, with some specifically looking to the scholarship of application for a fitting framework from which to conduct clinical nursing research (Limoges & Acorn, 2016).

HISTORICAL PERSPECTIVE

Riley, Beal, Levi, and McCausland (2002) outlined the importance of the concept of scholarly practice for the nursing profession. Many nurse leaders have called for links between practice and scholarship (Diers, 1995; Meleis, 1987), and rather than espouse a model that emphasizes a purely academic approach to scholarship, they developed a model that emphasizes a practical approach to scholarship. Research on this domain explored clinical scholarship from the perspectives of practicing nurses (Riley & Beal, 2013; Riley, Beal, & Lancaster, 2008).

Although advanced practice nursing has explored the concept of novice nurse practitioner adjustment to the new role, there has been little in-depth exploration of the concept of clinical scholarship. Earlier work by Brykczynski (1989) addressed clinical judgment and nurse practitioner practice. Her research highlighted the essential elements involved in the day-to-day practice of nurse practitioners and provided additional understanding of the complexities of providing care in a variety of settings. The knowledge development embedded in the practice of advanced practice nursing and the role development processes identified in her study also added to the understanding of clinical scholarship for advanced practice. Advanced practice role transition and the importance of mentoring have continued to be studied in the advanced practice literature. However, these concepts have not been linked explicitly to the concept of clinical scholarship. The research on clinical scholarship with nurses that is identified in this chapter has important relevance for APRNs.

Model for Clinical Scholarship

In response to the need for greater understanding and perspectives on the meaning of scholarship in nursing, leading nurse educators developed the Universal Model of Nursing scholarship and identified four domains: *knowing, teaching, practice,* and *service* (Riley et al., 2002). This model is unique to nursing as a practice discipline; it is comprehensive in its design and identifies a range of scholarly activities relevant to nurses in a variety of settings. The Universal Model of Nursing scholarship identifies components of scholarship including service, education, knowledge development, and practice. This model on scholarly practice has been expanded to include practicing nurses' descriptions of scholarly practice (Riley & Beal, 2013; Riley et al., 2008; Riley et al., 2002). Although the research by Riley et al. has been conducted on practicing nurses, it has great potential for application to advanced practice nursing.

Definition of Scholarly Practice

Riley et al. (2008) offer a definition of "scholarly practice" based on their research that states, "Scholarly nursing practice is defined as a multidimensional way of thinking about practice that includes role attributes of *active learner, out-of-the-box thinker, passionate about nursing, available,* and *confident,* and the role processes of *lead, give care, share knowledge, evolve,* and *reflect*" (p. 17). These role attributes and processes are outlined in Figure 15.1. This diagram highlights the many dimensions of the role of clinical scholar and the complexities involved in role enactment.

Four themes emerge in the model: role identification in providing care, role evolution, reflective practice, and leadership. *Role identification* incorporates immersion in care, vigilance, and prioritizing the relationships involved in patient care. *Role evolution* includes the openness to learning from patients and families, advancing knowledge acquisition, and staying abreast of current evidence. The third theme of *reflection in practice* is reported as a multidimensional concept that allows nurses opportunities to consider anticipatory thinking about potential issues that could arise in practice. The fourth component of the model is identified as the nurse as a *leader* that was further developed in the areas of nurses looking to develop other nurses. This dimension of practice is often omitted in the discussions

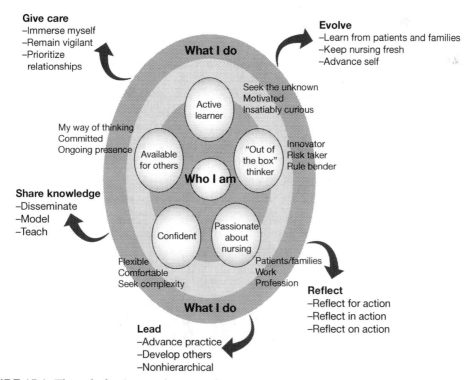

FIGURE 15.1 The scholar in nursing practice.
Source: Riley, J., Beal, J. A., and Lancaster, D. (2008). Scholarly nursing practice from the perspectives of experienced nurses. *Journal of Advanced Nursing, 61*(4), 425–435. doi:10.1111/j.1365-2648.2007.04499.x

of role development, and identifying this component of scholarly practice requires additional exploration.

Early career perspectives concerning clinical scholarship suggest that nurses identify a very complex process of role development (Riley & Beal, 2013). As nurses become comfortable with clinical competence and decision-making skills, they develop an awareness of what expert scholarly practice embodies and an awareness of a goal toward which they are working (Riley & Beal, 2013).

Experienced acute care nurses identified components of scholarly practice with themes that were different from those for less-experienced nurse. These nurses identified expert practice as involving less cognitive effort in the technical aspects of care, allowing for more focus on reflection and relationships with patients, families, and team members. Expert nurses view their professional identity as active learners, out-of-the-box thinkers, passionate about nursing, available, and confident. In addition, expert nurses characterized their roles as leading, caring, sharing knowledge with others, evolving, and reflecting on practice (Beal, Riley, & Lancaster, 2008).

Experienced nurses highlight the ongoing challenges faced in their role. Their descriptions of providing care reflected a process of developing relationships with patients and families as an essential component of providing expert care as well as vigilance in identifying patient needs. Reflection was characterized by reflection *on* action, reflection *in* action, and reflection *for* action. *Reflection on action* offered opportunities to critique clinical situations that had occurred to learn how to use their experiences to improve patient care. *Reflection in action* provided the opportunities to synthesize information about the patient while providing care. *Reflection for action* helped prepare for possibilities that might require action and provided an additional dimension to the concept of reflection (Beal et al., 2008).

The personal and professional characteristics that the nurses identified in their descriptions of novice and expert practice highlighted a dimension of practice that continues to enrich and inspire them to share with others, and to continually seek opportunities to further develop in their role. This research also provides additional depth to the understanding of the ongoing development of the roles of both the novice and expert nurse scholar. The refinement of these concepts of role attributes as well as processes is critical in our ongoing understanding.

The aforementioned model identifies the evolution of moving from technological practice to scholarly practice. The question remains: What is the scholarship of practice or scholarly practice? And what defines a nurse scholar? A "scholar" can be defined as a person who has done advanced study in a special field and is a learned person. "Other characteristics of scholars are that they typically know how to speak with authority, and are articulate in both written and oral communication" (Conrad & Pape, 2014, p. 88). An APRN who clearly articulates with authority fits the definition of a scholar.

As mentioned earlier, some nurse clinical scholars recommend that clinical nursing scholarship expand on and borrow from the traditions of the "scholarship of application." This type of scholarship is typically defined as a wide range of scholarly activities "in the sciences and humanities that involves translation of new knowledge to practical applications to solve problems of individuals and of society," which can include patient-oriented research (Shapiro & Coleman, 2000, pp. 895–898). Authors Limoges and Acorn argue that adopting the scholarship of application is especially critical to the next generation of nurse scholars. In a recent article on the scholarship of application in the clinical nursing context, Limoges and Acorn suggest that utilizing this framework will lend itself to uncovering and understanding clinical nursing concerns as a result of the tradition's emphasis on the three criteria for scholarship, practical problem solving, and rigor. The three criteria cited here for scholarship are documentation, peer review, and dissemination (Limoges & Acorn, 2016).

According to a literature review conducted by these authors, which focused on research completed between 1983 and 2015, there was little evidence of formal implementation of the scholarship of application in clinical nursing scholarship. Nevertheless, the authors report that they observed a parallel conversation and trajectory around translating knowledge gained from problem solving from the specific tradition of application within Boyer's model of scholarship and nursing research. They contend that the scholarship of application framework was originally discussed decades ago in close alignment with various elements of nursing research. For example, they note that clinical nursing scholarship is used to solve complex problems and requires expert knowledge, confidence, active learning, willingness to share findings, understanding of evidence-based practice, and creative problem-solving skills among nurse investigators—elements that are all supported by specific research from the field of nursing and correlate with the concept of Boyer's scholarship of application (Riley & Beal, 2013; Sigma Theta Tau International Clinical Scholarship Task Force, 1999; Wilkes et al., 2013). Thus, they observe that a renewed interest and discussion on the scholarship of application and clinical nursing scholarship are an important development in recent scholarly nursing dialogue to which the field should attend (Limoges & Acorn, 2016).

SCHOLARSHIP OF APRN PRACTICE

When scholarship of practice is discussed, most of the dialogue addresses faculty practice and its role in the tripartite mission of colleges and universities. Is faculty practice scholarship? The question has been the angst of many APRN faculty. To maintain APRN certification, the APRN faculty member must practice. The function of faculty practice is to maintain clinical competence, provide a source of professional development, and facilitate the linkage between theory and practice. Faculty practice is the bridge between the academic and clinical arenas (Honig, Smolowitz, & Larson, 2013; Premji et al., 2011).

Scholarship of practice also applies to the practicing APRN with or without an academic appointment. Scholarship of practice should be incorporated into the APRN professional role (Thomas, 2012). For APRNs to be taken seriously by the greater healthcare system, they must participate in the scholarship of practice. The question continues to arise: What is the scholarship of practice?

Scholarship of practice fits with Boyer's models (1990), the scholarship of integration and/or application. The scholarship of integration refers to the interpretation of research across disciplines. In other words, it answers the question, What does this mean? The scholarship of application "applies" the current evidence to real-world situations. This form of scholarship answers the question, How does this knowledge help individuals or institutions? (Boyer, 1990, p. 21).

The scholarship of practice requires building nursing knowledge, interpretation and/or application of the evidence, knowledge transfer, connecting academic research to practice, and practice-based research (Wilkes et al., 2013). Dissemination or knowledge transfer can take many forms, such as presentation at local, state, national, or international forums; scholarly writing or publication; web-based teaching modules; and staff education (Bosold & Darnel, 2012).

The scholarship of practice suggests that knowledge should come from collaboration between the researcher and clinician (Peterson, McMahon, Farkas, & Howland, 2005). Universities often fail to address those issues that are salient to the clinician and community (Crist, 2010). The relationship between the APRN and researcher is synergistic, and partnerships should be encouraged as well as developed. The role of the APRN is critical to guiding the researchers' questions, making the evidence relevant to the patient or community, and/or translating the evidence into practice.

With clarity of definitions and roles of the scholar and scholarship of practice, why do many APRNs not see themselves as scholars or not engage in scholarly activities? Most APRNs perhaps see themselves as "doers," not scholars (Lusk, 2014). Perhaps they lack the skill to conduct or translate research, feel their work is "not good enough," their writing skills are lacking, or the process takes too long. This mentality indirectly lessens APRNs' credibility in the healthcare system. Another concern for APRNs is that scholarship of practice often goes unrewarded in the clinical setting (Robert & Pape, 2011). Therefore, the motivation to become an active scholar is lacking.

So how does the APRN become a scholar? The APRN may have questions that arise from clinical practice, such as clinical situations, clinical guidelines, or policy issues. These questions can be examined with the current evidence. APRN graduates have the skills to interpret and evaluate current evidence and practice guidelines. The doctorate of nursing programs (DNPs) is designed to expand this knowledge to provide leadership for practice improvement, quality, and safety (Brown & Crabtree, 2013). An APRN who is unsure of his or her ability to evaluate research or outcomes or implement change can work with researchers. If an APRN is a preceptor, a student–practitioner research partnership under the guidance of a faculty researcher can be formed (Crist, 2010).

When an APRN institutes changes in practice, measures outcomes, serves as an expert in a particular area, or has learned the "tricks of the trade," these accomplishments should be shared with colleagues in both an informal and formal way. One way to share information is through publication. Publications can take the form of blogs, web-based activity, journals, and editorials in local papers, and so on. Perhaps the easiest way to begin the publication process is when one is in graduate school and uses the scholarly paper or DNP capstone project to develop a manuscript along with a faculty mentor.

In her recent chapter on clinical nursing scholarship and evidence-based practice, Dr. Catherine Tymkow also discusses the appropriateness of Boyer's model of scholarship for clinical nursing and describes the gaps in academic research models that do not make full use of nursing expertise and discovery. Tymkow states that, "The traditional definition of scholarship in academia did not account for the nuances and rigors of clinical practice knowledge and its application for problem solving and interactive, human engagement. Boyer's model, however, is well-suited to scholarship in nursing practice" (2014, p. 63). She goes on to argue that using this model in practice is essential for maximizing the potential of the research components of the advanced nursing practice degree, the Doctor of Nursing Practice (DNP), which she says was intended to address the gaps in clinical nursing scholarship (Tymkow, 2014).

Tymkow also argues that although randomized controlled trials with large numbers of participants are viewed as the gold standard for evidence-based interventions, many other qualitative and quantitative research processes and methods for conducting clinical nursing scholarship may be appropriate for addressing clinical questions. She cites various types of qualitative methods, including critical social theory research, ethnography, grounded theory studies, historical research, phenomenology, and philosophical research studies that have yielded results suitable for clinical nursing scholarship. In addition, Tymkow also cites quantitative methods and discusses in great detail the critical processes and concerns for conducting quantitative research in nursing. These include determining research question, purpose, context, design, data collection, analysis, interpretation of results, discussion of ethical issues, and synthesis of implications. Tymkow (2014) also specifically attends to crucial, persistent problems in scholarship overall that often end up impacting research, policy, and practice such as various types of bias, including gender and selection bias.

GUIDELINES FOR PUBLICATION AND PRESENTATION

This section provides the APRN with some tips for presentation and writing. Writing or presenting is a means to let your voice be heard. In an advanced practice role, the APRN must include professional writing and presenting as an integral part of his or her identity. By not valuing, practicing, and developing these skills while in graduate school, it is easy to slide down the slippery slope into a technical conceptualization of the role rather than professional ideation.

All APRNs will move from novice to expert; however, there are periods of transitions as one moves through the process of becoming an expert. For example, Bridges (1991) described a reorientation phase as a final step in transition. In reorientation, nurses in advanced practice roles redefine themselves as leaders. With this new identity, publishing and presenting are critical leadership actions. It is through dissemination that others' thinking and acting are influenced—and that is leadership.

Healthcare professionals read the professional literature and attend conferences for a reason, and one needs to identify such a reason. Begin with an issue or question from the reader's/audience's perspective. Ask, why would they want to know this? This may be a methodology, a population-specific intervention, a program, or clinical insight. The unique idea may relate to direct patient care, to a resource issue, or to collaboration within the unit or larger system of healthcare.

The writer/presenter persuades the reader/audience by writing or presenting in a simple and concise format. The goal is to have readers/audience become as interested as you are in the topic you are presenting. *Know your audience.* The content or topic will be presented differently for different audiences. For example, presenting to APRNs in a clinical arena may be different from presenting to a nurse educator/researcher or to a nonnurse audience.

Identify a journal or other forum for your topic. One should explore the journals and sources of information that are or were used in graduate school. Review the section "information to authors" or "manuscript guidelines." These guidelines are found in the print journals or online. If presenting at a conference, there is typically a conference theme. Reviewing topics and abstract guidelines is a must because the manuscript types or presentations that are accepted by the journal/conference are delineated (e.g., practice focus, research, literature reviews, policy, opinion pieces). Skimming articles in a recent issue or reviewing topics covered in a previous conference to examine style, tone, research base, and intended audience will help you decide whether the manuscript/presentation seems to fit. Finally, the journal's/conference's information for authors/presenters will identify the specific writing/presentation format (e.g., PowerPoint, poster, workshop, roundtable discussion).

Selecting a journal or conference that is peer reviewed is a basic criterion, especially for those in academic positions. In the peer-review process, two or three content and/or method experts provide a double-blind review to assist the journal editor or conference planners in making recommendations to the authors/presenters. The peer-review process ensures that a minimum standard of quality exists in the published literature or conference. For beginning writers/presenters, however, it may be advantageous to select local, state, or regional newsletters or other nonpeer-reviewed publications/conferences. Generally, there is a faster turnaround time to dissemination, and the submission process is less complex.

Once a conference or journal is selected, you need to organize your thoughts, and this can be done by drafting an outline of the major ideas you are interested in conveying to the reader/audience. The structure must be organized so that the reader/audience can move quickly and easily through the article or presentation. If the reader/audience is struggling to stay with you in format, language, or organization, the message may be lost no matter how notable the content; cognitive leaps and disorganization prevent the reader/audience from "getting it."

To help the reader/audience "get it," the use of transition is helpful. The first sentence of each paragraph should be designed as a bridge sentence; or link content together by articulating the connections. Do not assume the reader or audience has the same level of expertise that you have on the topic.

There are many handbooks for writers beginning the scholarly publication process. Dexter (2000) describes writing tips, including strategies to enhance clarity, precision, accuracy, logic, and depth. For beginning writers, the following may be helpful: (a) use an outline to plan and organize the paper; (b) after setting aside a manuscript, read it out loud (grammar problems, incomplete sentences, long sentences or paragraphs will be more easily heard than seen); and (c) paraphrase and use references precisely. In addition, Silvia (2007) has a bright and practical little book that stresses the need for a weekly writing schedule, how to address common writing barriers, and specific motivational tools. If a structured week-by-week approach appeals to you, Belcher's (2009) book helps academic authors overcome anxieties, learn a particular feature of a strong manuscript every week, and send their own work to a journal at the end of 12 weeks.

Collaborating with others or choosing a mentor is a strategy for beginners to bolster their confidence. By obtaining feedback from a coauthor/mentor, writing/presentation skills will expand. In addition, scheduled timelines with others provide structure, and brainstorming and dialogue enrich the process. However, multiple authors/presenters require consensus building, and blending different writing or presenting styles may be more time consuming. Another word of caution: Clearly determine author/presenter order (primary, secondary, etc.) at the outset, based on agreed-upon contributions and responsibilities.

Precise adherence to the manuscript guidelines or the organization's call for abstracts, particularly page limits or word counts, format, and content focus, is essential. A response from the journal editor after manuscript submission can vary from 6 weeks to nearly a year. Following the ethics of publishing, a manuscript can be submitted to only one journal at a time. The editor's response also may vary; he or she compiles the peer reviewers' appraisals and then typically decides to (a) publish as is, (b) reconsider after suggested revisions, or (c) not publish. Conference abstract submissions have deadlines, and they are either accepted or rejected. One strategy that increases your chances is to submit the abstract for podium or poster. This way a reviewer may say the abstract is not accepted for podium presentation but would be more appropriate for poster presentation.

With both manuscript and abstract submission, rejection is a possibility. Recognizing that everyone has a "pink slip" in their file, mentors are invaluable in helping one stand back up, dust oneself off, revise, reshape, and resubmit.

Delineating a professional development plan is part of the APRN's evolution as an emerging scholar. Career goals around employment, position, setting, and client population are highlighted in each individual plan. As one develops a scholarship of practice, it is helpful to develop an area of expertise early in one's advanced practice career. This area of expertise is then sustained throughout one's career and is the basis for a scholarship of practice.

SUMMARY

Many APRNs will blend clinical practice with academic roles (preceptor, researcher, or faculty). Regardless of whether the APRN is in practice or academe, the importance of scholarship cannot be ignored. Scholarship encompasses activities that support all the roles of an APRN and can include participation in quality improvement projects, engagement in clinical research, generation of new knowledge, evaluation of clinical practice, and many other activities. The basis of all scholarship is dissemination through publication or presentation (local, national, or international).

Scholarship of practice is the mechanism that moves the APRN from being a clinician to a scholar, and all APRNs have the ability; however, few will venture forward. Scholarship of practice in nursing is the foundation of teaching, research, and practice and give legitimacy to the profession.

ACKNOWLEDGMENT

The authors acknowledge the contributions of Cecelia R. Zorn who contributed to this chapter in the previous edition.

REFERENCES

American Association of Colleges of Nursing. (2016). Position statement: Defining scholarship for the discipline of nursing. Retrieved from http://www.aacnnursing.org/News-Information/Position-Statements-White-Papers/Defining-Scholarship

Beal, J., Riley, J., & Lancaster, D. L. (2008). Essential elements of an optimal clinical practice environment. *The Journal of Nursing Administration, 38*(11), 488–493. doi:10.1097/01.NNA.0000339475.65466.d2

Belcher, W. L. (2009). *Writing your journal article in twelve weeks: A guide to academic publishing success.* Thousand Oaks, CA: Sage.

Bosold, C., & Darnell, M. (2012). Faculty practice: Is it scholarly activity? *Journal of Professional Nursing, 28*(2), 90–95. doi:10.1016/j.profnurs.2011.11.003

Boyer, E. (1990). *Scholarship reconsidered: Priorities of the professoriate.* Princeton, NJ: The Carnegie Foundation for the Advancement of Teaching.

Bridges, W. (1991). *Managing transitions: Making the most of change*. Reading, MA: Addison-Wesley.

Brown, M. A., & Crabtree, K. (2013). The development of practice scholarship in DNP programs: A paradigm shift. *Journal of Professional Nursing, 29*, 330–337. doi:10.1016/j.profnurs.2013.08.003

Brykczynski, K. A. (1989). An interpretive study describing the clinical judgment of nurse practitioners. *Research and Theory for Nursing Practice, 3*(2), 75–104.

Conrad, P. L., & Pape, T. (2014). Roles and responsibilities of the nursing scholar. *Pediatric Nursing, 40*(2), 87–90.

Crist, P. A. (2010). Adapting research instruction to support the scholarship of practice: Practice-scholar. *Partnerships Occupational Therapy in Health Care, 24*(1), 39–55. doi:10.3109/07380570903477000

Dexter, P. (2000). Tips for scholarly writing in nursing. *Journal of Professional Nursing, 16*(1), 6–12. doi:10.1016/S8755-7223(00)80006-X

Diers, D. (1995). Clinical scholarship. *Journal of Professional Nursing, 11*(1), 24–30. doi:10.1016/S8755-7223(95)80069-7

Honig, J., Smolowitz, J., & Larson, E. (2013). Building framework for nursing scholarship: Guidelines for appointment and promotion. *Journal of Professional Nursing, 29*, 359–369. doi:10.1016/j.profnurs.2012.10.001

Limoges, J., & Acorn, S. (2016). Transforming practice into clinical scholarship. *Journal of Advanced Nursing, 72*(4), 747–753. doi:10.1111/jan.12881

Lusk, P. (2014). Clinical scholarship: Let's share what we are doing in practice to improve outcomes. [Editorial]. *Journal of Child and Adolescent Psychiatric Nursing, 27*, 1–2. doi:10.1111/jcap.12068

Meleis, A. (1987). Re-visions in knowledge development: A passion for substance. *Scholarly Inquiry for Nursing Practice: An International Journal, 1*(1), 5–19.

Peterson, E. W., McMahon, E., Farkas, M., & Howland, J. (2005). Completing the cycle of scholarship of practice: A model for dissemination and utilization of evidence-based interventions. *Occupational Therapy in Health Care, 19*(1/2), 31–46. doi:10.1300/J003v19n01_04

Premji, S. S., Lalani, N., Ajani, K., Akhani, A., Moez, S., & Dias, J. M. (2011). Faculty practice in a private teaching institution in a developing country: Embracing the possibilities. *Journal of Advanced Nursing, 67*(4), 876–883. doi:10.1111/j.1365-2648.2010.05523.x

Riley, J. M., & Beal, J. A. (2013). Scholarly nursing practice from the perspectives of early-career nurses. *Nursing Outlook, 61*(2), E16–E24. doi:10.1016/j.outlook.2012.08.010

Riley, J., Beal, J. A., & Lancaster, D. (2008). Scholarly nursing practice from the perspectives of experienced nurses. *Journal of Advanced Nursing, 61*(4), 425–435. doi:10.1111/j.1365-2648.2007.04499.x

Riley, J. M., Beal, J., Levi, P., & McCausland, M. P. (2002). Revisioning nursing scholarship. *Journal of Nursing Scholarship, 34*, 383–389. doi:10.1111/j.1547-5069.2002.00383.x

Robert, R. R., & Pape, T. M. (2011). Scholarship in nursing: Not an isolated concept. *Medical Surgical Nursing, 20*(1), 41–44.

Shapiro, E. D., & Coleman, D. L. (2000). The scholarship of application. *Academic Medicine, 75*(9), 895–898. doi:10.1097/00001888-200009000-00010

Sigma Theta Tau International Clinical Scholarship Task Force. (1999). Clinical scholarship resource paper. Retrieved from http://www.nursingsociety.org/about-stti/position-statements-and-resource-papers

Silvia, P. J. (2007). *How to write a lot: A practical guide to productive academic writing.* Washington, DC: American Psychological Association.

Thomas, T. (2012). Overcoming barriers to scholarly activity in a clinical practice setting. *American Journal of Health-System Pharmacy, 69,* 465–467. doi:10.2146/ajhp110290

Tymkow, C. (2014). Clinical scholarship and evidence-based practice. In M. Zaccagnini & K. W. White (Eds.), *The doctor of nursing practice essentials: A new model for advanced practice nursing* (2nd ed.). Sudbury, MA: Jones & Bartlett.

Wilkes, L., Mannix, J., & Jackson, D. (2013). Practicing nurses perspectives of clinical scholarship: A qualitative study. *BioMed Central Nursing, 12,* 21. doi:10.1186/1472-6955-12-21

Carole G. Traylor

LAUNCHING YOUR ADVANCED PRACTICE CAREER

Where your talents and needs of the world cross, there lies your vocation.

—Aristotle

The advanced practice registered nurse (APRN) needs to clearly understand what the designation "advanced practice" means. Advance practice nursing incorporates both providing care and prescribing care (Barnes, 2014). It encompasses an expanded range of competencies in a clinically focused specialty to improve health outcomes for patients and populations (Hamic, Hanson, Tracy, & O'Grady, 2012). Current health trends provide wide opportunities for the APRN to find the right option for a new healthcare career. During the educational program for an advanced nursing degree or certificate, students have the opportunity to experience clinical care in a wide variety of settings. These experiences enable the new graduate to reflect on what type of practice may be the right one for a clinical home. This chapter investigates ideas, approaches, suggestions, and recommendations to consider when beginning the transition from the RN role to a new clinical role as an APRN. It also includes some pitfalls to avoid when seeking a new employment opportunity.

The Patient Protection and Affordable Care Act (ACA, U.S. Department of Health and Human Services [DHHS], 2010) recognized APRNs as a valuable resource in meeting the healthcare needs of the American population, particularly in rural and underserved areas. The Institute of Medicine's (IOM's), *The Future of Nursing: Leading Change, Advancing Health* (2011) identified and outlined vital roles for nurses for a more effective and efficient healthcare system and opportunity. These included the following:

- Reconceptualize the role of nursing within the context of the entire healthcare system
- Expand the capacity of nursing education to produce an adequate number of well-prepared nurses to meet current and future demands

- Develop innovative solutions related to professional education and healthcare delivery by focusing on the delivery of nursing services
- Attract and retain well-prepared nurses in multiple care settings

These goals provide a framework for change at the national, state, and local level. A subsequent report, *Assessing Progress on the Institute of Medicine Report on the Future of Nursing*, reiterates that APRNs provide high-quality care with good patient outcomes, including fewer hospitalizations and emergency room visits (National Academies of Sciences, Engineering & Medicine, 2016). This report continues to include recommendations for removing barriers so that APRNs are able to practice to the full extent of their education and training.

UNDERSTANDING THE MARKETPLACE

There continues to be a growing market for APRNs in varied roles. Because there is a different focus on care depending on the type of APRN (nurse practitioner [NP], clinical nurse specialist, nurse-midwife, or nurse anesthetist), employment opportunities are diverse. Healthcare trends have resulted in the expansion of telehealth resulting in new and creative roles for the APRN. Table 16.1 lists trends that impact employment and role expectations.

Thinking about how the APRN can thrive in today's healthcare environment can help narrow the scope of employment possibilities. Completing a self-reflection and a professional self-inventory are helpful to identify the type of practice and job description that would be ideal. Some individuals are interested in large organizations that employ many APRNs, whereas

---

TABLE 16.1   Current Trends in Healthcare

- Efforts to control healthcare cost
- Consumer and payer demands for high-quality, accessible, equitable, effective, safe, and individualized care
- Increased competition in the marketplace
- Use of evidence-based systems to guide clinical interventions and analyze outcomes
- Increased competition among providers for market share
- Reduced or increased accountability for use of acute care services
- Increasing focus on primary care
- Greater demand for chronic care services, especially for an aging population
- Development of service models to address increasing ethnic diversity
- Increased efforts to develop interdisciplinary team care models
- Rapid growth of medical and pharmaceutical technology
- Increased use of alternative, complementary, and nontraditional therapies
- Expansion of electronic information systems for service delivery, outcomes analysis, and cost control
- Contraction of the overall job market, with increasing competition for desirable positions

others prefer a smaller, independently owned practice. An APRN-owned practice may be more suitable to some, whereas an interdisciplinary practice that incorporates different healthcare providers, such as physicians, physician assistants, mental health counselors, nutritionists, and APRNs, may be more appealing to others. Reflection on strengths and limitations of different types of healthcare organizations, while considering the desired physical attributes in a working environment, types of support needed for success, and prioritizing which items are most important, is helpful. Completing these types of exercises gives the individual a better idea of what is important to the APRN candidate and thereby allows a more focused new job search. Table 16.2 is a sample of self-reflection questions.

In the book, *What Color Is Your Parachute?* (2018), Richard Bolles offers a variety of tools to conduct a self-inventory. Proceeding with a professional self-inventory focusing on the APRN role will help the candidate become more confident in the type of position that is appealing to begin this new career. Table 16.3 focuses on a professional self-inventory exercise that further assists the job seeker in finding the ideal position.

If tuition payback is a high priority, exploring a position in a program that offers reimbursement might be helpful. Some entities to consider are: Indian Health Service, U.S. Public Health Service, National Health Service Corps, Nurse Corps Loan Repayment Program, and Community Health Centers.

HOW TO STAND OUT

Be familiar with the current marketplace where opportunities for employment exist.

TABLE 16.2 Sample of Self-Reflection Questions

Critical reflective questions to ask may include:
What are my skills and abilities?
What do I enjoy doing?
What are my beliefs and values about work, my practice as an APRN, and my role in organizations where I work?
What are my needs?

Identify:
Abilities and skills: clinical, caregiving, communication, teaching, consultation, research, leadership, organization, computer proficiency, mentoring, writing, political action, achievements (and failures)
Interests: desirable professional activities, acquiring new skills, entrepreneurial activities
Values (principles or qualities that guide life and work): career, family, friends, work–life balance, spiritual, physical, emotional, social justice, organizational transparency, veracity (Listing and prioritizing values can be helpful.)
Needs: desired levels of control, power, salary, independence, security, recognition, creativity, achievement (Consider satisfiers and dissatisfiers in prior work situations.)
Characteristics: physical, emotional, intellectual (relevant to career and job performance), physical limitations, endurance, stress tolerance, enthusiasm, creativity, sensitivity, learning ability/style

---

TABLE 16.3   Professional Self-Inventory

- What are my strengths as an APRN? What is special about me as an APRN?
- What are my weaknesses, and how am I working to improve them? What skills or knowledge do I need to develop further?
- What type of APRN job am I looking for?
- What do I enjoy most about working as an APRN? Least?
- Where do I want to live? What things are important about the place where I live? How much am I willing to travel for work?
- With what kinds of people do I like to work? What kinds of people are difficult for me?
- What things are stressful to me in my work? What do I need to manage stress?
- Am I comfortable working with a lot of autonomy? Would I prefer working closely with others? How much supervision is best for me?
- How many hours a day am I willing to work? How much call? How much weekend?
- Evening and night service? How many holidays?

TABLE 16.4   Clinical and Professional Issues

- Standards for practice in clinical or specialty area
- Regulations affecting advanced practice, including licensure, certification, prescriptive privileges, institutional credentialing, and collaborative practice
- Reimbursement patterns and regulations
- Healthcare services provided and needed in the setting or community
- The presence of and services offered by competitors, either other APRNs or disciplines such as physicians, physician assistants, social workers
- Communication skills, including professional networking and negotiation skills
- The employer's perception and utilization of APRNs

Table 16.4 lists clinical and professional issues that need to be considered during the early stages seeking a new position at the advanced practice level.

There are many facets to launching a new advanced practice career. With the expansion of the Internet and social media, searching for the right candidate or position has changed. Now employers can search a prospective name on the Internet, checking out Facebook, LinkedIn, Twitter, YouTube, and other sites, to get a sense of who the candidate is before actually meeting the individual. Therefore, it is important that any information about you on various media sources should be accurate and appropriate. When considering what is posted about you on the Internet, is this something you would want a prospective employer to read?

Although some may think a résumé, curriculum vitae (CV), or portfolio are outdated tools, they still offer a collective summary of a candidate's qualifications in a chronological order of pertinent facts relevant to position expectations and responsibilities (Bolles, 2018). Because the APRN is changing roles, giving the employer some perspective by describing clinical activity in the student role is often helpful. Table 16.5 lists components

TABLE 16.5   Content of Résumé or CV

- Personal contact information
- Formal education most recent first
- Possible inclusion of GPA
- Student clinical experiences—where and what kind of experience
- Pertinent work experience
- Licensure
- Certification
- Awards and honors
- Publications
- Professional affiliation
- Languages—written/spoken
- Community service
- References available upon request

CV, curriculum vitae; GPA, grade point average.

that are recommended in this type of document. Preparing the document in a descriptive and concise manner is desirable.

A cover letter should accompany the well-prepared and polished document. This letter is an opportunity for the candidate to let the reader know what position one is seeking and why the candidate is interested in the position. The content of the cover letter is intended to create an interest on the part of the employer and thus a desire to interview the candidate. Briefly describing how one meets the critical elements of the position is helpful in securing a personal interview. Expanding on some aspects of the position using the employer's keywords increases the strength of the cover letter (Holland, 2012). A sample cover letter is located in Table 16.6.

Taking time to prepare for a personal interview is helpful to insure the best possible outcome. The attributes a candidate discusses and demonstrates in an interview give the employer an insight into what type of employee the candidate might be (Holland, 2012). If the interviewer has not previously worked with APRNs, sharing the legal definition of what advanced practice nursing means from the state's statute can clarify the job description and expectations of the role. Table 16.7 gives a sample of a definition from the state of Florida.

Reviewing a list of attributes, such as being a team player, liking to initiate solutions to problems, good at prioritizing, or organized in work performance, reflects the candidate's philosophy and work ethic, and gives the individual some preselected discussion points when asked "What are your strengths?" during the interview (Bolles, 2018, pp. 152–154). Conversely, it allows the candidate an opportunity to explain some areas that previously have been challenging and what changes have been made to correct the deficiencies if asked about weaknesses. Using the word "challenges" rather than "weaknesses" gives a positive spin on the aspects that needed some focused attention and improvement. Be wary of the "tell me about yourself"

TABLE 16.6 Sample Cover Letter

February 20, 2018

Director
Community Health Services
Craig, CO 81626

Dear Director:
I am excited about the expansion of the outpatient services for both children and adults in our community and the interest in hiring nurse practitioners to provide care.

I am a 2015 graduate of the State University with a Master of Science degree with a primary care pediatric nurse practitioner option. During my education, I had excellent clinical experiences in pediatric primary care medical sites working with APRNs and physicians.

In addition to over 500 clinical hours in primary pediatric care, I had additional clinical experiences in pediatric cardiology and dermatology. I also spent 1 month providing care to medically fragile children attending summer camp where I managed the children's medical plan of care and served as camp nurse.

Since graduation, I have been employed as the on-site healthcare provider with full prescriptive authority at the International Boarding School providing acute and chronic care management for high school students attending the school. During the summer, I spend 6 weeks at the summer camp for medically fragile children.

I enjoy working with adolescents and their families. I have directed two quality improvement projects that established interventions to track immunizations in the adolescent population and provided education for families and staff members about new immunization recommendations.

I am out-going and am comfortable addressing difficult medical issues with parents and patients. With my experience, I am an ideal nurse practitioner candidate for the new adolescent out-patient clinic.

I have enclosed a copy of my résumé for your review. I look forward to meeting you at the upcoming interview.
Sincerely,
Carole G. Traylor
Carole G. Traylor, MSN, CPNP-PC
Encl

TABLE 16.7 Definition of Advanced Practice of Nursing in Florida

"Advanced registered nurse practitioner" means any person licensed in this state to practice professional nursing and certified in advanced or specialized nursing practice, including certified registered nurse anesthetists, certified nurse midwives, and nurse practitioners.
Citation: Fla.Stat.Ann. §464.003(3)

TABLE 16.8 Common Interview Questions

- What type of position are you interested in?
- Could you tell me about yourself?
- What are your strengths? Your weaknesses?
- What do you know about our company?
- What would you do in this situation (typical situation described)?
- Why are you leaving your present job?
- What are your professional or career goals?
- What do you enjoy most about work? Least? Why?
- Why should we hire you for this position?
- What salary do you expect?
- What questions do you have about this position? This company?

question. Often a candidate hesitates and does not know what to address (Bolles, p. 58). Identifying traits associated with excellence prior to the interview gives the candidate the opportunity to demonstrate one's ability to achieve desired outcomes in a healthcare setting. Written notes about work attributes and success can help the candidate focus on presenting key points about effectiveness during an interview. Table 16.8 lists common interview questions. Having answers ready for these common questions during the interview can demonstrate to the employer that the interviewee is articulate and prepared.

Identifying an area of expertise that would enhance patient care for a specific population within a healthcare setting may be useful. For example, becoming an expert in insulin pump management would be an asset for the practice and patients with diabetes. References are often requested; therefore, prepare a list of three to five individuals including correct titles, credentials, and contact information including the individuals' professional email addresses to share at the interview. After the interview, sending a thank you note to everyone involved with the visit including the secretary or receptionist may be helpful to keep your interview in the forefront of other applicants. This demonstrates that the candidate has good people skills and offers an opportunity to reiterate one's interests and strengths (Bolles, 2018). Organizing documents in a portfolio may be helpful. Table 16.9 lists appropriate documents to include in a portfolio (Buppert, 2018, p. 49).

There are other market tasks associated with selecting the ideal position. Many APRNs are unfamiliar with the art of negotiating. Discussing salary and other compensations are often difficult to talk about. However, unless the position is in a large established organization, the individual will need to consider salary and other aspects of the position that can be negotiated in the contract. Status needs to be agreed on. Will the APRN be an employee where the employer pays salary and taxes or an independent contractor where the individual is paid but taxes will not be paid (Brown & Dolan, 2016)? Other compensation issues include payment of malpractice insurance, incentives, and bonuses. Is administration time built into a work

TABLE 16.9 Portfolio Documents

- Current résumé and/or curriculum vitae
- Official transcripts of all academic programs after high school
- Copies of nursing licenses and certifications
- Current list of references with addresses, phone numbers, and email addresses
- Malpractice insurance policies
- Records of continuing education attendance
- Reprints of publications
- Abstracts or brochures documenting conference presentations
- Newspaper or media recognition
- Evidence of honors or awards
- Prior references, recommendations, and performance evaluations
- A sample job description listing desirable job functions and benefits
- Examples of clinical and leadership achievements such as patient education programs/tools, specialized physical examination skills, quality improvement projects, and research utilization projects
- Professional organization memberships
- Health records, particularly immunization status pertinent to APRN employment

TABLE 16.10 Benefits to Consider

- Paid vacation days
- Paid sick days
- Paid holidays
- Retirement benefits (type, employer contribution, and vesting)
- Health insurance (individual and family coverage, portability, preexisting condition coverage, pregnancy coverage, prescription coverage, optical and dental coverage, long-term care options)
- Life insurance, short- and long-term disability insurance
- Malpractice insurance (occurrence or claims made, gap, or tail coverage requirements)
- Licensing and certification fee reimbursement (RN, APRN, DEA, CPR, and ACLS, etc.)
- Orientation period (duration and content)
- Continuing education (travel, fees, meals, lodging)
- Tuition reimbursement or waivers
- Professional membership dues
- Subscriptions to texts/journals
- Office and supplies: private office, computer, email/Internet access, medical supplies/equipment, computer upgrades and apps such as UpToDate or Epocrates or similar apps, cell phone, pager, parking
- Mileage reimbursement
- Interview and relocation expense reimbursement
- Profit sharing
- Retention of intellectual property rights (e.g., create and/or publish patient education tool or device)

ACLS, advanced cardiopulmonary life support; CPR, cardiopulmonary resuscitation; DEA, Drug Enforcement Agency.

schedule? Discussion of expectation of services to be performed needs to be within the scope of practice of the APRN applicant. Considerations of benefits are a large part of the employment package. Table 16.10 lists benefits to consider when negotiating the contract (Brown & Dolan, 2016).

The contract negotiations also include length of term of employment, cause for termination, and noncompete clauses. The complexity of a contract for the APRN requires that the applicant become familiar with all aspects of the contract. In Carolyn Buppert's book, *Nurse Practitioner's Business Practice and Legal Guide* (2018) describes the components of a business contract in detail and can help the applicant work through the tedious contracting process. Because of the nature of business contracts within a healthcare entity, the applicant may want to consider having an attorney review the contract prior to signing (Dillon & Hoyson, 2014).

TRANSITIONING TO A NEW ROLE

After the APRN has accepted the position, the individual now can envision the future. The future for the APRN is more than changing jobs; it is accepting the charge to change nursing practice in a new and exciting way. It is a chance to influence the lives of patients, families, and communities by rendering exceptional care while treating, teaching, and instilling health ideals in very tangible ways.

No transition is easy. Understanding the stages and emotional adjustment that comes with each step of the process provides insight into what to expect along the journey of role transition. At times, the learning curve may be steep and emotions intense.

The process of becoming an APRN begins during the educational experience and continues with first position as an APRN. As the student moves through the educational requirements and clinical experiences, a sense of the new role begins to emerge.

Certain components of transition must be experienced to be successful in the process. In William Bridges's book, *Managing Transitions: Making the Most of Change* (1991), he reiterates, "a transition is not a trip from one side of the street to the other but rather a journey" (p. 37). There are three distinct components that are fundamentally necessary to make the journey a success. To begin anew, one must let go of the old. As one leaves the role of the RN to become an APRN, letting go often evokes feelings like those experienced during grieving. Leaving previous professional colleagues and a familiar work environment often produces feelings of sadness. The fear of the unknown in a new role may instill a sense of anxiety about the role. Feeling insecure in the role may be reflected in a wide variety of feelings including anger. The disorientation of transition may evoke a sense of loss.

After letting go of the old, one moves into a new phase, which is a time to see oneself with new eyes and begin to experience the new role and how the new role fits within the organization. As one achieves the transition, establishing learning opportunities to increase knowledge and skill will help the new APRN become successful in this new role. This challenges the APRN to take time away from the chaos of change and reflect on the transition to gain strength in the new role and develop competency in it. The shift from only implementation of care to be the decision maker and orchestrator of the plan of care can be daunting.

Brown and Olshansky (1998) discussed a similar process in going from "limbo to legitimacy" (p. 46). Their work establishes four categories of transition. The first is a *state of laying the foundation*. This is the time when the APRN has finished school and has not yet completed the necessary steps to secure employment. This stage includes recovering from school and pursuing certification and licensing and conducting a self-reflection inventory and a professional self-inventory. Stage 2, *launching*, is at the beginning of the first position and continues for a minimum of 3 months (Brown & Olshansky, 1998). The underpinning of this stage is the early transition from expert RN to the novice APRN in a clinical setting. It is hard work. This stage often creates feelings of anxiety and insecurity due to role confusion between the comfort places of being an expert to stepping back into a novice role that is just emerging. Over time, the transition process moves into Stage 3, *meeting the challenge* (Brown & Olshansky, 1998), which is a time when the APRN's expectations become more realistic and the individual gains more skill and confidence. Internal support systems help the new APRN deal with the daily challenges of the current healthcare system. Stage 4, the final stage, is the *broadening of the perspective*. It occurs when the APRN develops greater self-esteem and a secured feeling of legitimacy (Brown & Olshansky, 1998).

Research has explored the "imposter syndrome," which is often manifested during the transition to a new role. This concept initially identified by Chance and Imes (1978) recognized high-achieving individuals who reported experiencing intellectual phoniness. Since that time, additional research has further investigated this phenomenon. Rose O. Sherman, EdD, RN, FAAN, asked the following question at an American Nurses Association manager workshop, "How many of you feel like imposters?" (Sherman, 2013)? Many attendees feared they could not live up to others' expectations and felt like they were frauds. Individuals

TABLE 16.11 Action Steps

---

1. Enlist the help of a trusted mentor to discuss your feelings about imposter syndrome.
2. Pay attention to your own self-talk and consider whether your thoughts are empowering or disabling.
3. Make a list of the strengths you bring to the role and what you contribute.
4. Accept that perfection and the need to "know it all" are both unrealistic and can be personally costly.
5. Recognize that there are times when you will be on a steep learning curve in a role and need to further develop your competencies. Be honest about what you know and what you do not know and utilize the experts on your unit or in your organization.
6. Be willing to be uncomfortable and move through your fear.

Robinson-Walker, C. (2011). The imposter syndrome. *Nurse Leader, 9*(4), 12–13. doi:10.1016/j.mnl.2011.05.003

experiencing self-doubt attempt to overcome these feelings through over-work while experiencing a fear of failure (Sherman). In addition to performance anxiety, this syndrome can lead to burnout and depression (Sherman, 2013). Catherine Robinson-Walker, a nurse leader, delineates six action steps to overcome there feelings of inadequacy, as outlined in Table 16.11 (Robinson-Walker, 2011).

In addition to the emotional transition, the APRN also experiences a concern about the lack of knowledge and skill. Although prepared academically, the myriad of patient presentations and required proficiency can be challenging for the new graduate. Becoming an expert occurs only over time as greater skill, knowledge, and experience are gained.

Patricia Benner, in *From Novice to Expert* (1984), describes the attributes of levels of proficiency in nursing. These levels are novice, advanced beginner, competent, proficient, and expert. Benner uses the Dreyfus model to explore the levels of proficiency (Benner, 1984, 2004). The Dreyfus model of skill acquisition incorporates situational performance and experiential learning to acquire nursing skills and knowledge that are reflected in the achievement of the nurse as she moves through the various stages (Benner, 2004). A novice with limited experience requires rules and guidelines to govern practice. A feeling of mastery does not occur until the competent level is achieved, but is still without speed and flexibility in practice (Benner, 2004). At the proficient level, the individual perceives the situation as a whole instead of separate equal parts. The expert demonstrates a deep understanding of the situation that becomes intuitive (Benner, 2004). Gaining skills and perspective allow the new APRN to move through the levels of proficiency. Transition in gaining proficiency begins with the movement from abstract principles to the use of concrete experiences in critical thinking. In addition, a change in perception now occurs when experiencing new clinical situations. This creates an action of becoming the involved performer from a previous position as the observer.

Based on the APRN's previous nursing experiences and clinical learning situations during advanced education, graduates move through these stages at different rates. Although the progression is incremental, it may not necessarily be linear or step wise, nor may all individuals attain an expert level (Poronsky, 2013). Mentoring and supporting the APRN during these developmental stages is critical to successfully achieving the expert level of knowledge and experience.

In a qualitative study, authors identified an overarching theme of the essence of nursing as a vital foundation for achieving this transition (Spoelstra & Robbins, 2010). Their work further addressed subthemes that reflected the importance of building a framework for nursing practice. Their findings suggested that the role of the APRN was to provide patient care based on empirical evidence through collaboration and consultation with both nursing colleagues and other healthcare professionals (Spoelstra & Robbins, 2010). The importance of direct patient care was another theme emerging from their study. Attributes that demonstrate this theme in practice included seeing the patient from a holistic view while demonstrating expert clinical thinking and skillful performance (Spoelstra & Robbins, 2010). Developing patient partnerships allows the APRN to provide creative approaches for health and illness management. The final subtheme identified was the importance of exemplifying professional practice responsibilities. The manifestation of this theme was reflected in improved patient outcomes using evidence-based practice, role modeling, effective communication, and collaboration in multidisciplinary teams. The findings in this qualitative study exemplify the core competencies and expectations of the APRN as set forth by national professional nursing organizations and accrediting bodies for advanced practice educational programs.

Transition is both a personal and professional change. It requires letting go of what is comfortable and known and moving toward a place of unknowns and discomfort.

To successfully evolve into this new nursing role, one must spend time in self-reflection to determine what current attributes support this new role. This is a time to reflect on previous nursing experiences and gain insight into what types of patient relationships have been the most meaningful (Szanton, Mihaly, Alhusen, & Becker, 2010). It is also a time to imagine a new role. Having a grasp of one's strengths and weaknesses is part of this, but self-reflection is more important. APRNs report that patient relationships are embedded in their overall job satisfaction

In *Reinventing You* (Clark, 2013), the author recommends discerning what type of image one projects as a key component in carving out a new role and direction. There are many ways to go about investigating your image, for example, asking colleagues to share their perceptions of your image and having friends describe you in three words (2013). Becoming more cognizant of who you are and the image you project allows you to identify areas that need attention to achieve the professional APRN image you wish to attain.

THE MENTORING ROLE

Mentorship is a relationship between a novice and an expert (Hill & Sawatzky, 2011). Having a supportive mentor can help the new APRN validate that feelings of inadequacy are normal. The mentor can help the APRN move into the new role. Whether being assigned a mentor or selecting one, a mentor gives the novice direction and reassurance in a supportive environment. Having a mentor helps the novice learn to bridge the gap between school knowledge and experience and the working world (2011). A good mentor is enthusiastic and seeks out learning opportunities for the new novice. Because many APRNs are in positions that require some implementation of the medical model of care, a mentor can help the novice keep the nursing focus while assuming the clinician and diagnostician roles (2011).

Hart and Bowen (2016) conducted a study surveying 698 practicing NPs and asked about their perception of preparedness for practice after completing their APRN education. Although many of the respondents felt somewhat prepared, there was much interest in postgraduate residencies or fellowships. The respondents also reported that a formal mentorship and a formal orientation could influence the success of transition from the RN role to the APRN role. Educating students about the process of transitioning to the APRN role will better prepare them for what to expect. Encouraging students to contemplate expectations of a mentor can help establish the novice mentor relationship and meet the challenges of transition (Hill & Sawatzky, 2011).

Just as competence, confidence, and judgment were frequent questions at the onset of the NP movement, they remain critical elements to the success of the implementation of the APRN role for the present and future. Successful APRNs can convey confidence in their expertise to their patients and other healthcare providers (Gasalberti, 2014).

Remaining active in professional nursing organizations keeps new graduates informed of changes in the nursing arena as they begin to develop their new role. Opportunities for participation and leadership roles within organizations can help the APRN carve out a unique place in nursing practice. National meetings and workshops provide wide ranges of networking with APRNs with immeasurable experience and who are committed to the goals of advanced practice nursing. Staying connected with nursing colleagues gives the new graduate an opportunity to investigate solutions for identified problems in this new role. APRNs can become integral members of the healthcare team by participating in the development of quality tools, as well as monitoring and analyzing patient outcomes (Stanley, 2011).

The advanced practice movement has been paved by revolutionaries and reactionaries demonstrating the values and goals of professional nursing as evidenced by the contributors to the *Nurse Practitioner Pioneers—Celebrating 50 Years of Role Development* (Edmunds, 2015). Colleagues before you and those who will follow strengthen the APRN role and nursing's critical position in today's healthcare arena. It is now time to actualize your vision and contribute to the knowledge and action of nursing as an advanced practice nurse.

SUMMARY

As APRNs finish advanced education, the goal becomes promotion of their careers as APRNs.

Marketing is an important factor to consider moving forward in finding the position that complements your envisioned APRN role. Often this requires "selling oneself," which may be difficult in the beginning; however, using self-reflection to identify goals, APRNs' specific contributions to healthcare delivery, and realizing the potential of the APRN role are key elements to incorporate in marketing. For entrepreneurs in advanced nursing practice, realizing the new models of care will be the foundation of marketing. In essence, when launching your career as an APRN, understand the world of healthcare is yours to take and make it the way you want it to be.

The people who get on in this world are the people who get up and look for circumstances they want, and if they can't find them, make them! (George Bernard Shaw)

ACKNOWLEDGMENT

The author acknowledges the contributions of Shirley Van Zandt to this chapter in the previous edition.

REFERENCES

Barnes, H. (2014). Nurse practitioner role transition: A concept analysis. *Nursing Forum, 50*(3), 137–146. doi:10.1111/nuf.12078

Benner, P. (1984). *From novice to expert*. Reading, MA: Addison-Wesley.

Benner, P. (2004). Using the Dreyfus model of skill acquisition to describe and interpret skill acquisition and clinical judgment in nursing practice and education. *Bulletin of Science, Technology and Society, 24*, 188–199. doi:10.1177/0270467604265061

Bolles, R. (2018). *What color is your parachute?* Berkeley, CA: Ten Speed Press.

Bridges, W. (1991). *Managing transitions: Making the most of change*. Reading MA: Addison-Wesley.

Brown, L. A., & Dolan, C. (2016). Employment contracting basics for the nurse practitioner. *The Journal for Nurse Practitioners, 12*, e45–e51. doi:10.1016/j.nurpra.2015.11.026

Brown, M., & Olshansky, E. (1998). Becoming a primary care nurse practitioner: Challenges of the initial year of practice. *Nurse Practitioner, 23*(7), 46. doi:10.1097/00006205-199807000-00004

Buppert, C. (2018). *Nurse practitioner's business practice guide and legal guide*. Burlington, MA: Jones & Bartlett.

Chance, P., & Imes, S. (1978). The imposter phenomenon in high achieving women: Dynamics and therapeutic intervention. *Psychology: Theory, Research and Practice, 15*, 241–247.

Clark, D. (2013). *Reinventing you*. Boston, MA: Harvard Business Review Press.

Dillon, D., & Hoyson, P. (2014). Beginning employment: A guide for the nurse practitioner. *The Journal for Nurse Practitioners, 10*, 55–59. doi:10.1016/j.nurpra.2013.09.009

Edmunds, M. (2015). Let us celebrate 50 years of NP success. *Journal for Nurse Practitioners, 11*(6), A23–A24. doi:10.1016/j.nurpra.2015.04.003

Gasalberti, D. (2014). Developing a professional self-confidence to last a lifetime. *The Journal for Nurse Practitioners, 10*(8), 630–631. doi:10.1016/j.nurpra.2014.05.019

Hamic, A., Hanson, C., Tracy, M., & O'Grady, E. (2012). *Advanced practice nursing: An integrative approach*. St Louis, MO: Elsevier.

Hart, A., & Brown, A. (2016). New nurse practitioners' perceptions of preparedness for and transition into practice. *The Journal of Nurse Practitioners, 12*(8), 545–551. doi:10.1016/j.nurpra.2016.04.018

Hill, L., & Sawatzky, J. A. (2011). Transitioning into the nurse practitioner role through mentorship. *Journal of Professional Nursing, 27,* 161–167. doi:10.1016/j.profnu+rs.2011.02.004

Holland, R. (2012). *Cracking the new job market: The 7 rules for getting hired in any economy.* New York, NY: Amacom.

Institute of Medicine. (2011). *The future of nursing: Leading change, advancing health.* Washington, DC: The National Academies Press. doi:10.17226/12956.

National Academies of Sciences, Engineering, and Medicine. (2016). *Assessing progress on the Institute of Medicine report on the future of nursing.* Washington, DC: National Academies Press. doi:10.17226/21838

Poronsky, C. (2013). Exploring the transition from registered nurse to family nurse practitioner. *Journal of Professional Nursing, 29*(6), 350–358. doi:/10.1016/j.profnurs.2012.10.011

Robinson-Walker, C. (2011). The imposter syndrome. *Nurse Leader, 9*(4), 12–13. doi:10.1016/j.mnl.2011.05.003

Sherman, R. (2013). Imposter syndrome: When you feel like you're faking it. *American Nurse Today, 8*(5), 57–61.

Spoelstra, S., & Robbins, L. (2010). A qualitative study of role transition from RN to APRN. *International Journal of Nursing Education Scholarship, 7,* 1–14. Retrieved from http://www.bepress.com/ijnes/vol17/art20. doi:10.2202/1548-923X.2020

Stanley, J. (2011). *Advance practice nursing: Emphasizing common roles.* Philadelphia, PA: F. A. Davis.

Szanton, S., Mihaly, L., Alhusen, J., & Becker, K. (2010). Taking charge of the challenge: Factors to consider in taking your first nurse practitioner job. *Journal of the American Academy of Nurse Practitioners, 22,* 356–360. doi:10.1111/j.1745-7599.2010.00522.x

U.S. Department of Health and Human Services. (2010). The Affordable Care Act, section by section: Title V. Heath care workforce. Retrieved from http://www.hhs.gov/healthcare/rights/law/index.html

INDEX

Printed in the United States
by Baker & Taylor Publisher Services